CLINICAL CASES in MEDICAL RETINA

MEDICAL RETINA

A Diagnostic Approach

CLINICAL CASES in MEDICAL RETINA

A Diagnostic Approach

JENNIFER I. LIM, MD, FARVO, FASRS
Marion H. Schenk Esq. Chair in Ophthalmology
UIC Distinguished Professor
Vice-Chair for Diversity & Inclusion
Director of Retina Service
Department of Ophthalmology
Illinois Eye and Ear Infirmary
University of Illinois at Chicago
Chicago, Illinois
United States

WILLIAM F. MIELER, MD, FARVO, FASRS, FACS
Cless Family Professor
Vice-Chairman of Clinical Affairs
UIC Distinguished Professor
Director Vitreoretinal Fellowship Training
Director of Ocular Oncology
Department of Ophthalmology & Visual Sciences
University of Illinois at Chicago
Chicago, Illinois
United States

ELSEVIER

Elsevier
1600 John F. Kennedy Blvd.
Ste 1800
Philadelphia, PA 191032899

Notice

Practitioners and researchers must always rely on their own experience and knowledge in evaluating
and using any information, methods, compounds or experiments described herein. Because of rapid
advances in the medical sciences, in particular, independent verification of diagnoses and drug
dosages should be made. To the fullest extent of the law, no responsibility is assumed by Elsevier,
authors, editors or contributors for any injury and/or damage to persons or property as a matter of
products liability, negligence or otherwise, or from any use or operation of any methods, products,
instructions, or ideas contained in the material herein.

Senior Content Development Manager: Somodatta Roy Choudhury
Executive Content Strategist: Kayla Wolfe
Senior Content Development Specialist: Priyadarshini Pandey
Publishing Services Manager: Shereen Jameel
Project Manager: Vishnu T. Jiji
Senior Designer: Patrick C. Ferguson

Printed in India

Last digit is the print number: 9 8 7 6 5 4 3 2 1

Working together
to grow libraries in
developing countries

www.elsevier.com • www.bookaid.org

Dedication

I dedicate this book to my students and colleagues who continue to journey with me in the diagnosis and management of medical retinal conditions and who generously share their knowledge and patient experiences to enable us to learn from each another. I dedicate this book to my parents, Drs. Diosdado and Amada Lim, who inspired me to become a physician and nurtured my innate curiosity. I dedicate this book to my daughter, Bernadette Miao, who is beginning her MD, PhD journey, and to my husband, John Miao, for his continued support and understanding of my career that enable projects such as this to be achieved.

Jennifer I. Lim, MD

I would like to dedicate this textbook to all of my students, residents, fellows, and colleagues over the years who have contributed to my continued ongoing curiosity of trying to resolve and help each and every patient who has presented with challenging and unique medical/surgical problems. I thank my parents, William F. and Dorothy Mieler, and my uncle, Harold F. Deutsch, PhD, who helped to nurture my medical curiosity. Special thanks also goes to my three sons, Michael, Andrew, and Daniel, and my stepdaughter, Sabrina Kang Derwent. A very special thanks also goes to my wife, Jennifer J. Kang-Mieler, PhD, for her ongoing support and unique perspective into the busy lives of academic physicians. Thanks will also go out to the eventual readership of the textbook, hoping to expand the horizons and learning of those who browse through these pages.

William F. Mieler, MD

CONTRIBUTORS

Aliaa Abdelhakim, MD, PhD
Assistant Professor of Ophthalmology
Columbia University Medical Center
New York, New York
United States

Néda Abraham, MS
International Fellow, Retina
Clinical Research Coordinator, Retina
Stein Eye Institute, UCLA
Los Angeles, California
United States;
Orthoptist
Explore Vision
Paris, France

Luis Acaba-Berrocal, MD
Resident
Ophthalmology
Illinois Eye and Ear
Chicago, Illinois
United States

Anita Agarwal, MD
Professor of Ophthalmology
Vanderbilt Eye Institute
Vanderbilt University
Nashville, Tennessee;
West Coast Retina
San Francisco, California
United States

Michael T. Andreoli, MD
Vitreoretinal Surgeon
Ophthalmology
Northwestern Medicine
Naperville, Illinois
United States

Karl N. Becker, MD
Voluntary Attending
Division of Ophthalmology
Cook County Health;
Uveitis and Medical Retina Fellow
Illinois Eye and Ear Infirmary
University of Illinois College at Chicago
Chicago, Illinois
United States

Norbert M. Becker, MD
Director Uveitis Clinic (Retired)
Division of Ophthalmology
Cook County Health
Chicago, Illinois
United States

Sanjeeb Bhandari, MD, ChM, PhD
Clinical Fellow
Division of Epidemiology and Clinical
    Applications
National Eye Institute/National Institutes
    of Health
Bethesda, Maryland
United States;
Associate
Faculty of Medicine and Health
The University of Sydney
Sydney, New South Wales
Australia

Arthi D. Bharadwaj, BS
Medical Student
Department of Ophthalmology
University of Illinois at Chicago
Chicago, Illinois
United States

Pooja Bhat, MD
Associate Professor of Ophthalmology
Ophthalmology and Visual Sciences
Illinois Eye and Ear Infirmary
University of Illinois at Chicago
Chicago, Illinois
United States

Geoffrey K. Broadhead, MBBS, PhD, FRANZCO
National Eye Institute
National Institutes of Health
Bethesda, Maryland
United States;
Department of Ophthalmology
The University of Sydney
Sydney, New South Wales
Australia

Kelly Bui, MD
Physician
Ophthalmology
The Polyclinic
Seattle, Washington
United States

R.V. Paul Chan, MD, MSc, MBA
Professor and Chair
Ophthalmology and Visual Sciences
Illinois Eye and Ear Infirmary
University of Illinois at Chicago
Chicago, Illinois
United States

Felix Chau, MD
Associate Professor of Ophthalmology
Ophthalmology
Illinois Eye and Ear Infirmary
University of Illinois at Chicago
Chicago, Illinois
United States

Connie J. Chen, MD
Associate Member
Ophthalmology
Virginia Mason Medical Center
Seattle, Washington
United States

Katherine G. Chen, MD, MS
Department of Ophthalmology
Illinois Eye and Ear Infirmary
University of Illinois at Chicago
Chicago, Illinois
United States

Emily Y. Chew, MD
Director of Division of Epidemiology
    and Clinical Applications
Division of Epidemiology & Clinical
    Applications
National Eye Institute/National Institutes of
    Health
Bethesda, Maryland
United States

Emily Cole, MD, MPH
Retina Fellow
Ophthalmology
University of Michigan
Ann Arbor, Michigan
United States

Ricky Z. Cui, MD
Clinical Associate
Department of Ophthalmology
Duke University Hospital
Durham, North Carolina
United States

Mark J. Daily, MD
Retinal Specialist
Wheaton Eye Clinic
Wheaton, Illinois
United States

Talisa E. de Carlo Forest, MD
Assistant Professor of Ophthalmology
Medical Director of Imaging
Ophthalmology
University of Colorado
Denver, Colorado
United States

Livia Della Mora, MD
Ophthalmologist
Ophthalmology
Ospedale Sant'Orsola Malpighi
Bologna, Italy

Maura Di Nicola, MD
Uveitis/Medical Retina Fellow
Ophthalmology
University of Illinois at Chicago
Chicago, Illinois;
Assistant Professor of Ophthalmology
Bascom Palmer Eye Institute
Miami, Florida
United States

Diana V. Do, MD
Professor of Ophthalmology, Vice Chair for
    Clinical Affairs
Ophthalmology
Byers Eye Institute
Stanford University
Palo Alto, California
United States

Shannon A. Donley, BS
Medical Scribe
West Coast Retina
San Francisco, California
United States

Amani A. Fawzi, MD
Cyrus Tang and Lee Jampol Professor of
  Ophthalmology
Feinberg School of Medicine
Northwestern University
Chicago, Illinois
United States

Gerald A. Fishman, MD
Professor Emeritus
Ophthalmology
University of Illinois at Chicago
Chicago, Illinois
United States

Meira Fogel-Levin, MD
Professor of Ophthalmology
The Goldschleger Eye Institute
Sheba Medical Center
Ramat Gan, Israel;
Professor of Ophthalmology
Stein Eye Institute
University of California–Los Angeles
Los Angeles, California
United States

Andrew W. Francis, MD
Physician
Vitreous and Retinal Surgery
Chicagoland Advanced Retina Care
Addison, Illinois
United States

K. Bailey Freund, MD
Clinical Professor of Ophthalmology
NYU Grossman School of Medicine
Partner
Vitreous Retina Macula Consultants
  of New York
New York, New York
United States

Hisashi Fukuyama, MD, PhD
Research Fellow
Ophthalmology
Northwestern University
Chicago, Illinois
United States;
Assistant Professor of Ophthalmology
Hyogo College of Medicine
Nishinomiya, Japan

Hashem Ghoraba, MD, MSc
Clinical Instructor
Ophthalmology
Byers Eye Institute at Stanford University
Palo Alto, California
United States

Manjot K. Gill, MD, FRCS(C), FASRS
Professor
Ophthalmology
Professor
Medical Education
Northwestern University
Chicago, Illinois
United States

Morton F. Goldberg, MD
Director Emeritus
Wilmer Eye Institute
Johns Hopkins University School of Medicine
Baltimore, Maryland
United States

Debra A. Goldstein, MD, FRCSC
Magerstadt Professor of Ophthalmology
Department of Ophthalmology
Northwestern University Feinberg School of
  Medicine
Chicago, Illinois
United States

Ninel Z. Gregori, MD
Professor of Clinical Ophthalmology
Bascom Palmer Eye Institute
University of Miami Miller School of
  Medicine
Miami, Florida
United States

Sandeep Grover, MD
Professor of Ophthalmology
Associate Chair, Ophthalmology
Director, Inherited Retinal Dystrophies
Ophthalmology
University of Florida
Jacksonville, Florida
United States

Michael J. Heiferman, MD
Assistant Professor of Ophthalmology
Ophthalmology and Visual Sciences
University of Illinois at Chicago
Chicago, Illinois
United States

Nancy M. Holekamp, MD
Director, Retina Services
Ophthalmology
Pepose Vision Institute
St. Louis, Missouri
United States

Robert A. Hyde, MD, PhD
Assistant Professor of Ophthalmology
Illinois Eye and Ear Infirmary, Department of
    Ophthalmology and Visual Sciences
University of Illinois at Chicago
Chicago, Illinois
United States

Alessandro Iannaccone, MD, MS, FARVO
Professor of Ophthalmology
Department of Ophthalmology, Duke
    Eye Center
Duke University Medical School
Durham, North Carolina
United States

Sayena Jabbehdari, MD, MPH
Retina Specialist
University of Arkansas Medical School
Little Rock, Arkansas
United States

Kanishka Jayasundera, MD, MS, FACS, FRCSC, FRANZCO
Assistant Professor of Ophthalmology
Department of Ophthalmology and Visual
    Sciences
University of Michigan Kellogg Eye Center
Ann Arbor, Michigan
United States

Mark W. Johnson, MD
Professor and Chief, Vitreoretinal Service
Department of Ophthalmology and Visual
    Sciences
University of Michigan
Ann Arbor, Michigan
United States

Katherine A. Joltikov, MD
Clinical Instructor
Department of Ophthalmology & Visual
    Sciences
University of Illinois at Chicago
Chicago, Illinois
United States

Irmak Karaca, MD
Clinical Fellow in Uveitis and Medical Retina
Instructor in Ophthalmology
International Council of Ophthalmology
    RRF-Helmerich Fellowship Scholar
Ophthalmology
Byers Eye Institute at Stanford University
Palo Alto, California
United States

Tiarnán D. L. Keenan, BM, BCh, PhD
Staff Clinician
Division of Epidemiology and Clinical
    Applications
National Eye Institute, National Institutes of
    Health
Bethesda, Maryland
United States

Daniel F. Kiernan, MD, FACS
Retina Specialist
The Eye Associates
Ophthalmology
Sarasota Memorial Hospital
Sarasota, Florida
United States

Eleni K. Konstantinou, MD
Medical Retina Fellow
Division of Epidemiology and Clinical
    Applications
National Eye Institute, National Institutes of
    Health
Bethesda, Maryland
United States

Byron L. Lam, MD
Bascom Palmer Eye Institute
University of Miami School of Medicine
Miami, Florida
United States

Gerardo Ledesma-Gil, MD
Attending Physician
Professor of Ophthalmology
Retina Department
Institute of Ophthalmology Fundacion Conde
  de Valenciana
Mexico City, Mexico

Angela S. Li, MD
Ophthalmology Resident
Duke Eye Center
Duke University
Durham, North Carolina
United States

Ashley Li, BS
Research Assistant
Ophthalmology
Massachusetts Eye and Ear Infirmary
Boston, Massachusetts
United States

Yanliang Li, MD, PhD
Postdoctoral Researcher
Kazlauskas Lab
University of Illinois College of Medicine
Chicago, Illinois
United States

Jennifer I. Lim, MD, FARVO, FASRS
Marion H. Schenk Esq. Chair in
  Ophthalmology
UIC Distinguished Professor
Vice-Chair for Diversity & Inclusion
Director of Retina Service
Department of Ophthalmology
Illinois Eye and Ear Infirmary
University of Illinois at Chicago
Chicago, Illinois
United States

Helen Liu, BS
Medical Student
Department of Medical Education
Icahn School of Medicine at Mount Sinai
New York, New York
United States

Ann-Marie Lobo, MD, MS
Associate Professor of Ophthalmology
Ophthalmology
University of Illinois at Chicago
Chicago, Illinois
United States

Thayze Martins, MD, MSc
Ophthalmologist, Retina Specialist
Department of Ophthalmology
Altino Ventura Foundation
Recife, Pernambuco
Brazil

Michael T. Massengill, MD, PhD
Ophthalmology Resident
Illinois Eye and Ear Infirmary
Chicago, Illinois
United States

William F. Mieler, MD, FACS, FARVO
Cless Family Professor
Vice-Chairman of Clinical Affairs
UIC Distinguished Professor
Director Vitreoretinal Fellowship Training
Director of Ocular Oncology
Department of Ophthalmology & Visual
  Sciences
University of Illinois at Chicago
Chicago, Illinois
United States

Rukhsana G. Mirza, MD, MS
Ryan-Pusateri Professor of Ophthalmology
Ophthalmology & Medical Education
Northwestern University
Chicago, Illinois
United States

Yasha Modi, MD
Associate Professor of Ophthalmology
NYU Langone Health
New York University
New York, New York
United States

Rose A. Moore, BS
Scribe
Retina
West Coast Retina
San Francisco, California
United States

Monique Munro, MD, FRCSC
Vitreoretinal Surgeon
Department of Surgery, Section of
  Ophthalmology
University of Calgary
Calgary, Alberta
Canada

Mina M. Naguib, MD
Fellow
Ophthalmology
New York University
New York, New York
United States

Quan Dong Nguyen, MD, MSc
Professor of Ophthalmology
Byers Eye Institute
Stanford University
Palo Alto, California
United States

Timothy W. Olsen, MD
Chair Emeritus
Ophthalmology
Emory University
Atlanta, Georgia;
CEO
iMacular Regeneration, LLC
Rochester, Minnesota
United States

Chris Or, MD
Clinical Assistant Professor of Ophthalmology
Stanford University
Palo Alto, California
United States

Paul R. Parker, MD, MSE
Ophthalmology Resident
Ophthalmology & Visual Sciences
University of Illinois at Chicago
Chicago, Illinois
United States

Jose(ph) Serafin Pulido, MD, MS, MPH, MBA
Larry Donoso Chair of Translational
   Ophthalmology
Translational Ophthalmology
Wills Eye Hospital,
Bryn Mawr, Pennsylvania;
Professor Emeritus
Ophthalmology and Molecular Medicine
Mayo Clinic
Rochester, Minnesota
United States

Meera S. Ramakrishnan, MD
Vitreoretinal Fellow
Ophthalmology
Vitreous Retina Macula Consultants of NY
New York, New York
United States

Edward L. Randerson, MD
Assistant Professor of Ophthalmology and
   Visual Sciences
Medical College of Wisconsin
Milwaukee, Wisconsin
United States

Mohammad Amr Sabbagh, MD
Ophthalmology Resident
Illinois Eye and Ear Infirmary
University of Illinois at Chicago
Chicago, Illinois
United States

SriniVas Sadda, MD
Professor-in-Residence
Ophthalmology
University of California–Los Angeles;
Director
Doheny Image Reading and Research
   Laboratory
Doheny Eye Institute
Los Angeles, California
United States

Ahmad Santina, MD
Research Fellow
Retina Disorders and Ophthalmic Genetics
Jules Stein Eye Institute
University of California–Los Angeles
Westwood, California
United States

David Sarraf, MD
Clinical Professor of Ophthalmology
Stein Eye Institute
Los Angeles, California
United States

Dana Schlegel, MS, MPH, CGC
Genetic Counselor
Department of Ophthalmology and Visual
   Sciences
University of Michigan Kellogg Eye Center
Ann Arbor, Michigan
United States

Carol Shields, MD
Director of Ocular Oncology
Professor of Ophthalmology
Ocular Oncology Service
Wills Eye Hospital
Philadelphia, Pennsylvania
United States

Nathan C. Sklar, MD
Research Assistant
Ophthalmology
Northwestern University Feinberg School of
    Medicine
Chicago, Illinois
United States

George Skopis, MD
Retina Fellow
Ophthalmology, Retina Service
Illinois Eye and Ear Infirmary
University of Illinois at Chicago
Chicago, Illinois
United States

Kent W. Small, MD
President
Ophthalmology
Molecular Insight Research Foundation
Glendale, California
United States

Stephen J. Smith, MD
Clinical Assistant Professor of Ophthalmology
Stanford University School of Medicine
Palo Alto, California
United States

Wendy M. Smith, MD
Associate Professor of Ophthalmology
Mayo Clinic
Rochester, Minnesota
United States

Lucia Sobrin, MD, MPH
Professor of Ophthalmology
Retina and Uveitis Services, Department of
    Ophthalmology
Massachusetts Eye and Ear Infirmary
Harvard Medical School
Boston, Massachusetts
United States

Jihun Song, MD, PhD
Associate Professor of Ophthalmology
Ophthalmology
Ajou University School of Medicine
Suwon, Republic of Korea

Sudarshan Srivatsan, MD
Ophthalmology Fellow
University of Utah School of Medicine
Salt Lake City, Utah
United States

Patrick C. Staropoli, MD
Ophthalmology
Bascom Palmer Eye Hospital
Miami, Florida
United States

Hassan N. Tausif, MD
Vitreoretinal Surgery Fellow
Ophthalmology
Northwestern University
Chicago, Illinois
United States

Sudip D. Thakar, MD
Ophthalmologist
Ophthalmology
Duke University
Durham, North Carolina
United States

Catherine J. Thomas, MD, MS, MHA
Attending Physician
Ophthalmology
Cook County Health
Chicago, Illinois
United States

Nita Valikodath, MD, MS
Vitreoretinal Surgery Fellow
Department of Ophthalmology
Duke University
Durham, North Carolina
United States

Camila V. Ventura, MD, PhD
Director
Department of Research
Altino Ventura Foundation;
Retina Specialist
Department of Ophthalmology
Altino Ventura Foundation and HOPE Eye
    Hospital
Recife, Brazil

Sushant Wagley, MD
Vitreoretinal Surgeon
Ophthalmology
Iowa Retina Consultants
West Des Moines, Iowa
United States

Daniel W. Wang, MD
Vitreoretinal Fellow
Vitreoretinal Surgery
Illinois Eye and Ear Infirmary
University of Illinois at Chicago
Chicago, Illinois
United States

Alexis Warren, MD
Vitreoretinal Fellow
Department of Ophthalmology–Retina
University of Illinois at Chicago
Chicago, Illinois
United States

Christina Y. Weng, MD, MBA
Professor of Ophthalmology
Fellowship Program Director, Vitreoretinal
    Diseases & Surgery
Department of Ophthalmology
Baylor College of Medicine
Houston, Texas
United States

Henry E. Wiley, MD
Staff Clinician
Division of Epidemiology and Clinical
    Applications
National Eye Institute
Bethesda, Maryland
United States

J.D. Wilgucki, MD
Assistant Professor of Ophthalmology
Loyola University Chicago Stritch School of
    Medicine
Chicago, Illinois
United States

Basil K. Williams Jr., MD
Associate Professor of Ophthalmology
Department of Ophthalmology
Bascom Palmer Eye Institute
Miami, Florida
United States

Lawrence A. Yannuzzi, MD
Professor
Clinical Ophthalmology
Columbia University School of Medicine
New York, New York
United States

Melissa Yao, BA
Medical Student
Department of Medical Education
David Geffen School of Medicine at UCLA
Los Angeles, California
United States

Madeleine Y. Yehia, MD
Uveitis and Medical Retina Fellow
Department of Ophthalmology and Visual
    Sciences
University of Illinois at Chicago
Chicago, Illinois
United States

Benjamin Young, MD, MS
Assistant Professor of Ophthalmology
Department of Ophthalmology, Kellogg Eye
    Center
University of Michigan Medical School
Ann Arbor, Michigan
United States

Ivy Zhu, MD
Vitreoretinal Fellow
Ophthalmology
Northwestern University
Chicago, Illinois
United States

PREFACE

Medical case conferences inspired us to create this compilation of interesting medical retina cases that are presented in a progressive didactic format. As retina specialists, we savor the challenge of determining the correct retinal diagnosis of unusual presentations of rarer and less common medical and surgical retinal conditions. We enjoy helping a patient by determining the diagnosis of the problem and doing our best to help resolve and address the issue(s). We enjoy deciphering the diagnosis of patients presented at retina case conferences, such as the Rabb Retina Case Conferences in Chicago and the case presentations at the Macula Society, the Retina Society and American Society of Retina Specialists (ASRS), the Club Jules Gonin (CJG), the Macula Symposium, the Atlantic Coast Conference, the Pacific Retina Club, the International Retina Imaging Society (IntRIS), EURETINA, and others.

Special thanks go to the Midwest Ocular Angiography Conference (MOAC), established in 1989 by William F. Mieler, MD, and now entering its 34th year, which dedicates an annual meeting to presentation and review of 75 to 110 challenging mystery cases. A very special thank you also goes out to the Gass Club, named in honor of J. Donald M. Gass, MD, which is now entering its 48th year and is designed in a similar fashion to present and discuss diagnostically challenging cases. I, William F. Mieler, have had the honor to organize and coordinate the Gass Club since 2008.

Thus the format of *Clinical Cases in Medical Retina* strives to recreate the stimulating setting of the clinic or case conference presentation, in which the reader will first evaluate the presenting symptom and clinical examination findings and then ask pertinent questions about the patient's history to create a differential diagnosis. As such, the chapter titles are purposefully symptom based and vague as to the actual diagnosis. Then the reader will be presented with ophthalmic imaging and laboratory results to reach a final diagnosis. Algorithms and key points are included in each chapter to assist the reader to think methodically and to amalgamate salient diagnostic tests/procedures that help one arrive at the correct diagnosis. For both instructive value and for quick reference, the cases are grouped by disease category into hereditary, degenerative, inflammatory, infectious, retinovascular, neoplastic, toxic, and idiopathic topics.

The cases represent actual patients who presented to general ophthalmology and retina clinics from our own institutions and from those of our national and international colleagues. The selected case presentations were chosen because, although less common, they are likely to be encountered in a clinician's day-to-day practice. If one is not at least aware of these challenging diagnoses, one would have a limited differential and never be able to make certain diagnoses. It is our hope that this book, which places less common medical retinal conditions into one easily searchable volume, will prove useful to the busy clinician who is presented with an unusual medical retina condition. We hope that this book will be a useful learning tool for vitreoretinal fellows, ophthalmology residents, and medical students in addition to comprehensive ophthalmologists in the diagnosis and appropriate workup for unusual medical retina conditions.

We are grateful to our contributors for sharing their cases, expertise, and time to write their chapters. Our contributors, internationally recognized medical retina experts, collaborated with their fellows, residents, and medical students in the creation of case studies. We hope that you will enjoy learning from them as much as we have in creating *Clinical Cases in Medical Retina*. We welcome your comments and remain hopeful that we achieved our goal in creating an entertaining and educational didactic case studies book for unusual medical conditions.

Jennifer I. Lim, MD, FARVO, FASRS
William F. Mieler, MD, FARVO, FASRS, FACS

CONTENTS

Hereditary Macular Conditions

CHAPTER 1

Yellow Macular Spots in a Child

Alessandro Iannaccone

History of Present Illness

A 12-year-old White female child presented around age 7 years with blurred vision, which could not be corrected with glasses, and mild visual distortion (metamorphopsia) of more recent onset. The remainder of the past and present medical history was unremarkable. She denied floaters, photopsias, photophobia, or nyctalopia.

OCULAR EXAMINATION FINDINGS

Visual acuity with correction was 20/25 in the right eye and 20/30 in the left eye. Intraocular pressure was normal. External and anterior segment examinations were unremarkable. Dilated fundus examination showed coin-shaped, egg yolk–like, yellowish elevated lesions in the center of the macula in both eyes (Fig. 1.1). The remainder of the fundus examination was normal, without evidence of any satellite lesions, flecks, atrophy, retinal pigment epithelium (RPE) mottling, or other fundus changes.

IMAGING

Spectral domain optical coherence tomography (SD-OCT) showed dome-shaped hyperreflective lesions under the fovea of each eye (Fig. 1.2), with moderate fragmentation of the ellipsoid zone (EZ) but overall intact external limiting membrane (ELM). No intraretinal or subretinal fluid was seen. Fundus autofluorescence (FAF) imaging showed discrete round hyperautofluorescent lesions in both eyes at the foveal level (Fig. 1.3). In the right eye, the lesion showed partial fragmentation superiorly of the hyperautofluorescence. In the left eye, the hyperautofluorescent lesion was more compact and discrete but exhibited a focal hypofluorescent foveal spot (target-like appearance).

Questions to Ask

- Does the patient have a family history of ocular conditions[1] or consanguinity?[2-3] This patient's 43-year-old mother reported a positive history of possible Best disease on her side of the family, with multiple reportedly affected individuals of both sexes and across three generations, but the mother also reported having a previously normal eye examination herself and reported having been told she was unaffected with the condition.
  - Yes
- Has the patient been diagnosed with any cancer to this date, particularly with a melanoma[4-5] or a teratoma?[6-7] Although at this young age the possibility of a paraneoplastic

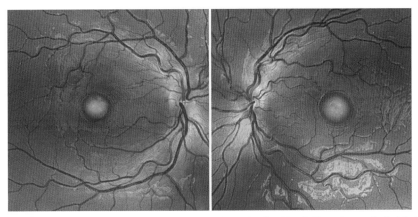

Fig. 1.1　Macular findings in the index case, showing elevated yellowish vitelliform (egg yolk–like) lesions. The remainder of the fundus examination is normal.

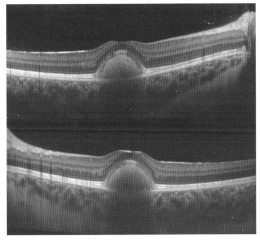

Fig. 1.2　Spectral domain optical coherence tomography of the index case, illustrating dome-shaped hyperreflective vitelliform lesions under the fovea of each eye seen ophthalmoscopically with moderate fragmentation of the ellipsoid zone but overall intact external limiting membrane.

acquired vitelliform maculopathy is very low, it cannot be 100% excluded. In young female patients a paraneoplastic retinopathy has been reported in conjunction with teratomas expressing, in those cases, retinal tissues that triggered the autoimmune reaction against the retina. Thus if this patient had a history of cancer or a teratoma, it would be important to exclude that the patient's cancer tissue did not exhibit RPE tissue within it (or other RPE-like antigens, particularly bestrophin) and that she did not exhibit antibestrophin auto-antibodies, which are present in patients with vitelliform paraneoplastic phenotypes and are usually associated with the same functional findings (see later) as in genetically determined vitelliform phenotypes.

■ No

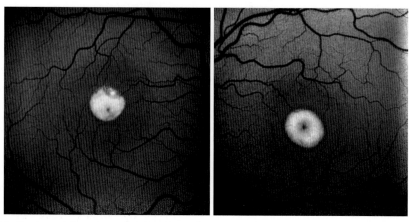

Fig. 1.3 Fundus autofluorescence imaging shows discrete round hyperautofluorescent lesions in both eyes at the foveal level.

Assessment

- This is a 12-year-old girl with no past ocular, medical, or surgical history to indicate or suggest an underlying teratoma or a malignancy, with a family history positive for possible Best disease on the maternal side but with a reportedly normal and unaffected mother. The patient demonstrates bilateral dome-shaped subfoveal macular vitelliform lesions on both SD-OCT and FAF.

Differential Diagnosis

- Autosomal dominant Best disease
- Autosomal recessive bestrophinopathy (ARB)
- Autosomal dominant macular pattern dystrophy (MPD) expressing a vitelliform phenotype
- Paraneoplastic acquired vitelliform maculopathy

Working Diagnosis

- Best disease
  - This condition is typically inherited in autosomal dominant fashion, and variable disease expression among family members with Best disease has been reported, although autosomal recessive variants (ARBs) of the disease are possible and can present with early-onset vitelliform lesions like the ones seen in our index case. Because the mother was reportedly unaffected, presently an autosomal recessive inheritance pattern cannot be excluded. Also, because MPDs can present with a macular vitelliform phenotype, especially the ones linked to the *PRPH2 (peripherin/RDS)* gene,[1,8] and family members presenting with a mild MPD phenotype can be asymptomatic well into their 60s,[1,9] presently it cannot be excluded that the mother of the index case may appear unaffected because she has not expressed the phenotype yet. The differential can be addressed clinically by functional testing with an electrooculogram (EOG), which would be expected to be pathological (Arden ratio <1.5) in either Best disease or patients with ARB but not in patients with MPD or in the parents of a patient with ARB.

Multimodal Testing and Results

- Fundus photos
  - As mentioned earlier, dilated fundus examination showed coin-shaped, egg yolk–like, yellowish elevated lesions in the center of the macula in both eyes (Fig. 1.1).
  - This presentation is equally common in bona fide dominant Best disease, ARBs, and MPDs expressing a vitelliform phenotype.[1,3] In the latter, neovascular exudative complications responsive to anti–vascular endothelial growth factor (VEGF) injections are common, but they can be seen also in patients with early-onset ARB.[3] Patients with dominant Best disease are not immune from this possible complication, but these frank exudative complications are far less common.
- SD-OCT
  - As illustrated earlier, dome-shaped hyperreflective lesions were seen under the fovea of each eye (Fig. 1.2), with moderate EZ fragmentation but an overall intact ELM, and no intra- or subretinal fluid.
  - This imaging modality is critical in establishing the clinical impression of the elevated subfoveal lesions, showing whether fluid is present, and ascertaining the state of the EZ and the ELM, but it does not permit a differential diagnosis.
- EOG
  - An EOG was obtained on the index case, but the patient was unreliable during the test, which requires tracking a moving light target correctly and repeatedly to measure the ocular standing potential (i.e., the steady flow of electricity being released by the eyes) and comparing reliably the lowest such potential in the dark (the "dark trough" [DT]) and the highest such potential once lights are turned on (the "light peak" [LP]). The mathematical rapport between the two values (LP/DT) is known as the *Arden ratio*.[10]
  - The unreliability of the EOG test in the index case yielded an Arden ratio greater than 3.0, which per se would have ruled out the diagnosis of either Best disease or an ARB but was potentially misleading. Thus to overcome the uncertainly in this case, we extended the investigation to the asymptomatic 43-year-old mother, who had visual acuity of 20/20 in both eyes and exhibited a minimal SD-OCT phenotype (Fig. 1.4) insufficient to support outright the diagnosis of dominant Best disease, as it would have been suggested by the positive history on her side of the family. However, she was able to perform an EOG correctly, and her Arden ratio was less than 1.0 (Fig. 1.5), which is diagnostic for a generalized RPE compromise and the diagnosis of either Best disease or an ARB. Because the positive family history of Best disease was present on her side, this outcome supported the working diagnosis of Best disease and an autosomal dominant inheritance pattern as the top diagnosis on the differential.
- Genetic testing
  - This needs to be obtained to confirm the working diagnosis and to establish correctly the reproductive risk for both the index case and her mother (particularly the autosomal dominant vs. recessive inheritance pattern). Because a reliable EOG could be obtained in the mother and was diagnostic for a condition linked to the *BEST1 (VMD2)* gene, a targeted genetic test for mutations in a single gene can be prospected without the absolute necessity to conduct a full inherited retinal disease (IRD) panel screen. Had the EOG not been obtained on the mother for whatever reason (e.g., unwilling, unavailable, deceased), then based on the "normal" EOG in the index case, a full IRD panel screen would have been necessary.

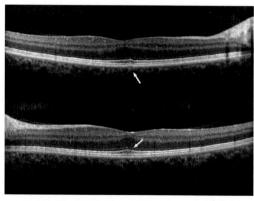

Fig. 1.4 Spectral domain optical coherence tomography of the mother of the index case, illustrating minimal changes in the foveal region.

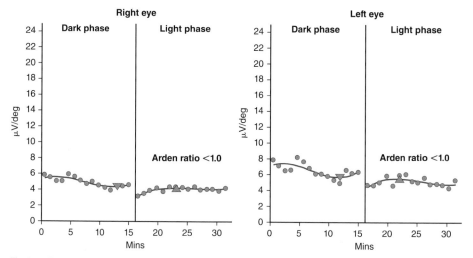

Fig. 1.5 Plots of the two eyes of the electrooculogram of the mother of the index case, showing a lack of "light peak" (LP) during the light-adapted phase of the test. Also, the dark-adapted phase does not show a true "dark trough" (DT) as it is normally seen. The resulting Arden ratio (LP/DT) was less than 1.0, fully diagnostic for a generalized retinal pigment epithelium dysfunction and strongly suggestive of dominantly inherited Best disease despite the minimal clinical disease expression.

■ In this case, both the index case and the mother tested positive for a single, heterozygous c.18 C>G, p.Tyr6Arg (T6R) point mutation in exon 2 of the *BEST1 (VMD2)* gene without any other changes in the second allele, thereby establishing in this patient and her family the diagnosis of autosomal dominant Best disease.

Management

■ Given that this patient was only mildly symptomatic and had visual acuity better than 20/30 in both eyes, the patient was observed, as was her asymptomatic mother, who had visual acuity of 20/20 in both eyes.

- Currently, no treatment is available for the vitelliform lesions of autosomal dominant Best disease.
- If an outright neovascular exudative complication occurs, these exudative manifestations have been shown to be responsive to anti-VEGF agents and should be treated if detected.

Follow-Up Care

- There are no previously established guidelines for follow-up.
- Our patient is followed on an annual basis, with the instruction to monitor the situation monthly with an Amsler grid to identify any change that may suggest a neovascular exudative complication and require management, in which case the patient would call our clinic immediately for evaluation.
- If the patient developed one such complication, more frequent follow-up would be indicated based on standard anti-VEGF treatment paradigms.

Algorithm 1.1: Algorithm for Differential Diagnosis for Best Disease

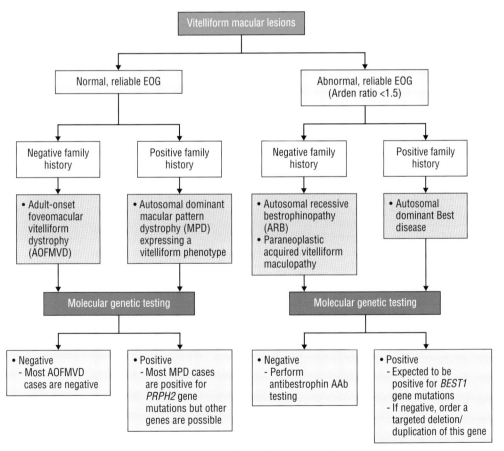

Algorithm 1.1 Algorithm for differential diagnosis for Best disease.

Key Points

- Consider either dominant or recessive *BEST1*-related disease in patients with vitelliform clinical presentations.

- Obtain an EOG to confirm the diagnosis, ideally on more than one family member, and, if normal, reroute the differential to a MPD presenting with a vitelliform lesion, which is genetically distinct (most often linked to *PRPH2* mutations).

- If the inheritance pattern cannot be established with certainty, order a deletion/duplication test of the *BEST1* gene because a second hard-to-detect change by standard testing may be present in the second allele and may point to a recessive inheritance rather than the more typical dominant one.

- If the patient presenting with this phenotype is older and/or has a history of cancer (or a teratoma), consider the paraneoplastic etiology and order antibestrophin autoantibody testing even if the EOG seems diagnostic for a *BEST1*-related disease, especially if genetic testing is negative. In the latter case, if the antibestrophin autoantibody testing is positive, then a cancer work-up would be indicated.

References

1. Iannaccone A. Genotype-phenotype correlations and differential diagnosis in autosomal dominant macular disease. *Doc Ophthalmol.* 2001;102:197-236.
2. Burgess R, Millar ID, Leroy BP, et al. Biallelic mutation of BEST1 causes a distinct retinopathy in humans. *Am J Hum Genet.* 2008;82:19-31.
3. Iannaccone A, Kerr NC, Kinnick TR, Calzada JI, Stone EM. Autosomal recessive best vitelliform macular dystrophy: report of a family and management of early-onset neovascular complications. *Arch Ophthalmol.* 2011;129:211-217.
4. Sotodeh M, Paridaens D, Keunen J, van Schooneveld M, Adamus G, Baarsma S. Paraneoplastic vitelliform retinopathy associated with cutaneous or uveal melanoma and metastases. *Klin Monbl Augenheilkd.* 2005;222:910-914.
5. Eksandh L, Adamus G, Mosgrove L, Andreasson S. Autoantibodies against bestrophin in a patient with vitelliform paraneoplastic retinopathy and a metastatic choroidal malignant melanoma. *Arch Ophthalmol.* 2008;126:432-435.
6. Suhler EB, Chan CC, Caruso RC, et al. Presumed teratoma-associated paraneoplastic retinopathy. *Arch Ophthalmol.* 2003;121:133-137.
7. Turaka K, Kietz D, Krishnamurti L, et al. Carcinoma-associated retinopathy in a young teenager with immature teratoma of the ovary. *J AAPOS.* 2014;18:396-398.
8. Fossarello M, Bertini C, Galantuomo MS, Cao A, Serra A, Pirastu M. Deletion in the peripherin/RDS gene in two unrelated Sardinian families with autosomal dominant butterfly-shaped macular dystrophy. *Arch Opthalmol.* 1996;114:448-456.
9. Wang X, Wang H, Sun V, et al. Comprehensive molecular diagnosis of 179 Leber congenital amaurosis and juvenile retinitis pigmentosa patients by targeted next generation sequencing. *J Med Genet.* 2013;50:674-688.
10. Constable PA, Bach M, Frishman LJ, Jeffrey BG, Robson AG, International Society for Clinical Electrophysiology of Vision. ISCEV standard for clinical electro-oculography (2017 update). *Doc Ophthalmol.* 2017;134:1-9.

CHAPTER 2

Long-standing Photophobia, Reduced Visual Acuity, Myopia, and Dyschromatopsia in a Young Adult Male Patient

Alessandro Iannaccone

History of Present Illness

We present a case of a 34-year-old male patient with a chief report of long-standing photophobia associated with reduced visual acuity, myopia, and dyschromatopsia. His vision has never been perfect, although he states subjectively, "It's pretty good." He has been wearing a myopic correction most of his life with partial benefit to visual acuity. He denies night blindness or visual field loss, and he has never exhibited nystagmus.

OCULAR EXAMINATION FINDINGS

Best corrected visual acuity with a high myopic correction was 20/50 in the right eye and 20/64 in the left. Ocular motility was intact in all positions of gaze; there was no ptosis and no nystagmus. External and anterior segment examinations were unremarkable, with no evidence of corneal pannus, and there were no iris transillumination defects, evidence for ectropion uveae, or corectopia. Intraocular pressure was normal.

Dilated fundus examination (Fig. 2.1) showed myopic findings with a mild posterior staphyloma involving both the macula and the peripapillary region, and blunting of the foveal reflexes with fine foveal mottling of the retinal pigment epithelium (RPE). The optic disc exhibited a sloped cup and mild temporal peripapillary atrophy (crescent-like). Retinal vasculature was normal, and there were no peripheral findings. There were no macular or peripheral pigmentary deposits or flecks, macular tapetal-like golden metallic sheen, or evidence for diffuse hypopigmentation. All findings were symmetrical between the two eyes.

Questions to Ask

- Does the patient exhibit any systemic findings in association to the visual reports? It is important to ask a patient like this about any history of kidney problems, hearing loss, diabetes or prediabetes, heart problems (in particular, dilated cardiomyopathy or heart conduction defects), or extra digits on hands and/or feet (or other anomalies of the extremities). Both height and weight should be measured to check for short stature and/or obesity (body mass index > 30). Any one or more of these features may be associated with an eye problem as part of a syndromic condition.
  - No

9

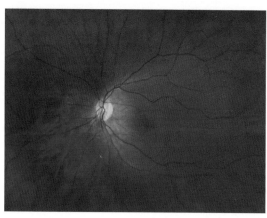

Fig. 2.1 Fundus photograph of the patient, mostly prominent for relatively nonspecific myopic findings and blunting of the foveal reflexes.

- What is the patient's refractive error? Myopic refraction in a male patient who reports long-standing photophobia, poor visual acuity, and dyschromatopsia is far more common in X-linked conditions such as blue cone monochromacy (BCM), X-linked cone dystrophy (XL-COD), X-linked cone–rod dystrophy (XL-CORD), and Bornholm eye disease (BED) (a condition characterized by the triad of X-linked myopia, deuteranopia, and cone dysfunction), whereas a hypermetropic refraction is far more common in patients with achromatopsia (ACHM) or another X-linked disorder, type 2 ("incomplete") congenital stationary night blindness (CSNB).[1-4] Other conditions associated with photophobia, poor visual acuity, and dyschromatopsia are not known to be more typically associated with any particular type of refractive error.
  - −6.75sph − 1.00 × 052 in the right eye and −6.75sph − 1.00 × 117 in the left eye
- Does the patient have a family history of ocular conditions, or is there consanguinity among his parents? A family history of a female sibling with similar reports in the absence of any other cases along the vertical family axis would suggest an autosomal recessive inheritance. Parental consanguinity would further support this possibility and would predict that any genetic etiology for the findings will be present in the homozygous state (same mutation inherited from each parent). A history of similar reports in his father would instead indicate male-to-male transmission and support an autosomal dominant inheritance pattern. If instead there were other male relatives affected with the same problem on the maternal side only and no instance of male-to-male transmission, with the mother being asymptomatic or exhibiting milder findings, this would suggest an X-linked recessive inheritance.
  - No. In this case, family history was not contributory, leaving the door open to both autosomal recessive and X-linked recessive inheritance.

Assessment

- This is a case of a 34-year-old male patient with a chief report of long-standing photophobia associated with reduced visual acuity, myopia, and dyschromatopsia, and with negative family history for other cases of similar reports in other relatives, who exhibits a largely normal fundus examination except for very clear foveal changes on macular spectral domain optical coherence tomography (SD-OCT).

Differential Diagnosis

- XL-COD
- XL-CORD
- BCM
- BED
- X-linked CSNB
- X-linked ocular albinism
- Autosomal dominant cone dystrophy
- Autosomal dominant PAX6-associated disease
- Autosomal recessive ACHM
- Autosomal recessive ocular albinism
- Autosomal recessive cone dystrophy
- Autosomal recessive cone–rod dystrophy
- Autosomal recessive CSNB

Because of the noted association of the myopic refractive defect with conditions that have an X-linked inheritance pattern, X-linked diagnoses are to be considered higher on the differential, but autosomal recessive inheritance cannot be fully ruled out in this case. Autosomal dominant inheritance (which is well-known to be associated with instances of incomplete penetrance and/or highly variable disease expressivity) also cannot be technically excluded and could also be an uncommon case of a de novo mutation, but at this moment there is nothing to support this possibility.

Working Diagnosis

- Based on the reports, the family history, and the refractive defect, the diagnoses XL-COD, XL-CORD, BCM, and BED are at this stage most and equally likely ones. Because there is no nystagmus, BCM (which is typically associated with it) is potentially the lowest on the differential at this stage.
- The possibility of a cone dystrophy–like variant of BCM, as they have been associated with particular genetic changes in the visual pigment locus control region, also exists and would be best compatible with the lack of nystagmus.

Multimodal Testing and Results

- SD-OCT
  - Despite the blunted foveal reflexes, but in line with the foveal RPE mottling seen on dilated fundus examination, SD-OCT (Fig. 2.2) showed a clearly identifiable and well-defined foveal pit in both eyes with an underlying area of focal loss of the ellipsoid zone (EZ), with hyporeflective EZ gaps (so-called cavitation lesions), and focal hypertransmission defects attributable to RPE loss. There were no intraretinal or subretinal hypo- or hyperreflective lesions, changes, or deposits. Despite the myopia, there was also no choroidal thinning. On horizontal SD-OCT scans, a downward slanting toward the disc of the retinal scan because of the staphyloma was also noticeable. Macular volume maps (not shown) were within normal limits.
- Macular fundus autofluorescence (FAF)
  - FAF (Fig. 2.3) was normal in both eyes except for a focal spot of foveal hypoauto-fluorescence and faint parafoveal hyperautofluorescence, seen bilaterally. Imaging findings are mostly compatible with XL-COD, BED, and BCM but do not allow us to differentiate between them. The diagnoses of either X-linked or autosomal recessive ocular albinism and of either X-linked or autosomal recessive CSNB are ruled out

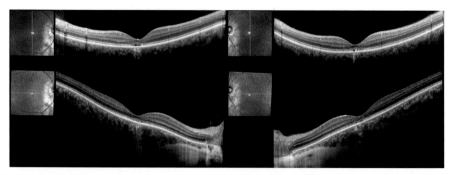

Fig. 2.2 Spectral domain optical coherence tomography of the index case illustrating the posterior staphyloma and the foveal findings.

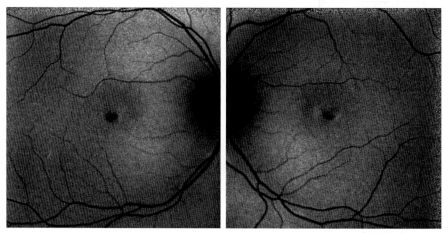

Fig. 2.3 Fundus autofluorescence imaging show subtle foveal changes, with a focal spot of foveal hypoautofluorescence and faint parafoveal hyperautofluorescence.

by these findings, because none of these conditions is expected to cause either EZ or FAF abnormalities.

- Full-field flash electroretinogram (ffERG)
  - ffERG testing showed (Fig. 2.4) normal dark-adapted rod-driven responses in both eyes, mildly reduced a-waves to dark-adapted mixed rod/cone-driven responses, and markedly but still clearly recordable light-adapted cone-driven responses. This finding further supports the working diagnoses of XL-COD, BED, and BCM but also does not allow us to differentiate between them. The diagnoses of either X-linked or autosomal recessive ocular albinism (in which the ffERG is typically normal) and of either X-linked or autosomal recessive CSNB (in which the rod-driven responses are typically completely or partially reduced vis-à-vis a much better preservation of the cone ones, and the mixed responses are characteristically electronegative due to a selective reduction of the mixed b-wave response) are further ruled out by these findings.
  - Therefore at this point, additional functional testing is needed to refine the differential for this patient.
- Color vision testing
  - The pseudoisochromatic Ishihara plates showed severe green color discrimination (deuteranopia) but essentially normal red color discrimination, and panel D-15 testing (a confrontation-based test) confirmed a dyschromatopsia exclusively along the green

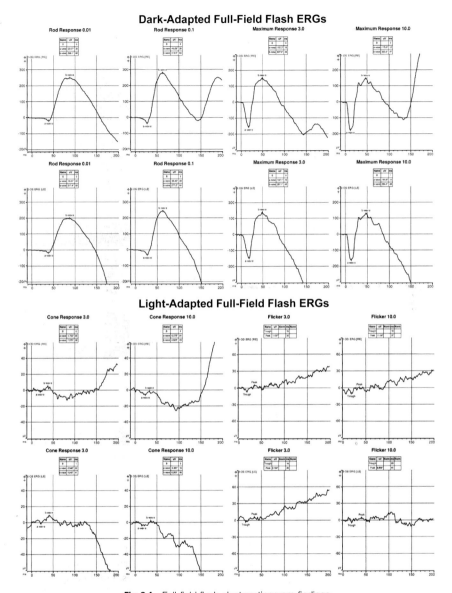

Fig. 2.4   Full-field flash electroretinogram findings.

(deutan) axis, with no apparent involvement of either the red (protan) or the blue–yellow axis. The regular alternating pattern of the test reveals its congenital nature (Fig. 2.5). Using additional, more refined pseudoisochromatic methods, such as the standard pseudoisochromatic plates (SPP)-1 (red–green axis) and SPP-2 plates (blue–yellow axis) and the Neitz Test of Color Vision (http://www.neitzvision.com/neitz-test/), which are both discrimination based, it was confirmed that there were profound defects along the green axis but that the red and blue–yellow axes were essentially intact.

- Perimetry
  - Consistent with the ffERG results, kinetic semiautomated perimetry was full in size in both eyes to all tested isopters.

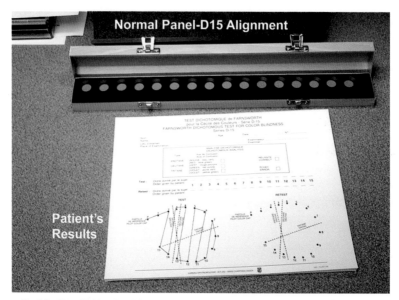

Fig. 2.5   Panel D15 color vision findings compared with a normal test result outcome.

- Despite the ffERG outcome, microperimetry using white-on-white, Goldmann size-III stimuli across the central 10 degrees was normal at all tested loci except for foveally, where a small but dense scotoma was found.
- Automated perimetry (Humphrey 30–2 testing) with short-wavelength automated perimetry, which uses blue–purple (440-nm), Goldmann size-V stimuli presented on a bright yellow background, this patient exhibited a near-normal outcome, corroborating the impression derived from color vision testing that the blue-light sensitive (S) cones of this patient were preserved. The outcome of color vision and perimetry testing concurred to suggest that this patient most likely has either BCM or its partial variant, BED.
- Molecular genetic diagnostic testing
  - This was obtained because all findings pointed in the direction of a genetic disorder and identified in this case a novel point mutation (c.260C>T, p.P87L) in the OPN1LW gene on the X chromosome. This gene encodes for the long wavelength–sensitive (green) cone pigment and is predicted to have a deleterious effect on the resulting protein. This finding supports at the molecular level the diagnosis of BED and reveals further (as it has been reported also in association to other gene changes in the cone photopigment gene cluster)[1-9] that BED is essentially a BCM variant with cone dystrophy-like manifestations, explaining why it was so difficult to discriminate between classical BCM and another type of X-linked cone dysfunction syndrome. Neither BED nor BCM is associated with rod compromise, thus this test outcome establishes that there is no threat to night vision in this patient.

Management

- Gene therapy for BCM and related disorders affecting the cone visual pigment gene cluster are being developed, but no treatment is available currently.
- Because BED is of the BCM family, which is only minimally progressive, no treatment needs to be pursued. However, because progression to macular atrophy is possible in both BED and classical BCM and is partially present in this patient, it would not be inappropriate to recommend dietary supplements that have been associated with neuroprotective

benefits to retinal cones both in preclinical and clinical studies, such as *N*-acetylcysteine,[10-12] although it is not presently clear whether the same oxidative stress–based mechanisms at play in dystrophies like retinitis pigmentosa would be involved also in BED and related disorders.

Follow-up Care

- There are no previously established guidelines for follow-up.
- Our patient is being followed approximately on an annual basis.
- If the patient demonstrates progression on SD-OCT, chromatic perimetry, and/or ffERG, treatment as recommended earlier would likely be indicated.

Algorithm 2.1: Algorithm for Differential Diagnosis for BED/BCM/X-Linked Cone Dystrophy

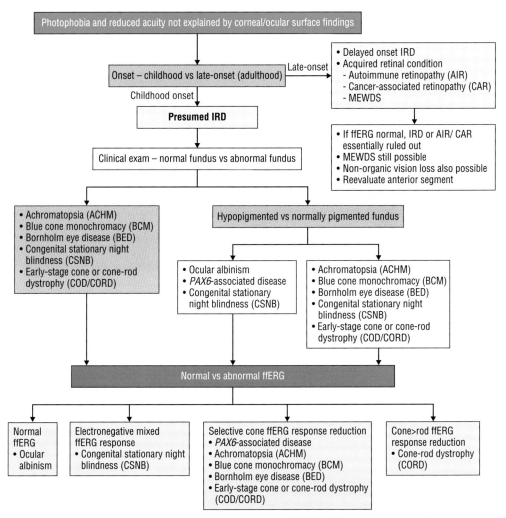

Algorithm 2.1 Algorithm for differential diagnosis for BED/BCM/X-linked cone dystrophy.

Key Points

- Consider BED, BCM, and one of the related cone dysfunction syndromes in patients with photophobia, high myopia, color vision defects, and reduced acuity.
- Although ffERG is essential in excluding several other diagnoses, in this case color vision testing was truly essential in suggesting most strongly the rarer diagnosis of BED, which is a variant of BCM, and not typical BCM (in which both the red and green color vision axes are compromised, whereby there is also nystagmus and poorer visual acuity).
- Molecular genetic diagnostic testing was decisive in confirming the diagnosis and should always be obtained when a retinal dystrophy is suspected.
- Patients with BED tend to have better visual acuity than patients with BCM or XL-COD but need to be followed with functional and imaging studies.

References

1. Young TL, Deeb SS, Ronan SM, et al. X-linked high myopia associated with cone dysfunction. *Arch Ophthalmol.* 2004;122:897-908.
2. McClements M, Davies WI, Michaelides M, et al. Variations in opsin coding sequences cause x-linked cone dysfunction syndrome with myopia and dichromacy. *Invest Ophthalmol Vis Sci.* 2013;54:1361-1369.
3. Aboshiha J, Dubis AM, Carroll J, Hardcastle AJ, Michaelides M. The cone dysfunction syndromes. *Br J Ophthalmol.* 2016;100:115-121.
4. De Silva SR, Arno G, Robson AG, et al. The X-linked retinopathies: physiological insights, pathogenic mechanisms, phenotypic features and novel therapies. *Prog Retin Eye Res.* 2021;82:100898.
5. Michaelides M, Johnson S, Bradshaw K, et al. X-linked cone dysfunction syndrome with myopia and protanopia. *Ophthalmology.* 2005;112:1448-1454.
6. McClements ME, Neitz M, Moore AT, Hunt DM. Bornholm eye disease arises from a specific combination of amino acid changes encoded by exon 3 of the L/M cone opsin gene. *Invest Ophthalmol Vis Sci.* 2010;51(13):2609.
7. Patterson EJ, Wilk M, Langlo CS, et al. Cone photoreceptor structure in patients with X-linked cone dysfunction and red-green color vision deficiency. *Invest Ophthalmol Vis Sci.* 2016;57:3853-3863.
8. Greenwald SH, Kuchenbecker JA, Rowlan JS, Neitz J, Neitz M. Role of a dual splicing and amino acid code in myopia, cone dysfunction and cone dystrophy associated with L/M opsin interchange mutations. *Transl Vis Sci Technol.* 2017;6:2.
9. Holmquist D, Epstein D, Olsson M, et al. Visual and ocular findings in a family with X-linked cone dysfunction and protanopia. *Ophthalmic Genet.* 2021;42:570-576.
10. Lee SY, Usui S, Zafar AB, et al. N-acetylcysteine promotes long-term survival of cones in a model of retinitis pigmentosa. *J Cell Physiol.* 2011;226:1843-1849.
11. Campochiaro PA, Iftikhar M, Hafiz G, et al. Oral N-acetylcysteine improves cone function in retinitis pigmentosa patients in phase I trial. *J Clin Invest.* 2020;130:1527-1541.
12. Kong X, Hafiz G, Wehling D, Akhlaq A, Campochiaro PA. Locus-level changes in macular sensitivity in patients with retinitis pigmentosa treated with oral N-acetylcysteine. *Am J Ophthalmol.* 2021;221:105-114.

CHAPTER 3

Bilateral Progressive Severe Loss of Vision and Obesity

Daniel W. Wang ▪ Kanishka Jayasundera ▪ Jennifer I. Lim
▪ Benjamin Young ▪ Dana Schlegel ▪ Helen Liu

History of Present Illness

A 26-year-old man with severe obesity and mild intellectual impairment presents with gradually progressive, severe vision loss of both eyes. He denies floaters, ocular pain, flashes, and other ocular symptoms.

OCULAR EXAMINATION FINDINGS

Visual acuity was hand motion (HM) in both eyes with no improvement with pinhole. Pupils were equal in size and reactive to light without an afferent pupillary defect. Intraocular pressure was 16 mm Hg in both eyes. Anterior segment examination demonstrated 1+ posterior subcapsular cataracts of both eyes but was otherwise unremarkable. Dilated fundus examination of both eyes showed waxy optic nerve pallor with diffuse midperipheral pigmentary degeneration with mottling and scattered bone spicules. The vessels appeared to be mildly attenuated (Figs. 3.1 and 3.2).

Questions to Ask

- Does the patient have a family history of retinal disorders/dystrophies? Several retinal dystrophies such as retinitis pigmentosa have inheritance patterns and may lead to advanced vision loss at a young age.
  - Not known
- Does the patient have postaxial polydactyly?
  - Yes. The patient was born with extra digits and underwent surgery in early childhood (Fig. 3.3).
- What medications does the patient take? Medications such as phenothiazines may concentrate in the retinal pigment epithelium and in some cases may manifest as a pigmentary retinopathy.
  - None
- Does the patient have associated hearing loss? Hearing loss is a highly prevalent symptom in similar conditions such as Alström syndrome or Usher syndrome, whereas hearing loss is not as common in Bardet-Biedl syndrome (BBS).
  - No
- Does the patient have a history of diabetes? Although obesity is a cardinal feature of BBS, diabetes is not common. Diabetes insipidus generally is more common with Alström syndrome.
  - No

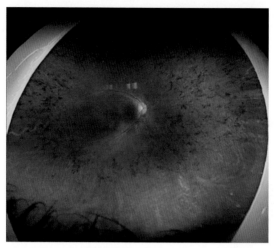

Fig. 3.1 Color fundus photograph reveals mild pallor of the optic disk along macular atrophy and scattered bone spicules that extend up to the midperiphery. There is prominent vascular attenuation.

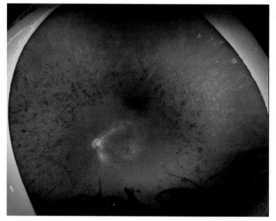

Fig. 3.2 Fundus photograph demonstrates a healthy disk appearance along with central geographical atrophy. Scattered bone spicules are noted in the midperiphery along with vascular attenuation within the posterior pole.

Assessment

This is a case of a 26-year-old man reporting with severe, chronic vision loss in the context of retinal dystrophy with associated obesity, intellectual impairment, polydactyly, and unknown family history.

Differential Diagnosis

- BBS
- Laurence-Moon syndrome

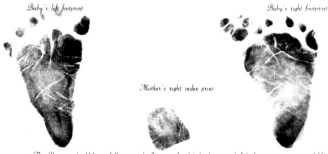

FAMILY HISTORY

Father's full name _____
Birthplace _____ Date _____
Mother's maiden name _____
Birthplace _____ Date _____
Residence at time child was born _____
Sex of child _____ Weight at birth _____ pounds _____ ounces. Length _____ inches

Baby's left footprint   Baby's right footprint

Mother's right index print

This Document should be carefully preserved. It is your family's heirloom record of the facts pertaining to your child's birth. The law requires that the original certificate (not this document) be filed with the Vital Statistics Office at _____ from which an official copy may be obtained.

Fig. 3.3 Birth certificate of the patient demonstrating polydactyly of the right and left foot.

- Retinitis pigmentosa
- Usher syndrome
- Alström syndrome
- Joubert syndrome
- Leber congenital amaurosis
- Senior-Loken syndrome

Working Diagnosis

- BBS

BBS is a clinical diagnosis. Diagnosis is confirmed in patients that meet at least four primary features (Fig. 3.4) or three primary and two secondary features of BBS.

PRIMARY FEATURES

1. Retinal degeneration
2. Truncal obesity
3. Intellectual impairment
4. Postaxial polydactyly
5. Hypogonadism
6. Renal abnormalities

SECONDARY FEATURES

1. Speech delay
2. Developmental delay

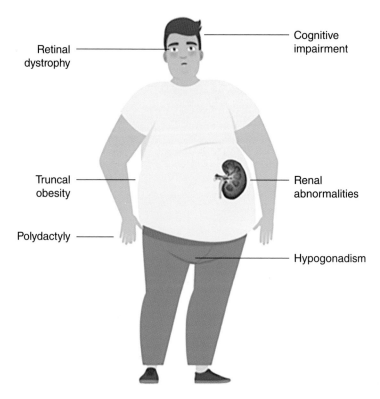

Fig. 3.4   Common clinical features of Bardet-Biedl syndrome.

3. Diabetes mellitus
4. Orodental abnormalities
5. Cardiovascular anomalies
6. Brachydactyly/syndactyly
7. Ataxia/poor coordination
8. Anosmia/hyposmia

Multimodal Testing and Results

- External examination
  - Most patients exhibit early obesity, polydactyly, and have intellectual impairment. Hypogonadism is also part of the major diagnostic criteria, and delayed puberty is frequently reported. Patients with BBS also show significant renal involvement.[1,2]
- Optical coherence tomography (OCT)
  - Generalized thinning of the retina with widespread photoreceptor outer/inner segment attenuation is appreciated in both eyes (Figs. 3.5 and 3.6). OCT scans in BBS patients typically show thinning in and around the fovea with varying severity of paracentral thinning and normal nerve fiber layer around the optic nerve.[3] Deletions and complete absence of the outer structure of the foveal area are common.[3] Other features observed in BBS patients on OCT include internal limiting membrane wrinkling and deposits adjacent to and anterior to Bruch's membrane.[2]

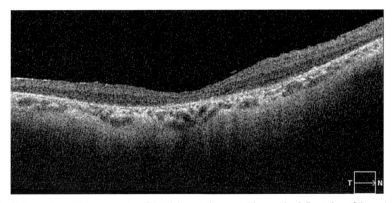

Fig. 3.5 Optical coherence tomography of the right eye demonstrating marked disruption of the outer retinal layers and prominent foveal atrophy.

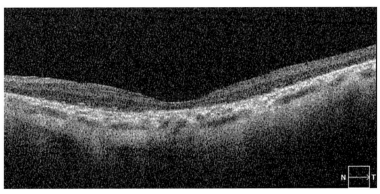

Fig. 3.6 Optical coherence tomography of the left eye demonstrating significant foveal atrophy along with loss of the outer retinal layers.

- Electroretinogram (ERG)
  - ERG will generally show a mixed rod–cone dystrophy, manifesting as diminished a- and b-waves in both scotopic and photopic conditions. Given the heterogeneity in the severity of retinal disease, studies have shown ERG is more sensitive than clinical examination findings, such as vision loss, and can detect abnormalities as early as age 5 years.[4]
- Autofluorescence
  - Both eyes demonstrate scattered areas of hypofluorescence corresponding to the observed peripheral pigmentary changes. Additionally, there is an ovoid area of hypofluorescence in the macula of both eyes (Figs. 3.7 and 3.8).

Management

Although there is no treatment, a multidisciplinary approach is required to address concomitant disease manifestations such as hypertension, metabolic syndromes, and diseases secondary to organ systems involved with BBS. Annual assessments of weight, blood pressure, lipid profile, liver function tests, and blood glucose level are recommended. Genetic counseling is also recommended. Current research on the treatment of BBS retinopathy includes BBS gene therapy, which shows immense promise when treating BBS retinopathy at the early stages, and genome

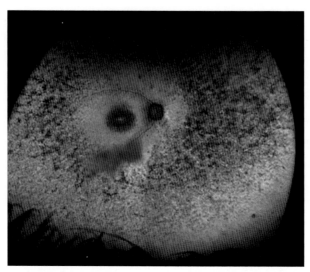

Fig. 3.7 Fundus autofluorescence image of the right eye showing a circular area of hypoautofluorescence in the macular region along with a granular pattern of hypoautofluorescence in the midperiphery corresponding to the bone spicules visualized on fundus examination. Artifact from a posterior capsular cataract is noted.

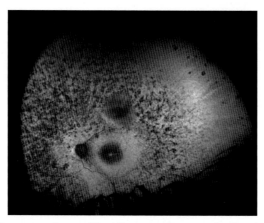

Fig. 3.8 Fundus autofluorescence image of the left eye revealing a prominent central area of geographical hypoautofluorescence. A granular pattern of hypoautofluorescence is appreciated throughout the midperiphery and posterior pole. Artifact from a posterior capsular cataract is noted.

editing.[1] Given the severity of visual dysfunction, referral to low-vision services is indicated. Ophthalmological evaluation for assessment of strabismus, nystagmus, and decreased visual acuity is needed.

Follow-up Care

There are no previously established guidelines for follow-up. The patient is to be followed annually. Based on the certainty of blindness for the patient, early educational planning is crucial. This includes instruction on Braille, mobility training, adaptive living skills, computing skills, and/or the use of large-print reading materials while vision is still present.

Algorithm 3.1: Algorithm Showing Differential Diagnosis for Retinopathy

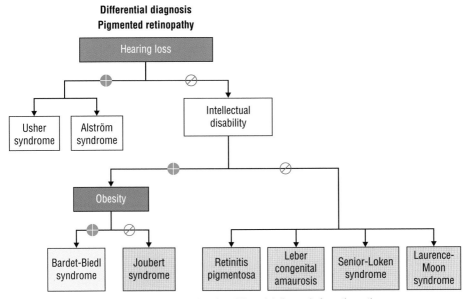

Algorithm 3.1 Algorithm showing differential diagnosis for retinopathy.

Key Points

- Bardet Biedl Syndrome, retinitis pigmentosa, obesity, syndrome

References

1. Forsythe E, Beales PL. Bardet-Biedl syndrome. *Eur J Hum Genet.* 2013;21(1):8-13.
2. Priya S, Nampoothiri S, Sen P, Sripriya S. Bardet-Biedl syndrome: genetics, molecular pathophysiology, and disease management. *Indian J Ophthalmol.* 2016;64(9):620-627.
3. Morjaria R, Khan H, Said M, et al. OCT characteristics associated with Bardet-Biedl syndrome (BBS) retinopathy. *Invest Ophthalmol Vis Sci.* 2019;60(9):1569.
4. Berezovsky A, Rocha DM, Sacai PY, Watanabe SS, Cavascan NN, Salomão SR. Visual acuity and retinal function in patients with Bardet-Biedl syndrome. *Clinics (Sao Paulo).* 2012;67(2):145-149.

CHAPTER 4

Bilateral Peripheral Retinal and Macular Schisis in a Young Boy

George Skopis ■ Madeleine Y. Yehia ■ Jennifer I. Lim

History of Present Illness

A 13-year-old boy presents to the retina clinic for blurry vision in both eyes. The patient's mother states that the patient has been on topical dorzolamide for many years prescribed by another ophthalmologist. The patient denies flashes, floaters, or nyctalopia.

OCULAR EXAMINATION FINDINGS

Best corrected visual acuity was 20/50 in the right eye and 20/150 in the left eye. Intraocular pressures were 12 mm Hg. The anterior segment examination was normal in each eye. Dilated fundus examination revealed a spoke wheel–like cystic appearance emanating from the fovea of each eye. In addition, there were inferotemporal smooth, dome-shaped retinal elevations in both eyes.

Questions to Ask

- What is the patient's refraction: is the patient myopic? Patients with myopia and staphyloma can develop myopic foveomacular schisis.
  - No
- Does the patient have a history of inflammatory eye disease? Uveitis may present with cystoid macular edema that may mimic retinoschisis.
  - No
- Does the patient have a past medical history of systemic disease? Conditions such as diabetes mellitus and hypertension are common causes of macular edema (diabetic macular edema, retinal vein occlusion with macular edema) that resemble retinoschisis.
  - No
- Does the patient have any family history of vision loss? Assessing the patient's family history of eye disease, vision loss or consanguinity is important when considering inherited forms of retinoschisis, retinitis pigmentosa, and enhanced S-cone syndrome.
  - Yes, the patient's two maternal uncles have a history of vision loss in childhood. The patient's mother in unaffected.

Assessment

- This is a case of a 13-year-old boy with positive family history of childhood vision loss in maternal uncles presenting with bilateral vision loss demonstrating bilateral macular schisis on optical coherence tomography (OCT).

Differential Diagnosis

- Myopic foveomacular schisis: as indicated earlier, patient was emmetropic
- Traumatic retinoschisis: patient had no known history of trauma
- Retinitis pigmentosa
- Vitreomacular traction: more commonly seen in older patients when posterior vitreous detachments are evolving
- Cystoid macular edema of any cause: pseudophakia, retinal vascular
- Optic pit: no pit in our patient
- Inherited retinoschisis: autosomal recessive, autosomal dominant, or X-linked
- Medication induced (taxanes, niacin)
- Enhanced S-cone syndrome
- Degenerative retinoschisis: usually seen in older patients

Workup and Diagnosis

- Further history revealed the patient's mother has two brothers who have had severe vision loss since childhood. The patient's mother denied any other family members with known ocular history or vision loss.
- Genetic testing was performed, and the patient was found to have a pathogenic deletion in the RS1 gene.
- A diagnosis of X-linked retinoschisis was made.

Multimodal Testing and Results

- Fundus photograph
  - Bilateral, spoke wheel–like folds seen emanating from the fovea are indicative of macular schisis and are the hallmark feature of X-linked retinoschisis[1] (Fig. 4.1). Vitreous hemorrhage and retinal detachment are the major vision-threatening complications.[2]

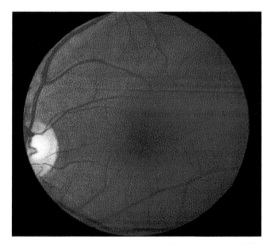

Fig. 4.1 A color fundus photograph of the left eye showing subtle, spoke wheel–like pattern emanating from the fovea. (Reproduced with permission from Tantri A, Vrabec TR, Cu-Unjieng A, Frost A, Annesley WH Jr, Donoso LA. X-linked retinoschisis: a clinical and molecular genetic review. *Surv Ophthalmol.* 2004; 49(2):214-230, fig. 2.)

Retinal neovascularization or bridging retinal vessels (Fig. 4.2) adjacent to schisis cavities may contribute to vitreous hemorrhage.

- Peripheral schisis is present in approximately 50% of patients and is usually located in the inferotemporal quadrant[3] (Fig. 4.3).
- OCT
    - In patients with X-linked retinoschisis, the foveomacular schisis cavities may occur in multiple layers of the retina. The retina nerve fiber layer, inner nuclear layer, or outer nuclear layer may be affected[4] (Fig. 4.4).
    - It has been shown that increased inner retinal foveal thickness and decreased perifoveal inner retinal thickness correlate with worse vision in patients with X-linked retinoschisis.[5] Overall retinal thickness decreases with age,[5] indicating collapse of the schisis cavities and subsequent atrophy, which can lead to diagnostic dilemma in older patients (Fig. 4.5).

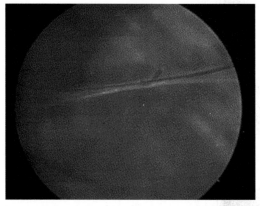

Fig. 4.2 Color fundus photograph showing a bridging vessel at the edge of a schisis cavity. These bridging vessels can be responsible for the vitreous hemorrhage seen in peripheral retinoschisis. (Reproduced with permission from Tantri A, Vrabec TR, Cu-Unjieng A, Frost A, Annesley WH Jr, Donoso LA. X-linked retinoschisis: a clinical and molecular genetic review. *Surv Ophthalmol.* 2004;49(2):214-230, fig. 3.)

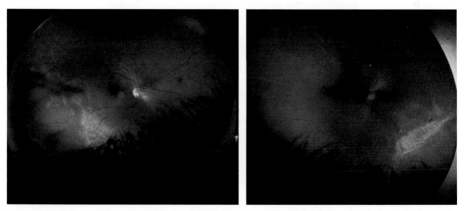

Fig. 4.3 Wide-field fundus photographs of the right and left eye showing schisis cavities in the classic inferotemporal quadrant.

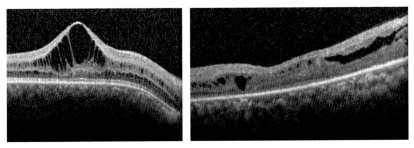

Fig. 4.4 Spectral domain optical coherence tomography of the right and left eye. Schisis cavities are seen in the inner and outer retina of both eyes.

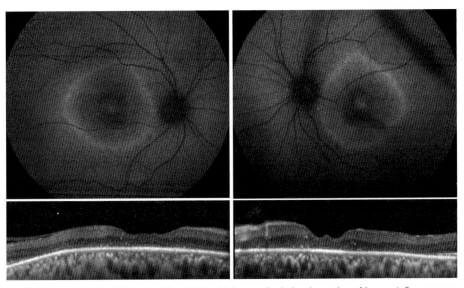

Fig. 4.5 Fundus autofluorescence of the right and left eyes *(top)* showing a ring of hypoautofluorescence surrounding the fovea and a ring of hyperautofluorescence more peripherally in the macula. Spectral domain optical coherence tomography of a 63-year-old man with X-linked retinoschisis *(bottom)* showing collapse of cystic and schisis cavities with resulting outer retinal atrophy. (Reproduced with permission from De Silva SR, Arno G, Robson AG, et al. The X-linked retinopathies: physiological insights, pathogenic mechanisms, phenotypic features and novel therapies. *Prog Retin Eye Res.* 2021;82:100898, fig. 16C–F.)

- OCT angiography (OCT-A)
  - Characteristic vascular abnormalities have been identified using OCT-A for patients with X-linked retinoschisis. Irregular foveal avascular zone and loss of flow at the deep capillary plexus in the distribution of the schisis cavities[6] has been described.
- Electroretinogram (ERG)
  - An "electronegative" ERG is the characteristic finding in patients with X-linked retinoschisis, although a normal ERG does not rule out X-linked retinoschisis.[7] An electronegative ERG occurs when the a-wave is of greater amplitude than the b-wave in the dark-adapted retina.[7]

- Genetic testing
  - X-linked retinoschisis is caused by mutations in the RS1 gene, which codes for the retinal protein retinoschisin.[8] The X-linked nature of inheritance means that females are almost always asymptomatic carriers and males will manifest the disease.
  - There are rare reports of females displaying clinical findings, including examination, ERG, and imaging consistent with X-linked retinoschisis.[9,10] As females possess two X chromosomes, a component of mosaicism or lyonization may lead to manifestation of disease in a patient population that would otherwise be asymptomatic carriers. One report shows that a female with a diagnosis of X-linked retinoschisis responded well to oral and topical carbonic anhydrase inhibitors, whereas her son had no improvement,[9] possibly indicating more mild disease that responds better to treatment. Females who display classic findings of X-linked retinoschisis may have an autosomal dominant or recessive inheritance pattern.

Management

- Genetic testing showing a mutation in the RS1 gene is necessary to clinch the diagnosis of X-linked retinoschisis.
- Genetic counseling should be discussed with the patient and family. Male patients should be counseled that they will pass the gene to all daughters but not to their sons. Daughters will almost certainly be asymptomatic carriers and have a 50% chance of passing the mutation; if passed to a daughter, she will be an asymptomatic carrier, but if passed to a son, he will be affected.
  - Our patient had genetic testing and was found to have a pathogenic deletion in the RS1 gene, diagnostic for X-linked hereditary retinoschisis.
- Carbonic anhydrase inhibitors have been shown to improve cystic and schisis changes on OCT and improve visual acuity.[11,12]
- Clinical trials involving gene therapy are in progress with promising results.[13]

Follow-up Care

- During early childhood the patient needs to be monitored closely and evaluated for amblyopia.
- Routine follow-up is recommended to monitor cystic and schisis changes, as well as response to carbonic anhydrase inhibitors.
- There is a chance for retinal detachment; strict retinal tear and retinal detachment return precautions should be extensively discussed.
- Over time, schisis cavities may collapse and lead to further retinal atrophy with worsened vision loss. The patient should be counseled about this possibility.

Key Points

- Consider X-linked retinoschisis in the differential diagnosis of cystic and schisis-like cavities in the macula of a child or adult.
- Both topical and systemic carbonic anhydrase inhibitors are helpful in treating OCT changes and in improving visual acuity.
- Genetic testing should be performed looking for mutations in the RS1 gene to clinch the diagnosis.
- A thorough past ocular history and family history will aid in the diagnosis of X-linked retinoschisis and may also help identify family members who may be asymptomatic carriers.

Algorithm 4.1: Diagnostic Flow Chart X-Linked Retinoschisis (XLR)

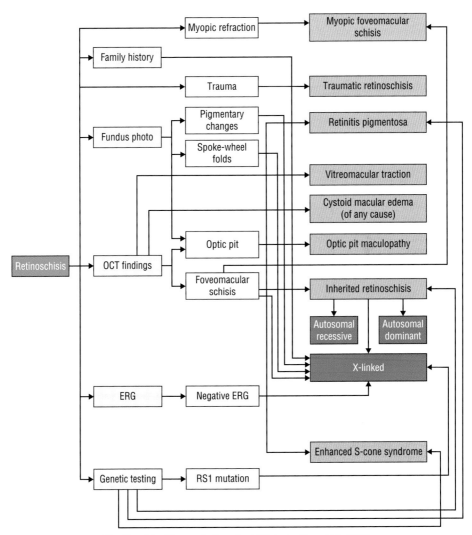

Algorithm 4.1 Diagnostic flow chart X-linked retinoschisis (XLR).

References

1. Rahman N, Georgiou M, Khan KN, Michaelides M. Macular dystrophies: clinical and imaging features, molecular genetics and therapeutic options. *Br J Ophthalmol*. 2020;104(4):451-460.
2. George ND, Yates JR, Moore AT. Clinical features in affected males with X-linked retinoschisis. *Arch Ophthalmol*. 1996;114(3):274-280.
3. Tantri A, Vrabec TR, Cu-Unjieng A, Frost A, Annesley Jr WH, Donoso LA. X-linked retinoschisis: a clinical and molecular genetic review. *Surv Ophthalmol*. 2004;49(2):214-230.
4. Yu J, Ni Y, Keane PA, Jiang C, Wang W, Xu G. Foveomacular schisis in juvenile X-linked retinoschisis: an optical coherence tomography study. *Am J Ophthalmol*. 2010;149(6):973-978.

5. Andreoli MT, Lim JI. Optical coherence tomography retinal thickness and volume measurements in X-linked retinoschisis. *Am J Ophthalmol.* 2014;158(3):567-573.
6. Han IC, Whitmore SS, Critser DB, et al. Wide-field swept-source OCT and angiography in X-linked retinoschisis. *Ophthalmol Retina.* 2019;3(2):178-185.
7. Molday RS, Kellner U, Weber BH. X-linked juvenile retinoschisis: clinical diagnosis, genetic analysis, and molecular mechanisms. *Prog Retin Eye Res.* 2012;31(3):195-212.
8. Sikkink SK, Biswas S, Parry NR, Stanga PE, Trump D. X-linked retinoschisis: an update. *J Med Genet.* 2007;44(4):225-232.
9. Ali S, Seth R. X-linked juvenile retinoschisis in females and response to carbonic anhydrase inhibitors: case report and review of the literature. *Semin Ophthalmol.* 2013;28(1):50-54.
10. Shimazaki J, Matsuhashi M. Familial retinoschisis in female patients. *Doc Ophthalmol.* 1987;65(3): 393-400.
11. Apushkin MA, Fishman GA. Use of dorzolamide for patients with X-linked retinoschisis. *Retina.* 2006;26(7):741-745.
12. Schmitt MA, Wang K, DeBenedictis MJ, Traboulsi EI. Topical carbonic anhydrase inhibitors in the long-term treatment of juvenile X-linked retinoschisis. *Retina.* 2022;42(11):2176-2183.
13. Mishra A, Sieving PA. X-linked retinoschisis and gene therapy. *Int Ophthalmol Clin.* 2021;61(4): 173-184.

CHAPTER 5

Congenital Blindness and Retinopathy in a Young Girl

Patrick C. Staropoli ▪ Byron L. Lam ▪ Ninel Z. Gregori

History of Present Illness

We present a case of a 5-year-old girl with an unremarkable past medical history referred for congenital blindness and retinopathy. There was no reported history of trauma, medication use, or premature birth. The maternal grandmother had a history of night blindness. The patient had a past medical history of positive immunoglobulin G serology for toxoplasmosis but no clinically significant infection.

OCULAR EXAMINATION FINDINGS

Visual acuities with correction were 20/400 in the right eye and 20/200 in the left eye. Intraocular pressures were normal. External examination revealed nystagmus. Anterior segment examination was unremarkable. Dilated fundus examination showed bilateral yellowish discoloration of the central macular region of both eyes, associated pigment clumping and mottling, diffuse pigmentary changes, and preserved paraarteriolar retinal pigment epithelium (RPE) (Fig. 5.1).

IMAGING

Optical coherence tomography (OCT) showed diffuse outer retinal atrophy and photoreceptor loss with extrafoveal thickened retina (Fig. 5.2A). Autofluorescence demonstrated diffuse hypoautofluorescence sparing periarteriolar areas, which appeared hyperautofluorescent (Fig. 5.2B). Full-field electroretinogram (ERG) revealed a nearly undetectable rod response and significantly reduced cone and combined rod–cone responses (Fig. 5.3).

Questions to Ask to Aid Diagnosis

- At what age did the parents first note visual impairment? Leber congenital amaurosis (LCA) is associated with visual impairment from birth or early life accompanied by nystagmus or roving eye movements.
  - The parents noted decreased visual attention and nystagmus soon after birth.
- What is the patient's refractive error? Hyperopia is commonly found in LCA, including CRB1-associated LCA, and is thought to result from impaired emmetropization, whereas myopia is characteristic of congenital stationary night blindness (CSNB).
  - $+3.75 + 2.00 \times 085$ in the right eye, $+1.50 + 2.00 \times 100$ in the left eye
- Does the patient have a family history of ocular conditions? Inheritance patterns can aid in the diagnosis of congenital blindness and are important for genetic counseling.
  - The patient's maternal grandmother had nyctalopia.

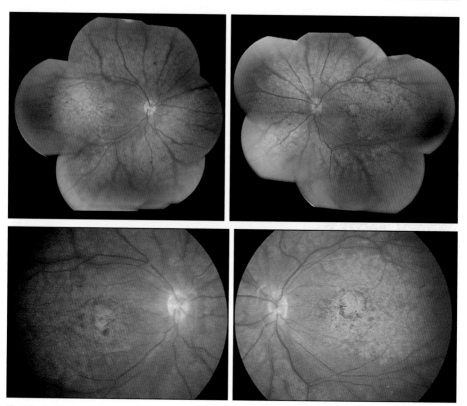

Fig. 5.1 A, Montage photographs of dilated fundus examination show bilateral yellowish discoloration of the central macular region of both eyes, associated pigment clumping and mottling, diffuse pigmentary changes, and preserved paraarteriolar retinal pigment epithelium. B, 30-degree photographs showing bilateral yellowish discoloration of the central macular region of both eyes with associated pigment clumping and mottling, and diffuse pigmentary changes.

- What is the pattern of fundus findings? Clinical phenotype can sometime correlate with the genetic mutation in LCA. GUCY2D, CEP290, CRB1, RDH12, and RPE65 are the most common LCA genotypes. RPE65-associated LCA (5–10% of LCA) typically has a blonde fundus and vascular attenuation.[1] GUCY2D (10–20% of LCA) presents with an essentially normal fundus but is associated with significant photophobia compared with most other LCA genotypes. CEP290 (15–20% of LCA) has a relatively normal fundus in infancy with variable visual acuity progressing to severe vision loss of finger counting or worse within the first decade. CRB1 (approximately 10% of LCA) demonstrates macular atrophy and paraarteriolar sparing of RPE. RDH12 (approximately 10% of LCA) typically has widespread RPE and retinal atrophy with minimal pigmentation in early childhood, dense bone-spicule pigmentation by adulthood, and early progressive macular atrophy with pigmentation and yellowing seen as excavation on OCT.[2] Vessel attenuation and disc pallor or drusen may also be present.[1]
  - Our patient's fundus demonstrates macular atrophy and paraarteriolar sparing of the RPE.
- Are there any syndromic features? Hearing loss can be associated with Usher and Alström syndromes, with the latter being associated with kidney dysfunction, obesity, diabetes mellitus, and cardiomyopathy. Renal anomalies, obesity, and diabetes are also seen in Bardet-Biedl syndrome; however, the presence of postaxial polydactyly, cognitive impairment, and

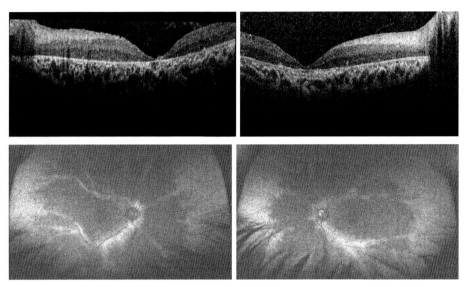

Fig. 5.2   A, Optical coherence tomography showed diffuse outer retinal atrophy and photoreceptor loss with extrafoveal thickened retina. B, Autofluorescence demonstrated diffuse hypoautofluorescence sparing peri-arteriolar areas, which appeared hyperautofluorescent.

hypogonadism differentiate Bardet-Biedl from Alström. Renal dysfunction is also observed in Joubert, Senior-Loken, and Saldino-Mainzer syndromes.[2] Joubert syndrome is associated with abnormal development of cerebellar vermis and brainstem resulting in the molar tooth sign on magnetic resonance imaging, whereas Saldino-Mainzer syndrome is associated with cone-shaped epiphyses of the hands, which can be seen on x-rays.[3]
  - No
- Are there any eye poking or stereotypic behaviors? Is there any presence of keratoconus from eye rubbing? Oculodigital reflex as a means of mechanically stimulating the retina is associated with LCA.
  - None

Assessment

- This is a case of a 5-year-old girl with congenital blindness in association with decreased photopic and scotopic ERG amplitudes, diffuse pigmentary changes, and preserved para-arteriolar RPE.

Differential Diagnosis

- LCA, which can be caused by multiple genes[1,2]
  - LCA, nonsyndromic
  - LCA with nephronophthisis
    - Joubert syndrome
    - Senior-Loken syndrome
    - Saldino-Mainzer syndrome
    - Alström syndrome
- Severe early childhood–onset retinal dystrophy (SECORD): better visual function compared with LCA despite early, progressive loss

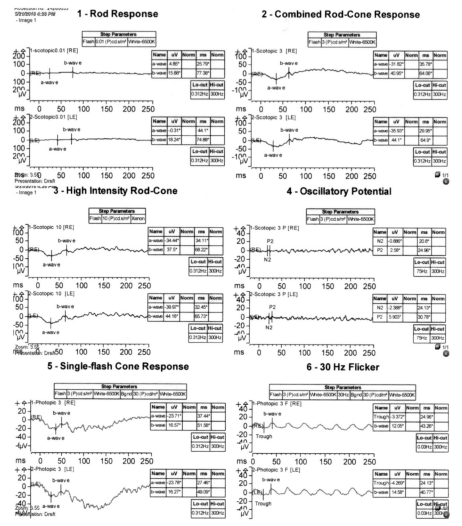

Fig. 5.3 Full-field electroretinogram revealed a nearly undetectable rod response and significantly reduced cone and combined rod–cone responses.

- Early-onset retinitis pigmentosa (RP): considered a milder form of LCA
- CSNB
- Achromatopsia: typically presents with day blindness, reduced visual acuity, photophobia, and nystagmus
- Blue-cone monochromatism: X-linked
- Metabolic[1,2]
  - Abetalipoproteinemia/Bassen-Kornzweig syndrome
  - Zellweger syndrome
  - Neonatal adrenoleukodystrophy
  - Infantile Refsum disease
- Infections (i.e., rubella or syphilis)

Working Diagnosis

- LCA: CRB1 phenotype given paraarteriolar RPE sparing

Multimodal Testing and Results

- Fundus photographs
  - Disease-causing CRB1 variants have been found in a wide range of phenotypes, including early-onset LCA or SECORD, RP with or without Coats-like vasculopathy, later-onset macular dystrophy, and even isolated autosomal recessive foveal retinoschisis.[4,5] Although fundus presentation can range from initially normal to pigmentary retinopathy, the characteristic fundus findings include macular atrophy, nummular RPE pigmentation, sparing of the paraarteriolar RPE, and possible presence of Coats-like reaction. As with other LCA/RP genotypes, optic disc abnormalities such as pallor and drusen may be seen. The CRB1 protein is a component of the outer limiting membrane and is involved in retinal development.[4]
- OCT
  - Our patient's OCT was notable for diffuse outer retinal atrophy with thickening of other retinal layers, a common finding in CRB1-associated LCA. Loss of normal retinal laminations and cystoid macular edema can also be present in a significant portion of patients.[4]
- Autofluorescence
  - Findings can vary depending on the CRB1 gene variant, with a variable amount of macular atrophy present. Widespread RPE atrophy leads to diffuse fundus hypoautofluorescence. A characteristic feature of CRB1-associated retinal dystrophy is spared RPE along the arterioles seen in our patient as preserved autofluorescence in a paraarteriolar distribution. This finding is characteristic of CRB1 mutation; however, its absence should not exclude CRB1 as a potential causative gene.[4,6]
- ERG
  - ERG was obtained, which showed nearly extinguished scotopic and severely decreased photopic responses, suggesting LCA.
- Genetic testing
  - Important in diagnosis, prognosis, and identifying gene therapy candidates. Our patient had genetic testing confirming a homozygous mutation in CRB1 (p.Cys948Tyr.2843 G>A).[7]

Management

- Our patient was entered into a gene therapy registry, referred to low-vision services, and provided with spectacle correction.
- It is also important to identify treatable conditions associated with LCA, including refractive error, cataract, keratoconus, and macular edema.
- Genetic counseling of the parents was provided considering CRB1-associated LCA is autosomal recessive and the risk of having another child with the same condition is 25%.
- The patient and family were referred to low-vision, educational, and social support resources.
- As of 2017, the U.S. Food and Drug Administration approved subretinal injection of voretigene neparvovec-rzyl (Luxturna Spark Therapeutics, Inc., Philadelphia, PA), for biallelic RPE65 mutation–associated LCA2.[8] Numerous other clinical trials are ongoing.
- Supplements, particularly vitamin A, have not been shown to be clearly beneficial and may be harmful in some conditions (i.e., ABCA4-associated inherited retinal disease).[9]

Follow-up Care

- Although there are no established guidelines, serial examinations, imaging, and genetic counseling are recommended.
- Carrier testing for family members and prenatal testing can be considered.
- If a patient exhibits syndromic features, further workup may include labs, renal ultrasound, hand x-ray, and evaluation by an internist.[10]

Algorithm 5.1: Algorithm for Differential Diagnosis of Congenital Blindness and Retinopathy

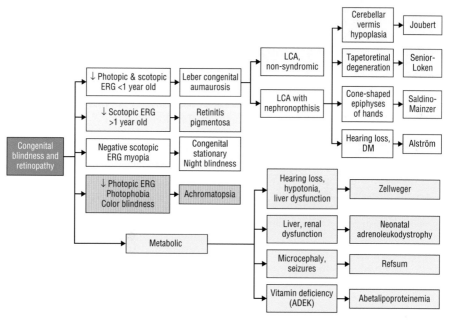

Algorithm 5.1 Algorithm for differential diagnosis of congenital blindness and retinopathy.

Key Points

- LCA should be considered in early, severe bilateral vision loss with poor scotopic and photopic responses on ERG.
- CRB1 mutation is found in up to 10% of LCA patients and is thought to affect neuronal development in the retina.[1,6] Sometimes this phenotype may demonstrate preservation of the paraarteriolar RPE.
- Visual prognosis is generally poor, and referral to low-vision services and genetic counseling is paramount.
- Genetic testing should be considered given the possibility of gene therapy or participation in clinical trials.

References

1. Kumaran N, Moore AT, Weleber RG, Michaelides M. Leber congenital amaurosis/early-onset severe retinal dystrophy: clinical features, molecular genetics and therapeutic interventions. *Br J Ophthalmol.* 2017;101(9):1147-1154. Erratum in: *Br J Ophthalmol.* 2019;103(6):862.
2. Senior B, Friedmann AI, Braudo JL. Juvenile familial nephropathy with tapetoretinal degeneration: a new oculorenal dystrophy. *Am J Ophthalmol.* 1961;52:625-633.
3. Giedion A. Phalangeal cone shaped epiphyses of the hands (PhCSEH) and chronic renal disease: the conorenal syndromes. *Pediatr Radiol.* 1979;8:32-38.
4. Bujakowska K, Audo I, Mohand-Saïd S, et al. CRB1 mutations in inherited retinal dystrophies. *Hum Mutat.* 2012;33(2):306-315.
5. Motta FL, Salles MV, Costa KA, et al. The correlation between *CRB1* variants and the clinical severity of Brazilian patients with different inherited retinal dystrophy phenotypes. *Sci Rep.* 2017;7:8654.
6. Lotery AJ, Jacobson SG, Fishman GA, et al. Mutations in the CRB1 gene cause leber congenital amaurosis. *Arch Ophthalmol.* 2001;119(3):415-420.
7. den Hollander AI, Heckenlively JR, van den Born LI, et al. Leber congenital amaurosis and retinitis pigmentosa with Coats-like exudative vasculopathy are associated with mutations in the crumbs homologue 1 (CRB1) gene. *Am J Hum Genet.* 2001;69:198-203.
8. Russell S, Bennett J, Wellman JA, et al. Efficacy and safety of voretigene neparvovec (AAV2-hRPE65v2) in patients with RPE65-mediated inherited retinal dystrophy: a randomised, controlled, open-label, phase 3 trial. *Lancet.* 2017;390(10097):849-860.
9. Schwartz SG, Wang X, Chavis P, et al. Vitamin A and fish oils for preventing the progression of retinitis pigmentosa. *Cochrane Database Syst Rev.* 2020;6(6):CD008428.
10. Fazzi E, Signorini SG, Scelsa B, Bova SM, Lanzi G. Leber's congenital amaurosis: an update. *Eur J Paediatr Neurol.* 2003;7(1):13-22.

CHAPTER 6

Progressive Nyctalopia and Tunnel Vision in a Young Man

Patrick C. Staropoli ■ Byron L. Lam ■ Ninel Z. Gregori

History of Present Illness

We present a case of a 17-year-old male patient with an unremarkable past medical history referred for progressive nyctalopia and tunnel vision first noted at age 2 years. There was no known family history, premature birth, maternal illness during pregnancy, or trauma.

OCULAR EXAMINATION FINDINGS

Visual acuity with correction was 20/50 in the right eye and 20/50 in the left eye. Intraocular pressures were 13 and 14 mm Hg in the right and left eye, respectively. Confrontational visual fields showed peripheral constriction. Color plates were 1/14 in both eyes. There was nystagmus and intermittent exotropia of six prism diopters. Anterior segment examination was unremarkable. Dilated fundus examination showed peripapillary atrophy, macular pigment mottling, vascular attenuation, and a blonde peripheral fundus with irregular pigmentation without bone spicules (Fig. 6.1).

IMAGING

Optical coherence tomography (OCT) showed peripheral outer retinal atrophy with relative preservation of the subfoveal inner segment/outer segment (IS/OS) junction (Fig. 6.2A). Fundus autofluorescence imaging was notable for a lack of the normal autofluorescence pattern and vascular attenuation (Fig. 6.2B). Visual field demonstrated significant bilateral constriction (Fig. 6.3). Full-field electroretinogram (ERG) revealed extinguished rod, cone, and combined rod–cone responses (Fig. 6.4).

Questions to Ask to Aid Diagnosis

- At what age did the parents first note visual impairment? Leber congenital amaurosis (LCA) is associated with visual impairment from birth or early life accompanied by nystagmus or roving eye movements.
  - Our patient was first noted to have difficulty navigating at night and bumping into objects at age 2 years.
- Does the patient have a family history of ocular conditions? Inheritance patterns can aid in the diagnosis of congenital blindness and are important for genetic counseling.
  - The patient has no known family history.
- Does the patient exhibit stereotypical behaviors? Depending on the causative gene, early and severe visual loss may be present. Oculodigital sign consisting of eye poking or rubbing to

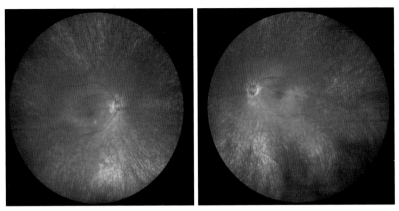

Fig. 6.1 Fundus photograph of the right and left eyes of this patient with Leber congenital amaurosis and biallelic RPE65 mutations. The fundus demonstrates peripapillary atrophy, macular pigment mottling, vascular attenuation, and a blonde peripheral fundus with irregular pigmentation without bone spicules.

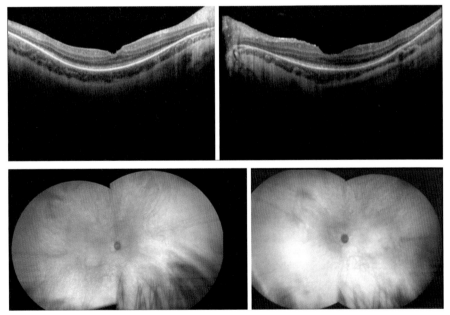

Fig. 6.2 A, Spectral domain optical coherence tomography showing peripheral outer retinal atrophy with relative preservation of the subfoveal inner segment/outer segment junction. B, Fundus autofluorescence demonstrating a lack of the normal autofluorescence pattern and vascular attenuation.

mechanically stimulate vision may be reported by the parents. The child may stare at lights and be terrified of being in the dark. Rarely, LCA may be associated with developmental delay, cognitive impairment, and oculomotor apraxia with difficulty initiating saccades.

- ■ Our patient reports only difficulty seeing in the dark and bumping into surroundings because of tunnel vision.
- ■ What is the pattern of fundus findings? Clinical phenotype can sometime correlate with the genetic mutation in LCA. GUCY2D, CEP290, CRB1, RDH12, and RPE65 are the

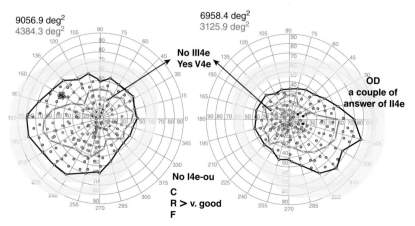

Fig. 6.3 Visual field testing demonstrating significant bilateral constriction.

most common LCA genotypes. RPE65-associated LCA (5–10% of LCA) typically has a blonde fundus and vascular attenuation.[1] GUCY2D (10–20% of LCA) presents with an essentially normal fundus but is associated with significant photophobia compared with most other LCA genotypes. CEP290 (15–20% of LCA) has a relatively normal fundus in infancy with variable visual acuity progressing to severe vision loss of finger counting or worse within the first decade. CRB1 (approximately 10% of LCA) demonstrates macular atrophy and paraarteriolar sparing of retinal pigment epithelium (RPE). RDH12 (approximately 10% of LCA) typically has widespread RPE and retinal atrophy with minimal pigmentation in early childhood, dense bone-spicule pigmentation by adulthood, and early progressive macular atrophy with pigmentation and yellowing seen as excavation on OCT.[1] Vessel attenuation and disc pallor or drusen may also be present.[2]

- Our patient's fundus shows no bone spicules and relative preservation of the macula, resembling the RPE65 phenotype.
- Are there any syndromic features? Hearing loss can be associated with Usher and Alström syndromes, with the latter being associated with kidney dysfunction, obesity, diabetes mellitus, and cardiomyopathy. Renal anomalies, obesity, and diabetes are also seen in Bardet-Biedl syndrome; however, the presence of postaxial polydactyly, cognitive impairment, and hypogonadism differentiate Bardet-Biedl from Alström. Renal dysfunction is also observed in Joubert, Senior-Loken, and Saldino-Mainzer syndromes.[3] Joubert syndrome is associated with abnormal development of cerebellar vermis and brainstem resulting in the molar tooth sign on magnetic resonance imaging, whereas Saldino-Mainzer syndrome is associated with cone-shaped epiphyses of the hands, which can be seen on x-rays.[4]
- No

Assessment

- This is a case of a 17-year-old male patient with progressive nyctalopia, nystagmus, bilateral visual field constriction, extinguished photopic and scotopic ERG amplitudes, and diffuse outer retinal and RPE atrophy.

Differential Diagnosis

- LCA, which can be caused by multiple genes[1]
  - LCA, nonsyndromic

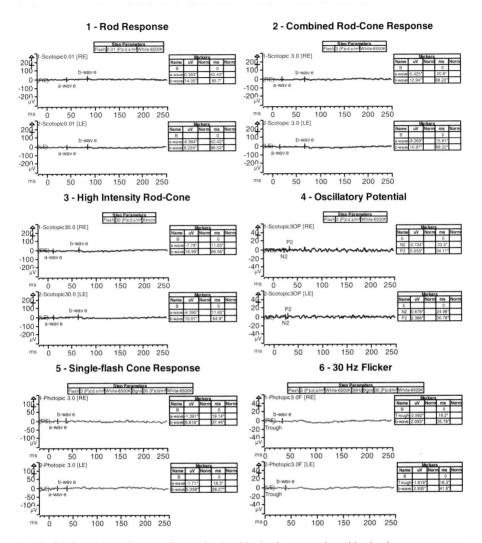

Fig. 6.4 Full-field electroretinogram disclosed extinguished rod, cone, and combined rod–cone responses.

- LCA with nephronophthisis
  - Joubert syndrome
  - Senior-Loken syndrome
  - Saldino-Mainzer syndrome
  - Alström syndrome
- Severe early childhood–onset retinal dystrophy (SECORD): better visual function compared with LCA despite early, progressive loss
- Early-onset retinitis pigmentosa (RP): considered a milder form of LCA
- Congenital stationary night blindness
- Achromatopsia: typically presents with day blindness, reduced visual acuity, photophobia, and nystagmus
- Blue-cone monochromatism: X-linked

- Metabolic[1]
  - Abetalipoproteinemia/Bassen-Kornzweig syndrome
  - Zellweger syndrome
  - Neonatal adrenoleukodystrophy
  - Infantile Refsum disease
  - Hyperthreoninemia
- Infections (i.e., rubella or syphilis)

Working Diagnosis

- LCA: retinal pigment epithelium–specific 65 kDa protein (RPE65) phenotype given diffuse RPE atrophy, vascular attenuation, and lack of autofluorescence

Multimodal Testing and Results

- Fundus photographs
  - In LCA, fundus findings can range from initially normal to a diffuse pigmentary retinopathy. Our patient demonstrated significant vascular attenuation, extensive peripheral retinal depigmentation, and relative central macular preservation.
- OCT
  - Our patient's OCT was notable for diffuse outer retinal atrophy with relative preservation of the IS/OS junction in the central macula, a finding that can be seen in RPE65-associated LCA with great variability depending on the severity of the causative mutation and the age of the patient. No clear relationship exists between the age of the patient and the genotype-phenotype correlation, as is common for inherited retinal diseases in general. GUCY2D may present with relatively preserved outer retinal structure and photoreceptor-associated layers on OCT with subfoveal cone loss. CRB1 is associated with retinal thickening and loss of normal lamination,[1] as well as cystoid macular edema.[5] RDH12 shows marked retinal thinning and excavation of the macula.[6]
- Autofluorescence
  - Findings vary depending on the mutation. For example, our patient demonstrated lack of normal autofluorescence pattern, a common finding in the RPE65 phenotype caused by interruption of the visual cycle and lack of lipofuscin within the RPE cells.[7] The GUCY2D gene results in normal fundus autofluorescence early with the appearance of areas of hypoautofluorescence and hyperautofluorescence as RPE degeneration progresses.[8] Meanwhile, the CRB1 phenotype has been described as hypoautofluorescence sparing paraarteriolar areas corresponding to preserved RPE along the arterioles.[5,9]
- ERG
  - ERG was obtained, which showed nearly extinguished scotopic and photopic responses, suggesting LCA or advanced RP and commonly seen with RPE65-associated retinal dystrophy. Interestingly, GUCY2D patients often show relatively preserved rod function (cone–rod disease) with a minority of patients showing reduced but detectable cone function.[1]
- Genetic testing
  - Important in diagnosis, prognosis, and identifying gene therapy candidates. Our patient had genetic testing confirming compound heterozygous mutations in the RPE65 gene (paternally inherited p.Tyr431Cys:c1292A>G and maternally inherited p.Glu364Lys: c1090G>A).[10]

Management

- Given our patient's biallelic RPE65 mutation–associated LCA2, our patient underwent gene therapy with subretinal injection of the U.S. Food and Drug Administration–approved voretigene neparvovec-rzyl (Luxturna Spark Therapeutics, Inc., Philadelphia, PA). The surgical procedure is shown in Fig. 6.5.
- Voretigene neparvovec-rzyl is a live, nonreplicating adenoassociated virus serotype 2 that has been genetically modified to express the human RPE65 gene, allowing the retinoid cycle to proceed with catalyzation of all-*trans*-retinyl ester to 11-*cis*-retinol.[11]
- The patient was pretreated with oral prednisone starting at 1 mg/kg per day (maximum 40 mg/day) 3 days prior to surgery with a taper for a total of 17 days per eye. The second eye surgery was performed 1 week later (the label states at least 6 days after the first eye).
- Genetic counseling of the parents was performed considering RPE65-associated LCA is autosomal recessive and the risk of having another child with the same condition is 25%.
- The patient and family were referred to available low-vision, educational, and social support services.

Follow-up Care

- The patient was seen postoperative day 1, week 1, month 1, month 3, month 6, and yearly for each eye with serial dilated examination, OCT, and visual field testing.
- Vision improved to 20/40 + 3 in the right eye by postoperative week 3 and remained stable at 20/50 in the left eye by postoperative week 4. Vision and OCT remained stable at 3.5 years of follow-up (Fig. 6.6).
- Carrier testing for other family members and prenatal testing can be considered.

Surgical Procedure for Subretinal Gene Therapy

The typical steps of subretinal voretigene neparvovec-rzyl delivery with optional balanced salt solution prebleb before the injection of the viral vector are shown in Fig. 6.5.[12]

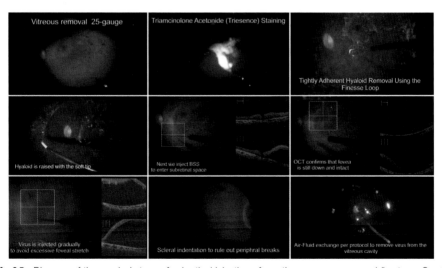

Fig. 6.5   Diagram of the surgical steps of subretinal injection of voretigene neparvovec-rzyl (Luxturna Spark Therapeutics, Inc., Philadelphia, PA) gene therapy. Step descriptions are shown.

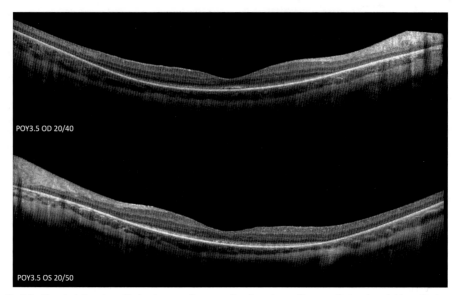

POY3.5 OD 20/40

POY3.5 OS 20/50

Fig. 6.6   Spectral domain optical coherence tomography at postoperative year 3 showing stable optical coherence tomography findings and final visual acuity of 20/40 + 3 in the right eye and 20/50 in the left eye.

Algorithm 6.1 Algorithm of Various Inherited Conditions Causing Nyctalopia With Poor Visual Acuity in Children

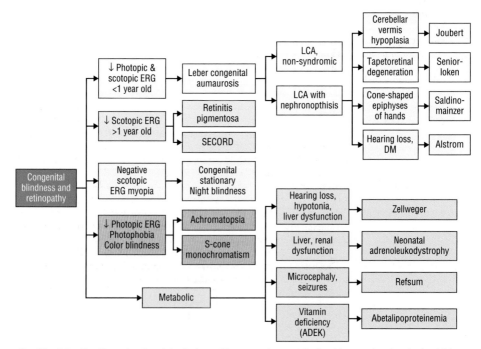

Algorithm 6.1   Algorithm of various inherited conditions causing nyctalopia with poor visual acuity in children.

Key Points

- LCA should be considered in early, severe, bilateral vision loss with nystagmus, nyctalopia, and poor scotopic and photopic responses on ERG.
- RPE65 mutation is found in approximately 5% to 10% of LCA patients.[13] This phenotype typically demonstrates a blonde fundus, vascular attenuation, and a diffuse lack of fundus autofluorescence.[1]
- RPE65-associated LCA patients are eligible for gene therapy with subretinal voretigene neparvovec-rzyl. Current clinical trial data demonstrate that it is a safe and effective therapy for visual improvement in select patients with viable retinal cells as determined by the OCT, and the effects of treatment persist to at least 4 years after surgery.[14]

References

1. Kumaran N, Moore AT, Weleber RG, Michaelides M. Leber congenital amaurosis/early-onset severe retinal dystrophy: clinical features, molecular genetics and therapeutic interventions. *Br J Ophthalmol.* 2017;101(9):1147-1154. Erratum in: *Br J Ophthalmol.* 2019;103(6):862.
2. Jacobson SG, Aleman TS, Cideciyan AV, et al. Identifying photoreceptors in blind eyes caused by RPE65 mutations: prerequisite for human gene therapy success. *Proc Natl Acad Sci U S A.* 2005; 102(17): 6177-6182.
3. Senior B, Friedmann AI, Braudo JL. Juvenile familial nephropathy with tapetoretinal degeneration: a new oculorenal dystrophy. *Am J Ophthalmol.* 1961;52:625-633.
4. Giedion A. Phalangeal cone shaped epiphyses of the hands (PhCSEH) and chronic renal disease: the conorenal syndromes. *Pediatr Radiol.* 1979;8:32-38.
5. Bujakowska K, Audo I, Mohand-Saïd S, et al. CRB1 mutations in inherited retinal dystrophies. *Hum Mutat.* 2012;33(2):306-315.
6. Mackay DS, Dev Borman A, Moradi P, et al. RDH12 retinopathy: novel mutations and phenotypic description. *Mol Vis.* 2011;17:2706-2716.
7. Lorenz B, Wabbels B, Wegscheider E, Hamel CP, Drexler W, Preising MN. Lack of fundus autofluorescence to 488 nanometers from childhood on in patients with early-onset severe retinal dystrophy associated with mutations in RPE65. *Ophthalmology.* 2004;111(8):1585-1594.
8. Bouzia Z, Georgiou M, Hull S, et al. GUCY2D-associated Leber congenital amaurosis: a retrospective natural history study in preparation for trials of novel therapies. *Am J Ophthalmol.* 2020;210:59-70.
9. Lotery AJ, Jacobson SG, Fishman GA, et al. Mutations in the CRB1 gene cause Leber congenital amaurosis. *Arch Ophthalmol.* 2001;119(3):415-420.
10. den Hollander AI, Heckenlively JR, van den Born LI, et al. Leber congenital amaurosis and retinitis pigmentosa with Coats-like exudative vasculopathy are associated with mutations in the crumbs homologue 1 (CRB1) gene. *Am J Hum Genet.* 2001;69:198-203.
11. Russell S, Bennett J, Wellman JA, et al. Efficacy and safety of voretigene neparvovec (AAV2-hRPE65v2) in patients with RPE65-mediated inherited retinal dystrophy: a randomised, controlled, open-label, phase 3 trial. *Lancet.* 2017;390(10097):849-860.
12. Davis JL, Gregori NZ, MacLaren RE, Lam BL. Surgical technique for subretinal gene therapy in humans with inherited retinal degeneration. *Retina.* 2019;39(suppl 1):S2-S8.
13. Cideciyan AV. Leber congenital amaurosis due to RPE65 mutations and its treatment with gene therapy. *Prog Retin Eye Res.* 2010;29:398-427.
14. Maguire AM, Russell S, Chung DC, et al. Durability of voretigene neparvovec for biallelic RPE65-mediated inherited retinal disease: phase 3 results at 3 and 4 years. *Ophthalmology.* 2021;128(10): 1460-1468.

CHAPTER 7

Rapid Progression of Vision Loss in a Child With Pigmentary Retinopathy

Sandeep Grover ▪ Gerald A. Fishman

History of Present Illness

A 9-year-old girl was referred for progressively decreasing central vision with additional impairment of both night and peripheral vision.

EXAMINATION FINDINGS

Best-corrected visual acuity was 20/150 in the right eye and 20/70 in the left eye. Eye examination showed normal anterior segment, cells in the vitreous humor, attenuated retinal arterioles, macular atrophy, epiretinal membranes, and diffuse hypopigmentation and pigment mottling in the inferior peripheral retina.

TESTS

Optical coherence tomography (OCT) showed a loss of photoreceptors in the macular zone and epiretinal membranes in both eyes (Fig. 7.1).

Goldmann kinetic perimetry showed a concentric visual field loss to a target III-4-e in both eyes.

Questions to Ask

- Is there a family history of retinal disease?
  - A third cousin, not examined by the authors, who was diagnosed with retinitis pigmentosa (RP) (not as severe as this proband).
- Is there a history of hearing loss from birth?
  - None observed (hearing loss would be present in Usher syndrome).
- Is there a history of developmental delay, polydactyly, or dental anomalies?
  - None observed (these would be seen in Bardet-Biedl syndrome).
- Is there a history of anosmia and ataxia?
  - None observed (these would be seen in Refsum disease).
- Is there a history of seizures, developmental regression, or behavioral changes?
  - None observed (all of these would be observed in Batten disease).

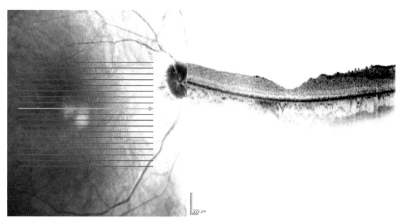

Fig. 7.1 Optical coherence tomography scans of the right eye through the macula show epiretinal membrane, loss of the ellipsoid zone, and foveal thinning.

Assessment

A 9-year-old proband with reduction in central, night, and peripheral vision was initially diagnosed as having a diffuse retinal pigmentary degeneration within the spectrum of RP or cone–rod dystrophy.

Differential Diagnosis

- RP (rod-cone dystrophy)
- Possibly a form of cone–rod dystrophy
- Batten disease

Working Diagnosis

Early-onset severe RP based on family history, night vision impairment, diffuse retinal degeneration, and severe visual field loss

Investigations

- OCT and Goldmann kinetic perimetry, as described earlier.
- Gene testing done with an inherited disease panel (248 genes) that showed a heterozygous pathogenic variant in the RPGRIP1L gene and one variant each in CC2D2A and PDZD7 genes of unknown significance.

Follow-up Care

Six months later, the patient was seen for rapidly deteriorating central vision (hand motion vision in each eye), developmental regression, and behavioral changes. The eye examination findings were similar to the initial visit.

The diagnosis of Batten disease was entertained, and the patient was referred to a pediatric geneticist. Exome testing confirmed the diagnosis of Batten disease showing two biallelic pathogenic variants in the PPT1 gene (c.223A>C [p.Thr75Pro] with a sequence change, and c.451C>T [p.Arg151*] that creates a premature translational stop signal) consistent with a diagnosis of autosomal recessive neuronal ceroid lipofuscinosis 1.

Management

1. There is no treatment at this point for reversing this condition, although some treatment trials are in progress.
2. Parents were counseled about the prognosis of the condition and mortality at an earlier age associated with the diagnosis.

Follow-up Care

Continued follow-up care was recommended with pediatrics and referred to neurology to evaluate for seizures and possibly electroencephalogram. One year later, the patient did develop seizures.

Key Points

1. Batten disease (NCL) is a heterogenous group of lysosomal storage diseases that cause rapid and progressive visual loss, behavioral changes, cognitive decline, and potential seizures.[1,2]
2. Batten disease, also known as neuronal ceroid lipofuscinoses (NCL), is inherited in an autosomal recessive pattern, and mutations have been described in ceroid lipofuscinosis neuronal (CLN) genes (CLN1–CLN8 and CLN10–CLN14).[2]
3. There is intracellular accumulation of an autofluorescent lipopigment in the neurons leading to their degeneration.[3]
4. Peripheral blood smears may show vacuolated lymphocytes (Fig. 7.2).
5. The most common finding on ultramicroscopy of dermal biopsy is the presence of curvilinear inclusions (Fig. 7.3).
6. Treatment trials are underway for brain-directed and eye-directed gene therapies for CLN3 and CLN6 mutations.[1,2]

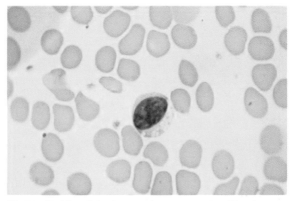

Fig. 7.2 Peripheral blood smear shows a vacuolated lymphocyte.

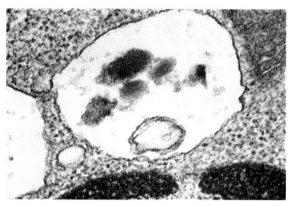

Fig. 7.3 Ultramicroscopy of dermal tissue shows the presence of curvilinear inclusions.

Algorithm 7.1: Algorithm for Differential Diagnosis of A Child With Pigmentary Retinopathy and Progressive Vision Loss

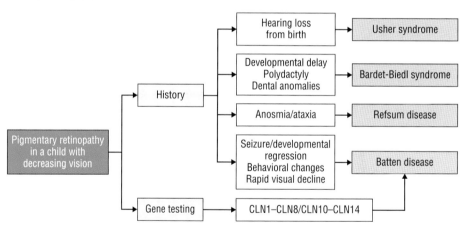

Algorithm 7.1 Algorithm for differential diagnosis of a child with pigmentary retinopathy and progressive vision loss.

References

1. National Institute of Neurological Disorders and Stroke. *Batten Disease Fact Sheet*. National Institutes of Health. NIH Publication No. 18-NS-2790. July 2018. Available at: https://catalog.ninds.nih.gov/sites/default/files/publications/batten-disease-other-neuronal-ceroid-lipofucinoses.pdf.
2. Murray SJ, Mitchell NL. Ocular therapies for neuronal ceroid lipofuscinoses: more than meets the eye. *Neural Regen Res*. 2022;17(8):1755-1756.
3. Goebel HH, Sharp JD. The neuronal ceroid-lipofuscinoses: recent advances. *Brain Pathol*. 1998;8: 151-162.

CHAPTER 8

Unilateral Tractional Retinal Detachment in a 6-Month-Old Female Infant With Erythematous Skin Lesions

Luis Acaba-Berrocal ■ Sudarshan Srivatsan ■ R.V. Paul Chan

History of Present Illness

We present a case of a 6-month-old female infant with an unremarkable birth history referred for evaluation of vitreous hemorrhage and retinal detachment (RD) in the left eye. Patient was born full term at 8 lbs 1.6 oz without supplemental oxygen use. Patient's family denied history of prior ocular conditions or ocular surgeries.

SYSTEMIC FINDINGS

Erythematous macular skin lesions were observed in bilateral lower extremities, and verrucous and pustular lesions were observed in upper extremities (Fig. 8.1).

OCULAR EXAMINATION FINDINGS

Vision was wink to light in both eyes. Intraocular pressure was normal to palpation. Pupils were round and reactive bilaterally. External examination was normal in both eyes. Anterior segment examination of the left eye demonstrated prominent iris vessels with 270 degrees of posterior synechiae, a shallow chamber, and a posterior lens opacity with overlying blood vessels (Fig. 8.2). Anterior segment evaluation of right eye was unremarkable. Fundus examination was unremarkable in the right eye. Fundus examination of the left eye revealed vitreous hemorrhage with no view of the posterior pole.

IMAGING

B-scan ultrasonography of the left eye showed a tractional RD (Fig. 8.3). Fundus photograph of right eye was notable for retinal pigment epithelium (RPE) hypopigmentation superiorly and a blunted foveal pit (Fig. 8.4). Fluorescence angiography of the right eye showed normal vascular filling and no areas of neovascularization or retinal ischemia. The foveal avascular zone in the right eye appeared to be enlarged (Fig. 8.5).

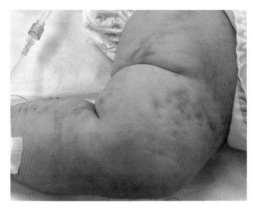

Fig. 8.1 External photograph showing erythematous macular skin lesions in lower extremity.

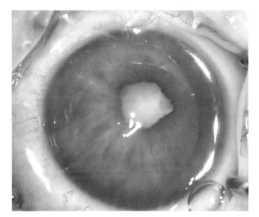

Fig. 8.2 External photograph of the left eye. Prominent iris vessels with 270 degrees of posterior synechiae, a shallow chamber, and a posterior lens opacity are noted.

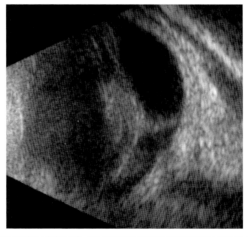

Fig. 8.3 B-scan ultrasonography of the left eye demonstrating a tractional retinal detachment. No masses are identified.

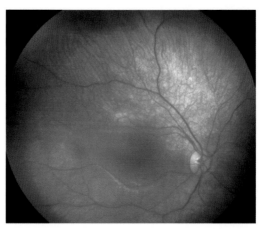

Fig. 8.4 Fundus photograph of right eye with retinal pigment epithelium hypopigmentation and a blunted foveal pit.

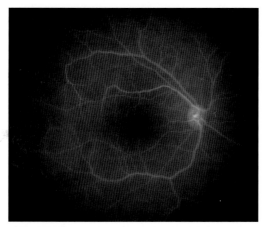

Fig. 8.5 Fluorescein angiography of the right eye showing an enlarged foveal avascular zone. There is normal vascular filling and no areas of neovascularization.

Questions to Ask

■ Was the patient born prematurely or with low birth weight? Retinopathy of prematurity is an important consideration in infant patients with evidence of retinal nonperfusion and RDs.
  ■ No

■ Does the patient have a family history of ocular or systemic conditions? A family history is important to differentiate between possible etiologies of abnormal retinal angiogenesis and RDs, such as familiar exudative vitreoretinopathy, sickle cell retinopathy, incontinentia pigmenti (IP), von Hippel–Lindau disease, X-linked juvenile retinoschisis, and Stickler syndrome.
  ■ Yes. Patient's mother had a family history of vision loss in infancy and amblyopia associated with skin lesions.

■ Is there a history of trauma? Trauma is associated with unilateral RD and retinal hemorrhages in infants.
  ■ No

- Does the patient have refractive error? Patients with Stickler syndrome have associated myopia.
  - No
- Is there a mass lesion on imaging or funduscopic examination? Masses or tumors are associated with retinoblastoma and von Hippel–Lindau disease.
  - No. The patient had no masses on B-scan ultrasonography.

Assessment

- This is a case of a 6-month-old female infant with an unremarkable birth history and erythematous skin lesions with a tractional RD in the left eye and enlarged parafoveal avascular zone.

Differential Diagnosis

- Retinopathy of prematurity
- Familiar exudative vitreoretinopathy
- Stickler syndrome–related rhegmatogenous RD
- Traumatic RD
- Retinoblastoma
- X-linked juvenile retinoschisis
- Von Hippel–Lindau disease
- Persistent fetal vasculature
- Eales disease

Working Diagnosis

- IP
  - IP or Bloch-Sulzberger syndrome is associated with progressive skin lesions, retinal nonperfusion, RPE defects, and RDs.[1-3] Although patients typically present with retinal peripheral nonperfusion, patients can present with tractional RDs.[1]

Multimodal Testing and Results

- Fundus photographs
  - Fundus examination is typically notable for absent foveal pit, hyper- or hypopigmented RPE defects, optic nerve atrophy, retinal/vitreous hemorrhages, and exudative or tractional RDs.[3,4]
- Optical coherence tomography (OCT)
  - Findings on OCT include retinal thinning of both inner and outer segments.[5]
- Fluorescein angiography (FA)
  - Our patient had evidence of an enlarged parafoveal avascular zone, which is typical of IP. Other signs common to IP not present in our patient include peripheral retinal nonperfusion, neovascularization, and retinal vessel occlusion.[1]
- Genetic testing
  - As an X-linked dominant disease, IP is associated with mutations in the NEMO/IKK gamma gene. Living male patients have the XXY genotype (Klinefelter syndrome). Diagnosis of IP was confirmed by genetic testing in our patient.[3]
- Laboratory testing
  - Eosinophilia may be present.
- Brain magnetic resonance imaging

- Evidence of vasoocclusion leading to cortical blindness, cerebral atrophy, corpus callosum hypoplasia, and hemorrhagic necrosis can be present.[3,6]

Management

- No cure exists.
- The focus is on treating symptoms.
- Consult with dermatology, neurology, and genetics to manage extraocular disease manifestations.
- The areas of peripheral avascularity are often treated with laser photocoagulation or cryotherapy in cases with evidence of neovascularization, vitreous traction, or vitreous hemorrhage.
- There is limited long-term data regarding the role of prophylactic laser ablation to prevent RDs.[1]
- RDs can be surgically repaired with pars plana vitrectomy and/or scleral buckle.
- Our patient underwent synechiolysis and lensectomy of the left eye. RD repair was deferred because of poor anatomical and visual potential.

Follow-up Care

- No established consensus guidelines for follow-up exist.
- One study of IP described retinal screening as soon as possible after birth, then monthly examinations until 4 months, then every 3 months until 1 year of age, then biannually until 3 years, and annually thereafter.[4]
- Follow-up includes examination under anesthesia (EUA) and FA.

Algorithm 8.1: Algorithm for Differential Diagnosis for Retinal Nonperfusion in Infants

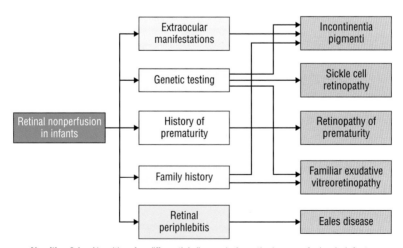

Algorithm 8.1   Algorithm for differential diagnosis for retinal nonperfusion in infants.

Key Points

- IP should be considered in infant patients with dermal, dental, and neurological manifestations along with retinal avascularity and RDs.
- Ablative therapy should be given to patients with evidence of neovascularization, vitreomacular traction, or vitreous hemorrhage.
- Tractional, exudative, or rhegmatogenous RDs can be surgically treated with pars plana vitrectomy and/or scleral buckle.
- Patients should be screened within the first few weeks of life and followed on a regular basis with outpatient examinations, EUA, and FA.

References

1. Chen CJ, Han IC, Tian J, Muñoz B, Goldberg MF. Extended follow-up of treated and untreated retinopathy in Iincontinentia pigmenti: analysis of peripheral vascular changes and incidence of retinal detachment. *JAMA Ophthalmol.* 2015;133(5):542-548.
2. Shields CL, Eagle RC, Shah RM, et al. Multifocal hypopigmented retinal pigment epithelial lesions in incontinentia pigmenti. *Retina.* 2006;26:328-333.
3. Weiss SJ, Srinivasan A, Klufas MA, et al. Incontinentia pigmenti in a child with suspected retinoblastoma. *Int J Retina Vitreous.* 2017;3:34.
4. Mangalesh S, Chen X, Tran-Viet D, et al. Assessment of the retinal structure in children with incontinentia pigmenti. *Retina.* 2017;37:1568-1574.
5. Goldberg MF. The blinding mechanisms of incontinentia pigmenti. *Ophthalmic Genet.* 1994;92:167-179.
6. Holmstrom G, Thoren K. Ocular manifestations of incontinentia pigmenti. *Acta Ophthalmol Scand.* 2000;78:348-353.

CHAPTER 9

Bilateral Peripheral Pigmentary Changes in a Woman

Connie J. Chen ■ Morton F. Goldberg

History of Present Illness

We present a 57-year-old woman with blurred central vision and mild impairment in night vision in both eyes. Her past ocular history is notable for bilateral cataract surgery and anterior chamber intraocular lenses at age 46. She denies metamorphopsia, scotomas, or constriction of peripheral visual field.

OCULAR EXAMINATION FINDINGS

Visual acuity was 20/25 in the right eye and 20/30 in the left eye. Intraocular pressures were normal. Retinal examination revealed coarse annular hyperpigmentation in the peripheral retina. No macular edema or atrophy was seen on clinical examination.

IMAGING

Fundus photographs of the macula and periphery were obtained (Fig. 9.1). Optical coherence tomography (OCT) was not obtained at initial visits, but at a follow-up 13 years later, central retinal pigment epithelial atrophy was noted, as well as development of perimacular drusen (Fig. 9.2).

Questions to Ask

- Does the patient have a family history of ocular conditions or consanguinity? The mode of inheritance could help distinguish different forms of inherited vitreoretinopathy. Enhanced S-cone (Goldmann-Favre) syndrome is an autosomal recessive disorder. Retinitis pigmentosa (RP) can be autosomal dominant, autosomal recessive, or X-linked. Autosomal dominant vitreoretinochoroidopathy (ADVIRC) typically involves family members affected in consecutive generations.
  - No consanguinity
- Does the patient have a nonsenile cataract or have a family history of nonsenile cataract? Premature development of cataract is seen in many inherited retinal conditions, including RP and conditions resulting from mutations in the *BEST1* gene.[1,2]
  - Yes. The patient had cataract extraction at age 46.
- If patient is phakic, what is the refractive error? In patients with *BEST1*-associated dystrophies, such as ADVIRC, there can be hypermetropia, nanophthalmos, microcornea, and associated angle closure glaucoma.
  - The patient is pseudophakic but does not have nanophthalmos, microcornea, or history of angle closure. Affected individuals in other ADVIRC pedigrees may demonstrate nanophthalmos and/or microcornea.[3,4]

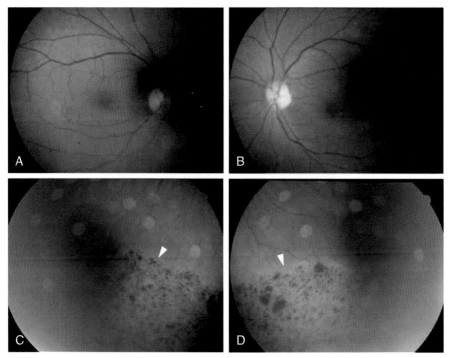

Fig. 9.1 Fundus photographs of patient at age 46 years revealed peripheral circumferential band of hyperpigmentation (C and D, *arrowheads*) beginning at the ora serrata and extending to a well-defined posterior boundary at the equator.

Assessment

This is a case of a 57-year-old woman with history of early presenile cataract and peripheral circumferential hyperpigmentation in the fundi.

Differential Diagnosis

- RP
- Enhanced-S cone (Goldmann-Favre) syndrome
- Microcornea, retinal dystrophy, cataract, and posterior staphyloma
- Wagner vitreoretinal degeneration
- ADVIRC

Working Diagnosis

- ADVIRC

Multimodal Testing and Results

- Fundus photographs
  - Fundus photographs revealed a peripheral circumferential band of hyperpigmentation and atrophy beginning at the ora serrata and extending posteriorly to a well-defined

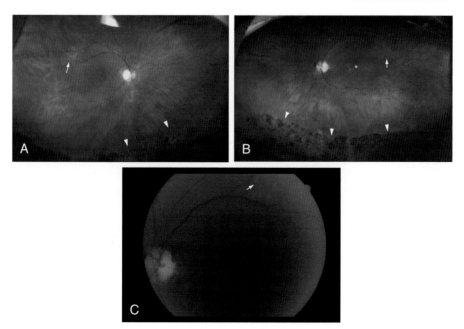

Fig. 9.2 Fundus photographs of patient at age 57 years show new areas of retinal pigment epithelial atrophy in the macula (B, *asterisk*) and perimacular drusen (A and B, *arrows*), which were not present a decade earlier. Peripheral annular hyperpigmentation and atrophic changes persist (A and B, *arrowheads*).

boundary at the equator (Fig. 9.1). This annual band of peripheral hyperpigmentation is highly characteristic of ADVIRC.

- Punctate, white intraretinal or preretinal deposits are often present. Retinal arteriolar narrowing and neovascularization can be seen. In rare instances, vitreous hemorrhage can cause substantial vision loss.[1,5]
- Fluorescein angiogram
  - Fluorescein angiography was not performed on this patient. In ADVIRC, angiography can show petaloid leakage from cystoid macular edema, retinal vascular incompetence, peripheral retinal avascularity, and/or leakage from rare retinal neovascularization.[5]
- OCT
  - In this patient, retinal pigment epithelial atrophy was observed on ophthalmoscopy and OCT at age 70.[6] Though not seen in this patient, macular edema has been described and can lead to significant visual impairment.[5]
- Electroretinogram (ERG)
  - The ERG revealed normal cone and rod function at age 46. Then, progressive decline in cone function occurred over the following decades.[6] ERG findings in ADVIRC can range from normal to severely reduced cone and rod function.[5,7]
- Electrooculogram (EOG)
  - Though not performed in our patient, EOG is usually significantly subnormal in ADVIRC patients,[3,7] presumably related to a mutation in the *BEST1* gene.
- Goldmann automated perimetry
  - Though not performed in our patient, Goldmann perimetry is often normal early but may demonstrate mild constriction over time.[7]

- Genetic testing
  - Genetic testing can be quite helpful in confirming the diagnosis of *BEST1*-related conditions, including ADVIRC.
  - ADVIRC is an autosomal dominant condition with causative missense mutations leading to altered splicing of the *BEST1* gene.[3,8-10]

Management

- Observation was recommended in this patient because no macular edema or retinal neovascularization was present.
- In patients with presenile cataract, cataract extraction may improve visual acuity and symptomatic glare.
- Macular edema may be treated with subtenon's and intravitreal or topical corticosteroids, as well as by nonsteroidal anti-inflammatory drugs and carbonic anhydrase medications.[8] Retinal neovascularization can be treated with panretinal photocoagulation or vitrectomy for eyes complicated by severe vitreous hemorrhage.

Follow-up Care

- There are no established guidelines for follow-up, though patients may be followed annually in the absence of retinal neovascularization or macular edema.
- If the patient is symptomatic or demonstrates progression on OCT or fundus examination, more frequent follow-up may be indicated.

Algorithm 9.1: Algorithm for Bilateral Peripheral Pigmentary Changes

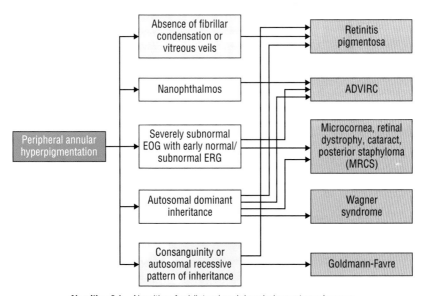

Algorithm 9.1 Algorithm for bilateral peripheral pigmentary changes.

Key Points

- Consider ADVIRC in patients with peripheral, annular pigmentation with a positive family history and presenile cataracts.
- Genetic testing may be helpful in confirming *BEST1* mutation.
- Early in the condition, visual acuity can be mildly impaired because of macular edema and mild cone dysfunction. In later decades, patients may experience significant vision loss secondary to progressive cone dysfunction and retinal pigment epithelial atrophy.[8,9]
- In rare cases, vitreous hemorrhage and retinal detachment can develop.

References

1. Traboulsi EI, Payne JW. Autosomal dominant vitreoretinochoroidopathy: report of the third family. *Arch Ophthalmol.* 1993;111(2):194-196.
2. Boon CJ, Klevering BJ, Leroy BP, Hoyng CB, Keunen JE, den Hollander AI. The spectrum of ocular phenotypes caused by mutations in the BEST1 gene. *Prog Retin Eye Res.* 2009;28(3):187-205.
3. Yardley J, Leroy BP, Hart-Holden N, et al. Mutations of VMD2 splicing regulators cause nanophthalmos and autosomal dominant vitreoretinochoroidopathy (ADVIRC). *Invest Ophthalmol Vis Sci.* 2004; 45(10):3683-3689.
4. Vincent A, McAlister C, Vandehoven C, Héon E. BEST1-related autosomal dominant vitreoretinochoroidopathy: a degenerative disease with a range of developmental ocular anomalies. *Eye (Lond).* 2011; 25(1):113-118.
5. Kaufman SJ, Goldberg MF, Orth DH, Fishman GA, Tessler H, Mizuno K. Autosomal dominant vitreoretinochoroidopathy. *Arch Ophthalmol.* 1982;100(2):272-278.
6. Chen CJ, Goldberg MF. Progressive cone dysfunction and geographic atrophy of the macula in late stage autosomal dominant vitreoretinochoroidopathy (ADVIRC). *Ophthalmic Genet.* 2016;37(1):81-85.
7. Lafaut BA, Loeys B, Leroy BP, Spileers W, De Laey JJ, Kestelyn P. Clinical and electrophysiological findings in autosomal dominant vitreoretinochoroidopathy: report of a new pedigree. *Graefes Arch Clin Exp Ophthalmol.* 2001;239(8):575-582.
8. Chen CJ, Kaufman S, Stöhr H, Weber BH, Goldberg MF. Long-term macular changes in the first proband of autosomal dominant vitreoretinochoroidopathy (ADVIRC) due to a newly identified mutation in BEST1. *Ophthalmic Genet.* 2016;37(1):102-108.
9. Goldberg MF, McLeod S, Tso M, et al. Ocular histopathology and immunohistochemical analysis in the oldest known individual with autosomal dominant vitreoretinochoroidopathy. *Ophthalmol Retina.* 2018;2(4):360-378.
10. Burgess R, MacLaren RE, Davidson AE, et al. ADVIRC is caused by distinct mutations in BEST1 that alter pre-mRNA splicing. *J Med Genet.* 2009;46(9):620-625.

CHAPTER 10

I Was Never Good at Ghosts in the Graveyard

Mark J. Daily

History of Present Illness

The patient is a 46-year-old practicing neurologist reporting difficulty with near vision. His fundus examination is abnormal, and upon questioning he says he has been told in the past that he has "some type of retinal condition" but no further evaluation was ever done. He says that as a youngster, he was never good at playing Ghosts in the Graveyard.

OCULAR EXAMINATION FINDINGS

Visual acuity with correction was 20/25 right eye and 20/20 left eye. Pupils were 4 mm and equally reactive. Motility was full. Visual fields were full but slow to confrontation. There were macular white flecks in each eye. The peripheral retina showed midperipheral rings of pigment atrophy and nummular pigment migration into the retina (Fig. 10.1). Goldmann fields demonstrated a midperipheral scotoma in the right eye. External and anterior segment examinations were normal, and intraocular pressures were 16 mm Hg in each eye.

IMAGING

Fluorescein angiography showed areas of hyperfluorescence in the midperiphery consistent with areas of pigment atrophy (Fig. 10.2). In the optical coherence tomography (OCT) images, the maculas were fairly normal, but the periphery of each retina showed extensive disruption of the outer layers (Fig. 10.3).

Questions to Ask

- Is the patient on any medications?
  - No
- Do any other family members have ocular reports of night blindness or hereditary eye conditions?
  - No

Assessment

A 46-year-old physician presented with good distance vision, a chief complaint of presbyopia, and, when asked, mild night blindness. Peripheral retinal atrophy and pigmentation is present in the fundus.

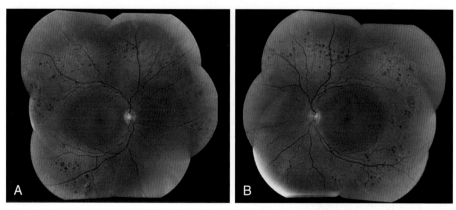

Fig. 10.1 Fundus photographs of right (A) and left (B) eyes. Note midperipheral atrophy and nummular pigmentation.

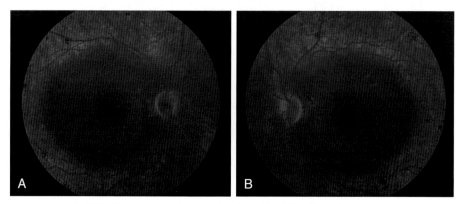

Fig. 10.2 Fluorescein angiograms showing midperipheral hyperfluorescence.

Differential Diagnosis

- Retinitis pigmentosa (RP)
- Medication toxicity, such as thioridazine retinopathy
- Enhanced S-cone syndrome

Working Diagnosis

- Enhanced S-cone syndrome

Genetic Testing

Genetic analysis at the Carver Nonprofit Genetic Testing Laboratory at the University of Iowa showed a missense mutation (Arg311Gln) and a splice site mutation (IVS1–2A>C) in the NR2E3 genes, consistent with a diagnosis of autosomal recessive enhanced S-cone syndrome.

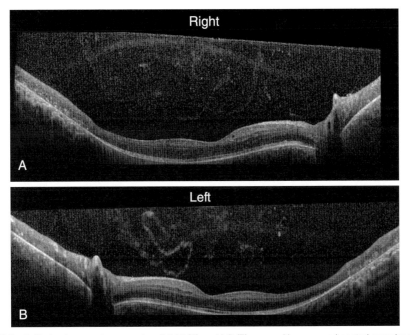

Fig. 10.3 Optical coherence tomography of right (A) and left (B) eyes, with preserved central macular areas and adjacent areas of retinal thinning nasally and temporally.

Multimodal Testing and Results

- Fundus photographs: Midperipheral symmetrical atrophy with nummular (not bone spicule–like) pigment migrations is seen. Flecks are present in the macular regions with sparing of the periphery in enhanced S-cone syndrome in contrast to retinitis pigmentosa, which shows peripheral bone spicule-like pigment changes.
- Fluorescein angiography: Hypofluorescence consistent with areas of pigment atrophy in the periphery are seen.
- OCT: Demonstrates sparing of the maculas with extensive outer retinal damage pericentrally and in the periphery.

Diagnosis

Molecular genetic analysis is available and necessary to confirm the correct diagnosis.

Enhanced S-Cone Syndrome

This condition, previously known as Goldmann-Favre syndrome, was identified in the 1990s[1] and contains mutations in the NR2E3 gene, which is a transcription factor important in embryonic development. These patients have 17 times more blue cones (S or "small wavelength" cones) than red (L or "large wavelength") or green (M or "medium wavelength") cones and few rods. Some patients develop schisis cavities in the periphery.[2] The combination of retinoschisis and pigmentary retinopathy was previously known as Goldmann-Favre Syndrome until recent advances in the genetic identification.

Management

No medical treatment is available, and though there is slow progression, there is considerable variability in the prognosis,[3] with some patients, such as this patient, maintaining excellent central acuity and mild field loss.

Follow-Up Care

The patient was prescribed reading glasses and will be seen annually for examination.

Algorithm 10.1: Algorithm Showing Diagnosis for Enhanced S-Cone Syndrome

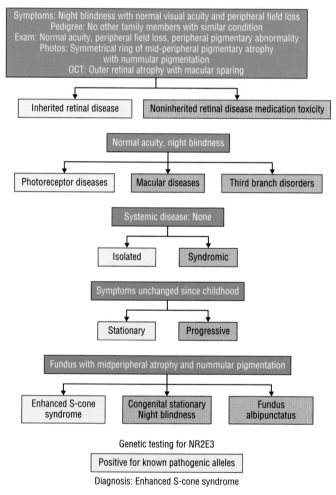

Algorithm 10.1   Algorithm showing diagnosis for enhanced S-cone syndrome.

Key Points

- Although the fundus was suggestive of the phenotype of RP, the peripheral retinal vessels were relatively preserved, and the pigment in the affected areas was round and nummular instead of bone spicule–like.
- This patient was able to complete medical school and practice medicine for 15 years despite having a degenerative retinal disease.

References

1. Jacobson SG, Marmor MF, Kemp CM, Knighton RW. SWS (blue) cone hypersensitivity in a newly identified retinal degeneration. *Invest Ophthalmol Vis Sci*. 1990;31(5):827-838.
2. De Carvalho ER, Robson AG, Arno G, Boon C, Webster AA, Michaelides M. Enhanced S-cone syndrome: spectrum of clinical, imaging, electrophysiological and genetic findings in a retrospective case series of 56 patients. *Ophthalmol Retina*. 2021;5(2):195-214.
3. Marmor MF. An examination of the propositus of enhanced S-cone syndrome 30 years after diagnosis. *JAMA Ophthalmol*. 2020;138(9):1004-1006.

CHAPTER 11

Bilateral Perifoveal Degeneration in a Woman

Hisashi Fukuyama ■ Amani A. Fawzi

History of Present Illness

A 47-year-old woman presented to our clinic with a chief report of "spots in vision." She denied other changes in her vision, flashes, or floaters and had no past history of ocular conditions or surgeries.

OCULAR EXAMINATION FINDINGS

Visual acuity with correction was 20/20 in both eyes. Intraocular pressures were normal. External and anterior segment examinations were unremarkable. Dilated fundus examination showed pigmentary changes in the perimacular areas in both eyes and a large cotton wool spot along the arcade.

IMAGING

Color fundus photography showed retinal pigment epithelium (RPE) hyperpigmentary changes and subtle yellow spots surrounding the macular area (Fig. 11.1). Optical coherence tomography (OCT) showed that the hyperpigmented areas corresponded to a hyperreflective dome-shaped lesion on the RPE (Fig. 11.2, *green arrow*), and the outer retina was markedly attenuated (Fig. 11.2, *yellow arrow*).

Fundus autofluorescence (AF) showed alternating hyper- and hypoautofluorescent lesions in the perifoveal area and nasal to the optic nerve (Fig. 11.3).

Questions to Ask

- Is there a previous history of ocular disease and/or relapsing vision loss? Previous history of subretinal fluid is associated with retinal pigment epitheliopathy abnormalities due to central serous chorioretinopathy (CSC)/pachychoroid disease. Geographical atrophy and RPE changes could also be observed in dry age-related macular degeneration (AMD) in older patients.
  - No
- What medications does the patient take? Pentosan polysulfate maculopathy may be associated with RPE and outer retinal atrophy.
  - Patient was on no medications and had no history of pentosan polysulfate usage.
- Is there a history of systemic medical illness? Inflammatory diseases, including syphilis and sarcoidosis, might be accompanied by ocular manifestations. A thorough history and review of systems are helpful. When multiple systems are affected without another obvious explanation, mitochondrial retinal disease should be suspected. Diabetes mellitus (DM),

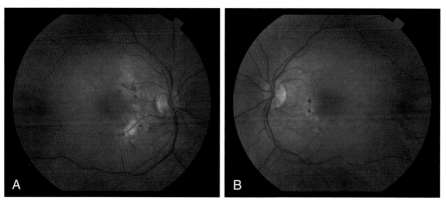

Fig. 11.1 Color fundus photographs of right eye (A) and left eye (B).

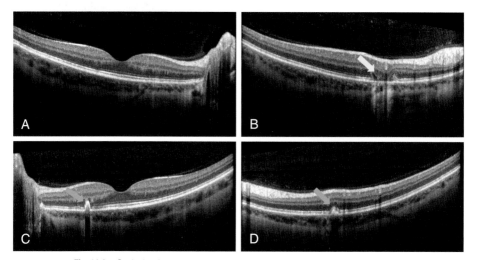

Fig. 11.2 Optical coherence tomography of right eye (A, B) and left eye (C, D).

especially maternally inherited, and clinical or subclinical hearing loss (maternally inherited diabetes and deafness [MIDD] syndrome) are the most common features associated with the A3243G mitochondrial mutation.

- Yes. She has a history of DM.

■ Does the patient have a family history of ocular conditions or consanguinity? A family history would be essential to ascertain inherited retinal disorders. MIDD and stroke-like episodes are caused by various mitochondrial DNA mutations. MIDD also has been shown to have a high correlation with pattern dystrophies.

- No history of ocular conditions.

Assessment

■ This is a case of a 47-year-old woman with no past ocular or surgical history demonstrating bilateral macular dystrophy and subretinal hyperreflective flecks on OCT and a ring of alternating hyper- and hypoautofluorescence surrounding the fovea. She has DM.

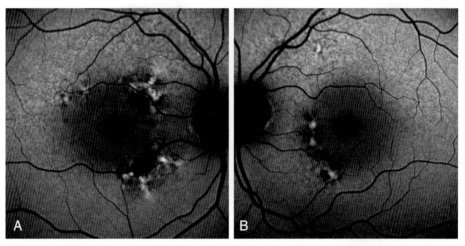

Fig. 11.3 Fundus autofluorescence images of right eye (A) and left eye (B).

Differential Diagnosis

- Syphilitic chorioretinitis
- Pseudoxanthoma elasticum maculopathy
- Pattern dystrophy: RDS peripherin/RDS gene
- Mitochondrial retinopathy
- Central areolar choroidal dystrophy
- AMD
- CSC/pachychoroid disease
- Pentosan polysulfate maculopathy

Working Diagnosis

- DNA testing revealed A3243G mitochondrial DNA point mutation.
- The diagnosis is m.3243A>G-associated maculopathy.

Multimodal Testing and Results

- Fundus photographs
  - On fundus examination, hyperpigmented lesions surrounding the macula are typically visualized involving the peripapillary retina (Fig. 11.1).[1,2]
- OCT
  - As mentioned earlier, OCT showed hyperreflective areas and outer retinal attenuation. OCT also showed ellipsoid zone and RPE thinning in areas without atrophy and outer retinal attenuation in areas of chorioretinal atrophy (Fig. 11.2).[3,4]

- Fundus AF
  - Our patients' AF showed alternating hyper- and hypoautofluorescence in the perifoveal area and nasal to the optic nerve. AF examination revealed hyperautofluorescence due to yellow-white spots/flecks (RPE thickening on OCT) and hypoautofluorescence due to atrophic changes (Fig. 11.3).[4]
- Genetic testing
  - Genetic testing of mitochondrial DNA identified a point mutation at locus 3243 that confirmed this disorder. Our patient has a history of DM at a young age. mtDNA genome sequencing and heteroplasmy analysis can now be effectively performed in blood, although it may be necessary to test other tissues in affected organs. Analysis in urine can selectively be more informative and accurate than testing in blood alone, especially in older individuals.[5]

Management

- Because this patient was asymptomatic and visual acuity was 20/20 in both eyes, the patient was observed.
- There is currently no effective treatment for m.3243A>G-associated maculopathy.

Follow-up Care

- There are no previously established guidelines for follow-up.
- Our patient is followed on a biannual basis.
- Our patient's visual acuity remains 20/20 but the area of perifoveal degeneration has progressed (Fig. 11.4).
- Natural history of m.3243A>G-associated maculopathy is unknown.
- One study reported two cases followed over 15 years; one patient lost two Snellen lines in both eyes, and another lost one line in one eye.[6]

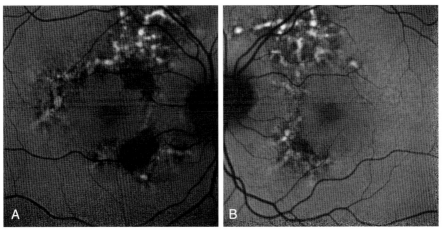

Fig. 11.4 Fundus autofluorescence images of right eye (A) and left eye (B) 5 years after initial visit.

Algorithm 11.1: Algorithm for Differential Diagnosis for Bilateral Perifoveal Degeneration

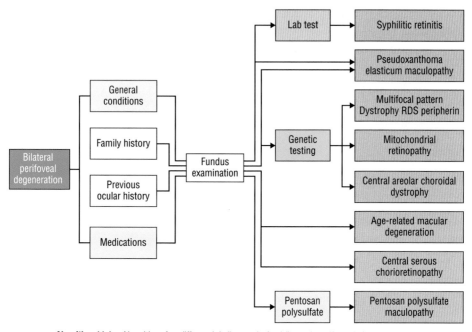

Algorithm 11.1   Algorithm for differential diagnosis for bilateral perifoveal degeneration.

Key Points

- MIDD macular atrophy spares the fovea; generally, multifocal RPE changes surround the macula. Peripapillary lesions may also be seen in m.3243A>G-associated maculopathy.
- A genetic test is the only way to definitively diagnose this disease.
- Consider m.3243A>G-associated maculopathy in patients with DM and hearing loss, especially when maternal inheritance is documented.

References

1. Coussa RG, Parikh S, Traboulsi EI. Mitochondrial DNA A3243G variant-associated retinopathy: current perspectives and clinical implications. *Surv Ophthalmol.* 2021;66(5):838-855.
2. Jones M, Mitchell P, Wang JJ, Sue C. MELAS A3243G mitochondrial DNA mutation and age related maculopathy. *Am J Ophthalmol.* 2004;138(6):1051-1053.
3. Daruich A, Matet A, Borruat FX. Macular dystrophy associated with the mitochondrial DNA A3243G mutation: pericentral pigment deposits or atrophy? Report of two cases and review of the literature. *BMC Ophthalmol.* 2014;14:77.
4. de Laat P, Smeitink JAM, Janssen MCH, Keunen JEE, Boon CJF. Mitochondrial retinal dystrophy associated with the m.3243A>G mutation. *Ophthalmology.* 2013;120(12):2684-2696.
5. Parikh S, Goldstein A, Koenig MK. Diagnosis and management of mitochondrial disease: a consensus statement from the Mitochondrial Medicine Society. *Genet Med.* 2015;17(9):689-701.
6. Ambonville C, Meas T, Lecleire-Collet A, et al. Macular pattern dystrophy in MIDD: long-term follow-up. *Diabetes Metab.* 2008;34(4 pt 1):389-391.

CHAPTER 12

Autosomal Dominant Radial Drusen

Alexis Warren ▪ William F. Mieler

History of Present Illness

A 38-year-old asymptomatic female patient with an unremarkable medical history was referred from an optometrist for bilateral drusen found on a routine eye examination. She denies blurry vision, scotomas, or metamorphopsia. She also denies any history of ocular conditions or ocular surgeries. Family history includes one brother with macular degeneration and father with documented drusen.

OCULAR EXAMINATION FINDINGS

Visual acuity with correction was 20/20 in both eyes. Intraocular pressure was normal. External and anterior segment examination was unremarkable. Dilated fundus examination showed radial drusen in the macula with dense and nearly confluent drusen nasal and abutting the disc in both eyes.

IMAGING

Optical coherence tomography (OCT) showed small bilateral deposits throughout the macula at the level of the retinal pigment epithelium (RPE) and Bruch membrane without intraretinal or subretinal fluid. Fluorescein angiography (FA) showed significant bilateral macular drusen with areas of hyperfluorescence consistent with atrophy (Figs. 12.1 and 12.2).

Questions to Ask

- At what age did the drusen present? Drusen onset can vary in these patients but can present as early as childhood, with most patients presenting by their third or fourth decade of life.
    - This patient first presented at 38 years of age.
- Does the patient have a family history of ocular conditions, macular degeneration, or drusen? Family history is important for inherited retinal diseases such as Sorsby macular dystrophy, North Carolina macular dystrophy, and malattia leventinese, which are all inherited in an autosomal dominant fashion.
    - Yes

Assessment

- This is a case of a 38-year-old asymptomatic female patient with good vision, no ocular or medical history, and a positive family history demonstrating an incidental finding of bilateral macular radiating drusen throughout the macula without choroidal neovascularization.

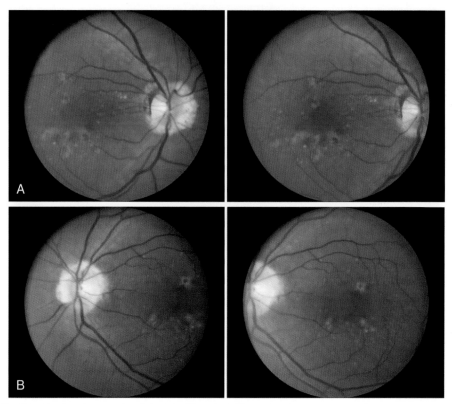

Fig. 12.1 Fundus photographs of the right (A) and left (B) eye showing bilateral macular drusen in a radial pattern. There is also round drusen nasal to the optic nerve in both eyes.

Differential Diagnosis

- Sorsby macular dystrophy
- North Carolina macular dystrophy
- Adult-onset foveomacular vitelliform dystrophy
- Stargardt disease
- Pattern dystrophy
- Basal laminar (cuticular) drusen
- Membranoproliferative glomerulonephritis type II

Working Diagnosis

- Malattia leventinese, autosomal dominant radial drusen (ADRD)

Multimodal Testing and Results

- Fundus photographs
  - On fundus examination, there are radiating and sometimes confluent drusen in the macula with the nasal portion being large and round and those in the temporal macula smaller and more elongated. The nasal drusen often abut the nasal portion of the optic nerve.[1]

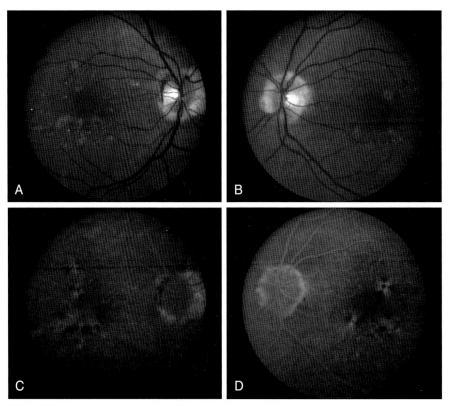

Fig. 12.2 Fluorescein angiography with early phases (A) and (B) highlighting the radial drusen. Late photographs (C) and (D) with evidence of atrophy without leakage or evidence of choroidal neovascularization.

- These patients can also present variably with RPE hyperplasia, choroidal neovascular membranes, and even geographical atrophy.[2]
- OCT
  - OCT of these patients often shows bilateral deposits throughout the macula at the level of the RPE and Bruch membrane.[2,3]
- FA
  - These images can highlight the radial drusen but even more so the associated RPE atrophy that can be masked clinically.
  - Late leakage in these photographs may also reveal areas of secondary choroidal neovascularization.[4]
- Fundus autofluorescence
  - These drusen often present with hyperautofluorescence unlike that present in age-related macular degeneration; however, progression of disease and RPE atrophy with hypoautofluorescence occurs.[5]
- Electroretinogram (ERG)
  - The full-field ERG is usually normal with an abnormal pattern ERG given the focal macular changes of this disease.[1]
- Genetic testing
  - This can be important in differentiating this disease from other autosomal dominant macular dystrophies. Malattia leventinese is often caused by a single-point mutation on

chromosome 2 in the endothelial growth factor–containing fibrillin-like extracellular matrix protein 1 (EFEMP1) gene.[6,7]

- OCT angiography (OCT-A)
  - Choroidal neovascularization may present eventually in these patients; however, historically this is less common than other forms of inherited macular dystrophies.
  - Interestingly, the aforementioned areas of confluent drusen may mask small areas of choroidal neovascular abnormalities, which may highlight the importance of OCT-A for identifying high-flow structures at the level of the choriocapillaris, likely consistent with choroidal neovascularization.[8]

Management

- Fortunately, this patient was asymptomatic, so no treatment was necessary. This patient was observed for several years with no significant progression of visually significant disease.
- Generally, these patients are relatively asymptomatic, unless there is choroidal neovascularization or significant atrophy.
- Those patients with choroidal neovascular membranes are often treated with anti–vascular endothelial growth factor intravitreal injections.

Follow-up Care

- Because this diagnosis often can be an incidental finding, there is no established guideline for follow-up for these patients.
- This disease can present variably, and follow-up should be tailored to the specific patient scenario. Large areas of confluent drusen may suggest the presence of risk of choroidal neovascularization and warrant closer follow-up.[8]
- If the patient has symptomatic scotomas or demonstrates rapid progression of drusen and atrophy, more frequent follow-up may be indicated.

Algorithm 12.1: Basic Algorithm for Macular Dystrophies

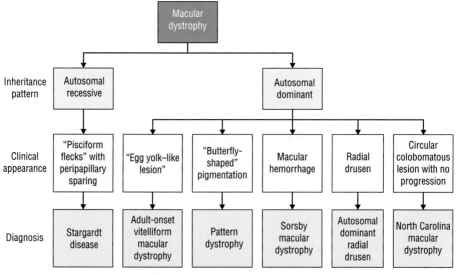

Algorithm 12.1 Basic algorithm for macular dystrophies.

Key Points

- In patients with bilateral macular deposits at a young age, an inherited macular dystrophy, like ADRD, should be considered.
- ADRD can have variable clinical features, but these patients typically present asymptomatically and often have relatively good vision.
- Genetic testing in these patients may help aid diagnosis and future family planning.
- Visual decline, if present, in these patients may be secondary to choroidal neovascularization and may warrant treatment with intravitreal injections.

References

1. Schachat AP, Wilkinson CP, Hinton DR, Sadda SVR, Wiedemann P. Macular dystrophies. In: Sadda S. V. R., Schachat A. P., Wilkinson C. P., et al., eds. *Ryan's Retina*. 6th ed. Elsevier; 2018.
2. Freund KB, Mieler WF, Sarraf D, Yannuzzi LA. Hereditary chorioretinal dystrophies. In: Freund KB, Sarraf D, Mieler WF, Yannuzzi LA, eds. *The Retinal Atlas*. 2nd ed. Elsevier; 2017.
3. Souied EH, Leveziel N, Letien V, Darmon J, Coscas G, Soubrane G. Optical coherent tomography features of malattia leventinese. *Am J Ophthalmol*. 2006;141(2):404-407.
4. Guigui B, Leveziel N, Martinet V, et al. Angiography features of early onset drusen. *Br J Ophthalmol*. 2011;95(2):238-244.
5. Tsang SH, Sharma T. Doyne honeycomb retinal dystrophy (malattia leventinese, autosomal dominant drusen). *Adv Exp Med Biol*. 2018;1085:97-102.
6. Stone EM, Lotery AJ, Munier FL, et al. A single EFEMP1 mutation associated with both malattia leventinese and Doyne honeycomb retinal dystrophy. *Nat Genet*. 1999;22(2):199-202.
7. Narendran N, Guymer RH, Cain M, Baird PN. Analysis of the EFEMP1 gene in individuals and families with early onset drusen. *Eye (Lond)*. 2005;19(1):11-15.
8. Serra R, Coscas F, Messaoudi N, Srour M, Souied E. Choroidal neovascularization in malattia leventinese diagnosed using optical coherence tomography angiography. *Am J Ophthalmol*. 2017;176:108-117.

Degenerative/Deficiency

CHAPTER 13

Bilateral Asymptomatic Pigmentary Retinopathy

Mohammad Amr Sabbagh ■ Robert A. Hyde

History of Present Illness

■ We present a case of a 57-year-old woman with a history of rheumatoid arthritis referred for establishment of care in the setting of chronic hydroxychloroquine use (10 years). She denied any central or peripheral vision loss, nyctalopia, ocular pain, photopsia, new floaters, or metamorphopsia. She also denied any past ocular history.

OCULAR EXAMINATION FINDINGS

■ Visual acuity without updated refraction was 20/40 in the right eye and 20/25 in the left eye (best corrected visual acuity was 20/20 in both eyes 1 year earlier). Intraocular pressures were normal. Pupils were symmetrical with no relative afferent pupillary defect in either eye. Slit lamp examination was unremarkable except for mild nuclear sclerotic cataracts. Dilated funduscopic examination showed a sharp foveal light reflex and dense scattered paravenous pigmentation in both eyes (Figs. 13.1 and 13.2).

IMAGING

■ Goldmann visual field showed regional constriction and scotomas corresponding to the areas of pigmentation. Optical coherence tomography (OCT) showed a normal fovea with a preserved ellipsoid zone in both eyes (Fig. 13.3). An area of outer retinal atrophy, corresponding to a focal hyperautofluorescent area on fundus autofluorescence (FAF) in the inferotemporal macula in the right eye, was noted (Figs. 13.4 and 13.5). Comparison of images to outside records from 3 years earlier appear stable.

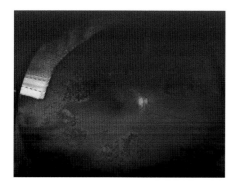

Fig. 13.1 Fundus photo (right eye).

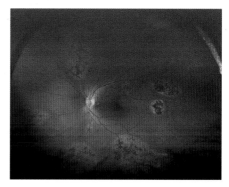

Fig. 13.2 Fundus photo (left eye).

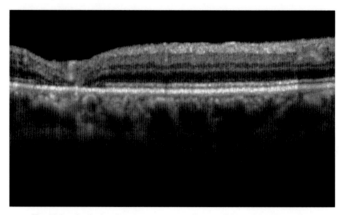

Fig. 13.3 Optical coherence tomography overlying area of atrophy.

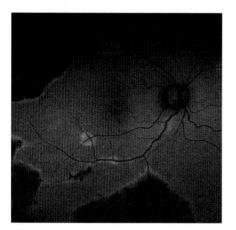

Fig. 13.4 Fundus autofluorescence (right eye).

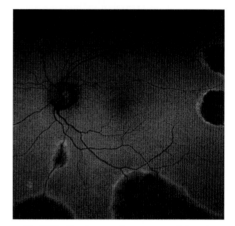

Fig. 13.5 Fundus autofluorescence (left eye).

Questions to Ask

- What is the patient's past medical history? Specifically, is there any history of a systemic inflammatory or infectious condition (e.g., sarcoidosis, syphilis, tuberculosis)?
  - Known history of rheumatoid arthritis, for which she has been taking hydroxychloroquine for over 10 years
- What medications is the patient currently taking or has taken in the past?
  - Hydroxychloroquine (4.3 mg/kg/day), which is not known to be associated with peripheral pigmentary retinopathy, but rather showing macular atrophy and pigment changes
  - Sulfasalazine
- Is there a family history of any ocular conditions?
  - No

Assessment

- This is a 57-year-old woman with a past medical history of rheumatoid arthritis treated with hydroxychloroquine for many years who presents with bilateral paravenous pigmentation on fundoscopy with corresponding defects on Goldmann visual field.

Differential Diagnosis[1]

- Retinitis pigmentosa (pericentral, sectoral, and typical)
- Helicoid peripapillary chorioretinal atrophy
- Serpiginous choroidopathy
- Angioid streaks
- Stickler syndrome
- Sarcoidosis
- Syphilis
- Tuberculosis

Working Diagnosis

- Pigmented paravenous retinochoroidal atrophy (PPRCA)

Multimodal Testing and Results

- Fundus photos[2]
  - Pigmentation along retinal veins in the form of either bone spicules, coarse pigment clumps, or fine pigment
  - Typically a bilateral process, though unilateral cases have been reported
  - Our patient had dense paravenous clumping of bone spicules in both eyes. Maculae appeared unremarkable in both eyes.
- Visual field[2,3]
  - Visual fields tend to be variable. They may be normal or may exhibit ring or paracentral scotomas, concentric constriction, or some combination thereof, typically corresponding to the areas of paravenous atrophy.
  - Goldmann visual fields were obtained for our patient, which showed constriction and scotomas that corresponded to the dense pigment clumping.
  - A Humphrey 10–2 visual field was also obtained in the setting of chronic hydroxychloroquine use, which was full in both eyes.
- OCT[4,5]
  - The macula tends to be spared in PPRCA. Hyperpigmented lesions exhibit hyperreflectivity with shadowing. Our patient also exhibited an area of outer retinal atrophy without clinically evident pigmentation.
- FAF[5]
  - It is common to have both areas of hypoautofluorescence (typically areas of clumped pigment), where the retinal pigment epithelium (RPE) is atrophic, and areas of hyperautofluorescence (indicating hyperactive RPE), as evident in our patient.
- Fluorescein angiogram (FA)[6]
  - A window defect would be expected in the presence of RPE atrophy, whereas blockage would be expected in areas of dense pigmentation.
- Indocyanine green angiography (ICG)[6]
  - Hypocyanescence that follows the same pattern as hypofluorescence on FA, but can often extend further out with ICG, indicating that ICG may be better at estimating the extent of atrophy than FA.
- Electroretinogram or electrooculogram[2,7]
  - Electrophysiologic data tend to be variable and nonspecific, ranging from normal to undetectable.
- Laboratory testing and imaging[2]
  - It is necessary to undergo systemic evaluation to help rule out potential infectious or inflammatory etiologies.

■ Testing includes (but is not limited to) chest x-ray; complete metabolic panel; erythrocyte sedimentation rate; C-reactive protein; QuantiFERON-TB Gold; angiotensin-converting enzyme; lysozyme; syphilis serologies; herpes simplex virus, herpes zoster virus, and cytomegalovirus serologies; and antinuclear antibodies.

Management

■ No specific treatment for PPRCA exists.[8]

Follow-up Care

■ PPRCA is mostly a nonprogressive or slowly progressive disease. Comparison to images taken 3 years earlier reveals stable appearance. Given no available treatment, longer follow-up intervals are usually adequate (sooner if the patient notes any changes).[8]
■ Given no evidence of hydroxychloroquine maculopathy, the patient was advised to continue treatment for now with close monitoring.

Algorithm 13.1: Algorithm for the Differential Diagnosis of Pigmented Paravenous Retinochoroidal Atrophy

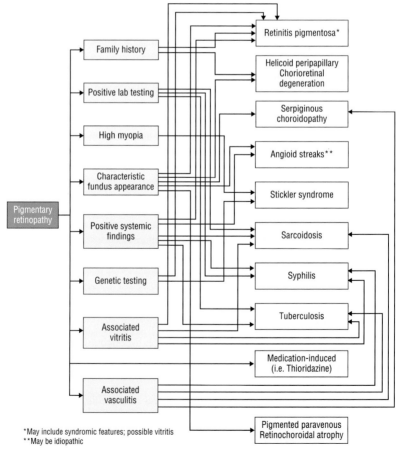

Algorithm 13.1   Algorithm for the differential diagnosis of pigmented paravenous retinochoroidal atrophy.

Key Points

- PPRCA is generally bilateral and is of unknown etiology.
- The majority of patients are asymptomatic with central vision spared. Dense clumps of pigmentation may cause visual field defects often unbeknownst to patients.
- PPRCA is typically nonprogressive or very slowly progressive with no available treatment. Once infectious/inflammatory etiologies have been ruled out, follow-up intervals can be extended.

References

1. Huang HB, Zhang YX. Pigmented paravenous retinochoroidal atrophy (review). *Exp Ther Med.* 2014;7(6):1439-1445.
2. Noble KG, Carr RE. Pigmented paravenous chorioretinal atrophy. *Am J Ophthalmol.* 1983;96(3):338-344.
3. Al-Husainy S, Sarodia U, Deane JS. Pigmented paravenous retinochoroidal atrophy: evidence of progression to macular involvement in a family with a 42-year history. *Eye (Lond).* 2001;15(pt 3):329-330.
4. Ghosh B, Goel N, Batta S, Raina UK. SD-OCT in pigmented paravenous retinochoroidal atrophy. *Ophthalmic Surg Lasers Imaging.* 2012;43(3):e41-e43.
5. Fleckenstein M, Charbel Issa P, Helb HM, Schmitz-Valckenberg S, Scholl HP, Holz FG. Correlation of lines of increased autofluorescence in macular dystrophy and pigmented paravenous retinochoroidal atrophy by optical coherence tomography. *Arch Ophthalmol.* 2008;126(10):1461-1463.
6. Yanagi Y, Okajima O, Mori M. Indocyanine green angiography in pigmented paravenous retinochoroidal atrophy. *Acta Ophthalmol Scand.* 2003;81(1):60-67.
7. Batioglu F, Atmaca LS, Atilla H, Arslanpençe A. Inflammatory pigmented paravenous retinochoroidal atrophy. *Eye (Lond).* 2002;16(1):81-84.
8. Choi JY, Sandberg MA, Berson EL. Natural course of ocular function in pigmented paravenous retinochoroidal atrophy. *Am J Ophthalmol.* 2006;141(4):763-765.

CHAPTER 14

Unilateral Macular Schisis With Blurred Vision in a Woman

Nancy M. Holekamp

History of Present Illness

A 44-year-old mildly symptomatic woman is referred for a "swollen retina" and vision that cannot be corrected better than 20/30 in her left eye. She has a past ocular history significant for high myopia. She is a frequent contact lens wearer, although dry eyes made her intolerant to contact lenses, and she underwent phakic intraocular lens (IOL) surgery in each eye 2 years earlier.

OCULAR EXAMINATION FINDINGS

Visual acuities with correction were 20/20 in the right eye and 20/30 in the left eye. Intraocular pressures were normal. Anterior segment examination showed bilateral phakic IOL and symmetrical mild nuclear sclerotic cataracts but otherwise was unremarkable. Dilated fundus examination of the right eye showed a myopic, tilted optic nerve with peripapillary atrophy. The right macula showed some mild hypopigmentation. Dilated fundus examination of the left eye showed a slightly myopic, tilted optic nerve. The left macula showed pigment mottling consistent with myopic macular degeneration (Fig. 14.1).

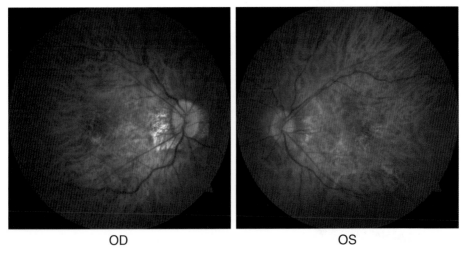

OD   OS

Fig. 14.1 Several features typical of degenerative myopia, including chorioretinal atrophy, peripapillary atrophy, posterior staphyloma, and lacquer cracks, may or may not be seen with myopic macular schisis.

IMAGING

Optical coherence tomography (OCT) of the right eye was normal for a myopic eye. OCT of the left eye showed intraretinal cyst-like changes in the outer retina (outer plexiform and outer nuclear layers) in the foveal and parafoveal regions. The foveal contour was irregular, but there was no epiretinal membrane (Fig. 14.2).

Questions to Ask

- What is the patient's refractive error? Myopic foveoschisis should be considered in the differential diagnosis for retinoschisis.
    - Refraction before phakic IOL surgery was −28.50 − 0.75 × 153 in the right eye and −29.50 − 0.25 × 009 in the left eye
- Does the patient have a family history of ocular conditions or consanguinity? A family history would be important to ascertain etiologies for retinoschisis such as congenital juvenile X-linked retinoschisis (CXLR), retinitis pigmentosa, or familial internal limiting membrane dystrophy.
    - No

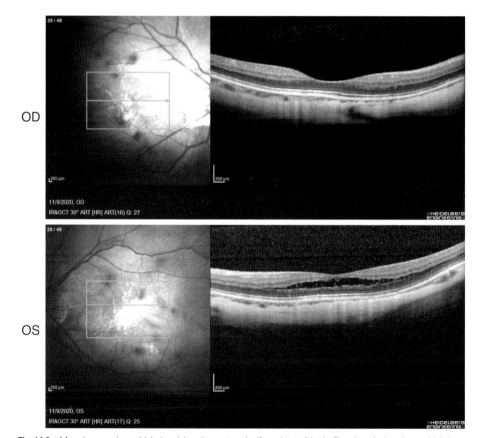

OD

OS

Fig. 14.2 Myopic macular schisis involving the outer plexiform layer (Henle fiber layer) showing a thick inner layer and thin outer layer.

- Does the patient have a history of trauma? Trauma has been associated with macular retinoschisis.
  - No
- What medications does the patient take? Medications such as niacin and taxanes can cause cystic macular edema that appears similar to retinoschisis.
  - None

Assessment

- This is a case of a 44-year-old woman with a past ocular history of high myopia and bilateral phakic IOL surgery demonstrating unilateral myopic macular schisis of mainly the foveal and parafoveal areas on OCT.

Differential Diagnosis[1]

- CXLR
- Stellate nonhereditary idiopathic foveomacular retinoschisis
- Myopic choroidal neovascularization
- Pseudophakic cystoid macular edema
- Epiretinal membrane
- Lamellar macular hole
- Degenerative retinoschisis
- Medication-associated retinoschisis (niacin, taxanes)
- Traction retinal detachment

Working Diagnosis

- Myopic macular schisis (also called myopic foveoschisis) in a highly myopic patient

Multimodal Testing and Results

- Fundus photos
  - On fundus examination, characteristic findings of high myopia can be seen, but the intraretinal cystic spaces typically cannot be appreciated.
  - Features typical of degenerative myopia, including chorioretinal atrophy, peripapillary atrophy, posterior staphyloma, and lacquer cracks, may or may not be seen.[1]
- OCT
  - As mentioned, OCT of the left eye showed cyst-like changes in the outer retina in the foveal and parafoveal regions along with an irregular foveal contour, even in the absence of any epiretinal membrane.[2]
  - The diagnosis of myopic macular schisis is almost impossible without OCT.
- Fluorescein angiography (FA)
  - FA does not show any late leakage or petaloid hyperfluorescence in the macula.[1]

Management

- Given that this patient was mildly symptomatic with visual acuity of 20/30 in the affected eye, the patient was observed.

- This condition has also been called myopic traction maculopathy, which is a misnomer. There are no tractional membranes present on the retinal surface. The condition does not respond well to vitrectomy with internal limiting membrane peel, and this intervention is associated with complications because of the severity of the myopia in most cases and should be avoided in eyes with good vision.
- Patients generally maintain a stable OCT appearance and relatively good and stable visual acuity for many years.[3]

Follow-up Care

- There are no previously established guidelines for follow-up.
- Our patient is followed on an annual basis. Vision and OCT in the left eye have been unchanged (Fig. 14.3).
- If the patient is symptomatic or demonstrates progression on OCT, more frequent follow-up is indicated. However, the bar for considering surgical intervention is very high.

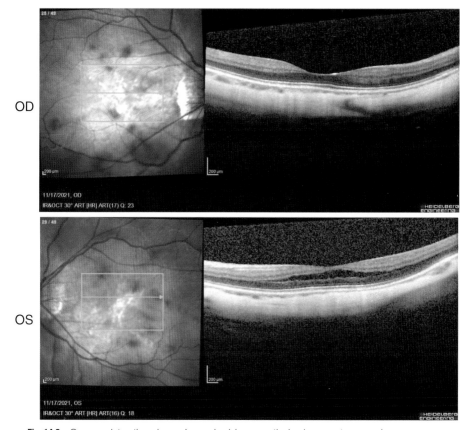

Fig. 14.3 One year later, there is no change in vision or optical coherence tomography appearance.

Algorithm 14.1: Algorithm Representing Myopic Macular Schisis

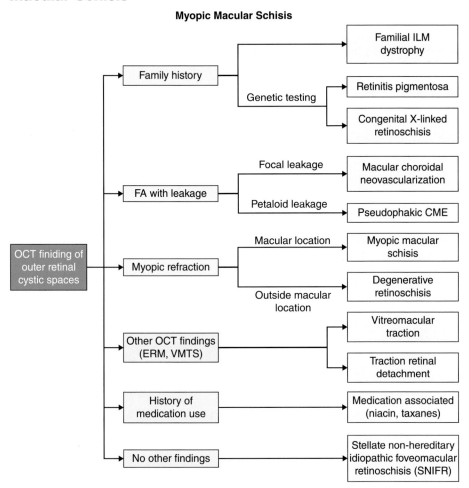

Algorithm 14.1   Algorithm representing myopic macular schisis.

Key Points

- Consider myopic macular schisis in patients with foveomacular retinoschisis with a negative family history or degenerative or acquired etiology who have a "high minus" refractive error.
- Patients tend to have moderately good vision and can be observed.
- Surgery is rarely indicated and is controversial.
- Patients should be followed on an annual basis and at shorter intervals if symptomatic or have progression on OCT.

References

1. Benhamou N, Massin P, Haouchine B, Erginay A, Gaudric A. Macular retinoschisis in highly myopic eyes. *Am J Ophthalmol.* 2002;133(6):794-800.
2. Sayanagi K, Morimoto Y, Ikuno Y, Tano Y. Spectral-domain optical coherence tomographic findings in myopic foveoschisis. *Retina.* 2010;30(4):623-628.
3. Wu Q, Li SW, Lu B, et al. Clinical observation of highly myopic eyes with retinoschisis after phacoemulsification. Article in Chinese. *Zhonghua Yan Ke Za Zhi.* 2011;47(4):303-309.

CHAPTER 15

Acute Vision Loss in an Elderly Patient Associated With Unilateral Intraretinal Blot Hemorrhage in the Macula

Ahmad Santina   Néda Abraham   SriniVas Sadda   David Sarraf

History of Present Illness

An 80-year-old female patient presented with acute vision loss in the left eye. She denied any associated pain, floaters, or photopsias. Past medical history was significant for hypertension, peripheral vascular disease, and chronic obstructive pulmonary disease.

OCULAR EXAMINATION FINDINGS

Visual acuity without correction was 20/20−2 in both eyes. Intraocular pressures were normal. External and anterior segment examination were unremarkable. Dilated fundus examination showed retinal pigment epithelium (RPE) mottling and macular drusen in both eyes with an isolated intraretinal macular blot hemorrhage nasal to the foveal center of the left eye (Fig. 15.1).

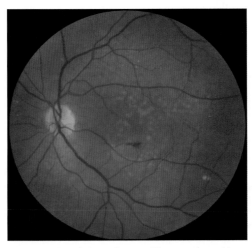

Fig. 15.1 Color fundus photograph of the left eye (from a different patient with age-related macular degeneration) shows the classic intraretinal blot hemorrhage associated with type 3 macular neovascularization.

IMAGING

Optical coherence tomography (OCT) of the right eye showed macular drusen and no evidence of intraretinal or subretinal fluid. OCT of the left eye showed a serous pigment epithelial detachment (PED) with a focus of intraretinal hyperreflectivity at the apex of the PED associated with the "steer sign"[1] and surrounding cystoid macular edema (CME) (Fig. 15.2). OCT angiography (OCTA) showed a corresponding intraretinal focus of microvascular flow at the apex of the PED of the left eye (Fig. 15.3).

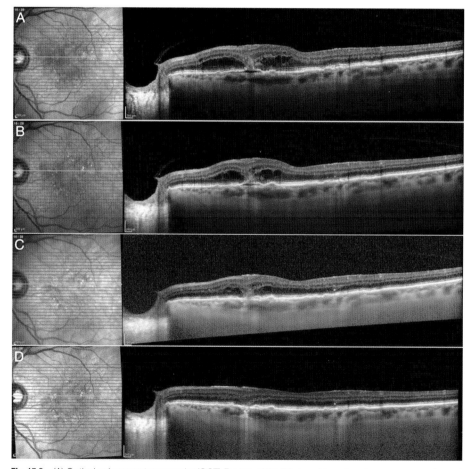

Fig. 15.2 (A) Optical coherence tomography (OCT) B scan of the left eye at baseline shows a serous pigment epithelial detachment (PED) associated with a focus of intraretinal hyperreflectivity (type 3 macular neovascularization [MNV]) at the apex of the PED and surrounding intraretinal fluid. Downward deflection or subsidence of the outer plexiform layer into the type 3 MNV (i.e., the "steer sign") can also be identified. Note the associated thin choroid, which was present in both eyes. (B–D) Tracked OCT B scans after a treat and extend protocol of anti–vascular endothelial growth factor therapy show collapse of the PED and essential resolution of both the type 3 lesion and the cystoid macular edema. There was commensurate improvement of the visual acuity in the left eye.

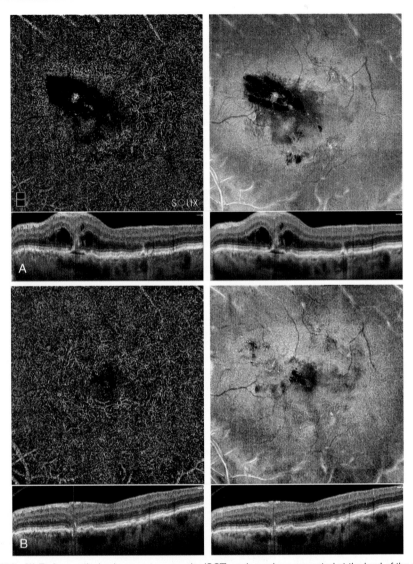

Fig. 15.3 (A) En face optical coherence tomography (OCT) angiography, segmented at the level of the outer retina, with corresponding en face structural OCT and with registered OCT B scan overlay of the left eye at baseline shows a tuft of microvascular flow (type 3 macular neovascularization [MNV]) at the apex of the serous pigment epithelial detachment (PED). The flow originates from the deep retinal capillary plexus and descends into the PED. (B) After anti–vascular endothelial growth factor therapy, there is collapse of the PED and essential resolution of the flow pattern of the type 3 MNV.

Questions to Ask

- Does the patient have any history of diabetes mellitus (DM)?
  - No. The patient denied DM. Macular hemorrhage and fluid may be the result of diabetic macular edema (DME), but in the absence of diabetic retinopathy in either eye, DME is a very unlikely etiology.

- Does the patient have a history of anemia or malignancy?
  - No. Anemia, thrombocytopenia, or malignancy (e.g., leukemia) can be the cause of retinal hemorrhage, but the unilateral presentation and the isolated focus of macular heme makes these etiologies very unlikely.
- Is the patient on any medications that can be associated with intraretinal fluid, such as niacin or taxanes?
  - No.
- Does the patient have a history of age-related macular degeneration (AMD)?
  - Yes. She endorsed a history of AMD in both eyes and noted that earlier she had received anti–vascular endothelial growth factor (VEGF) injections in each eye.

Assessment

- This is a case of an 80-year-old female patient with AMD who presented with a unilateral macular blot hemorrhage in the left eye and macular drusen in both eyes. A serous PED associated with CME in the left eye and thin choroid in both eyes were noted by cross-sectional OCT, and a focus of intraretinal microvascular flow was identified with OCTA in the left eye.

Differential Diagnosis

- Retinal angiomatous proliferation (RAP) or type 3 macular neovascularization (MNV)
- Choroidal neovascularization (types 1 and 2 MNV)
- Polypoidal choroidal vasculopathy (PCV)
- Perifoveal exudative vascular anomalous complex
- Macular telangiectasia
- CME due to vitreomacular traction or uveitis
- CME due to retinal vascular disease (e.g., diabetic retinopathy, retinal vein occlusion)

Neovascularization	Origin	OCT Location
Type 1	Choroid	Sub-RPE
Type 2	Choroid	Subretinal
Type 3	Deep retinal capillary plexus	Intraretinal
PCV	Choroid	Sub-RPE

Working Diagnosis

- Type 3 MNV

OCT Classification of Type 3 MNV[2]	Characteristic Findings
Precursor stage	Intraretinal hyperreflective focus
Stage 1	Intraretinal hyperreflective lesion + CME without outer retinal disruption ellipsoid zone/external limiting membrane disruption)
Stage 2	Stage 1 + outer retinal disruption +/− RPE disruption
Stage 3	Stage 2 + RPE disruption + extension of lesion through RPE associated with serous PED

Multimodal Imaging

- Fundus photograph
  - Spot or blot of intraretinal hemorrhage in the perifoveal region (Fig. 15.1) associated with a PED is a classic finding of type 3 MNV or RAP lesions.[3]
- OCT
  - Focus of intraretinal hyperreflectivity at the apex of a serous PED associated with the "steer sign" (i.e., downward deflection or subsidence of the outer plexiform layer [OPL]) and surrounding intraretinal fluid (Fig. 15.2)[1] are essential diagnostic features of type 3 MNV.
  - Eyes with a thin choroid and subretinal drusenoid deposits (i.e., reticular pseudodrusen) are at increased risk for type 3 MNV.[4,5]
- Fluorescein angiography (FA)
  - Focal hot spot of leakage and adjacent pooling into a serous PED can be appreciated with FA.[6]
- Indocyanine green angiography (ICGA)
  - Parafoveal hot spot can be identified with ICGA.[6]
- OCTA
  - A tuft or focus of microvascular flow can be identified with OCTA corresponding to the hyperreflective intraretinal lesion with cross-sectional and en face OCT (Fig. 15.3).[7,8]
  - The cross-sectional OCT/OCTA overlay can show the focus of flow originating from the deep capillary plexus and extending into the apex of the PED and into the sub-RPE compartment.[9]
  - Inner retinal feeder vessels into the intraretinal neovascular focus may also be detected. Feeder vessels may not regress after anti-VEGF treatment.[7,10]

Management

- Anti-VEGF injections were restarted in the left eye of this female patient with subsequent resolution of CME and collapse of the serous PED (Figs. 15.2 and 15.3).
- Type 3 MNV, especially early lesions, can be highly responsive to anti-VEGF therapy with brisk regression of the lesion and the fluid. Macular atrophy, however, is a frequent anatomical outcome.[3]
- Laser treatment to the hot spot with photodynamic therapy or argon photocoagulation are historical considerations; anti-VEGF injection therapy is now the gold standard of care.[6]

Follow-up Care

- Anti-VEGF therapy was administered on a treat-and-extend protocol with significant visual acuity and edema improvement in this case. Interval fluid-free periods of 16 to 20 weeks or longer may be obtained in some eyes with type 3 MNV when employing a treat and extend protocol.[11,12] An anti-VEGF regimen on an as-needed, or PRN, basis may also be considered given that type 3 MNV can be associated with long intervals of nonexudative inactivity.
- Close monitoring of the fellow eye should be performed for type 3 MNV development at every visit because of the high rate of bilateral involvement (100% occurrence of type 3 MNV in the fellow eye after 3 years).[13]
- Macular atrophy is a common complication.

Algorithm 15.1: Algorithm for Differential Diagnosis of Unilateral Intraretinal Macular Blot Hemorrhage With Cystoid Macular Edema

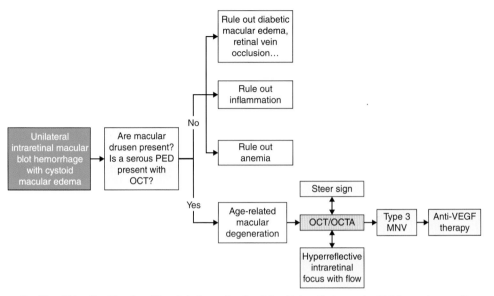

Algorithm 15.1 Algorithm for differential diagnosis of unilateral intraretinal macular blot hemorrhage with cystoid macular edema.

Key Points

- A unilateral intraretinal macular blot hemorrhage in an elderly patient with macular drusen, especially subretinal drusenoid deposits associated with a thin choroid (with OCT), is highly suspicious for neovascular AMD and type 3 MNV.
- Although intraretinal fluid and CME are common associations of retinal vascular (e.g., diabetic macular edema) and inflammatory diseases, intraretinal neovascularization in the setting of neovascular AMD should be definitively excluded.
- OCT signs of type 3 MNV include a focus of intraretinal hyperreflectivity at the apex of a serous PED.
- The "steer sign" or downward deflection or subsidence of the OPL toward a serous PED is very suggestive of type 3 MNV.
- OCTA (en face with cross-sectional overlay) can be valuable in confirming the presence of intraretinal neovascularization.
- Type 3 MNV, especially early lesions, respond very well to anti-VEGF injections.
- Treat-and-extend or as-needed protocol may be administered and long fluid-free intervals on OCT may be encountered, especially with the early lesions.
- The fellow eye is at high risk of type 3 MNV development, and close monitoring with OCT and OCTA is indicated.

References

1. Nagiel A, Sarraf D, Sadda SR, et al. Type 3 neovascularization: evolution, association with pigment epithelial detachment, and treatment response as revealed by spectral domain optical coherence tomography. *Retina.* 2015;35(4):638-647.
2. Su D, Lin S, Phasukkijwatana N, et al. An updated staging system of type 3 neovascularization using spectral domain optical coherence tomography. *Retina.* 2016;36:S40-S49.
3. Spaide RF. New proposal for the pathophysiology of type 3 neovascularization as based on multimodal imaging findings. *Retina.* 2019;39(8):1451-1464.
4. Kim JH, Kim JR, Kang Se W, Kim SJ, Ha HS. Thinner choroid and greater drusen extent in retinal angiomatous proliferation than in typical exudative age-related macular degeneration. *Am J Ophthalmol.* 2013;155:743-749, 749.e1-2.
5. Kim J, Chang Y, Kim J, Lee T, Kim C. Prevalence of subtypes of reticular pseudodrusen in newly diagnosed exudative age-related macular degeneration and polypoidal choroidal vasculopathy in Korean patients. *Retina.* 2015;35(12):2604-2612.
6. Yannuzzi L, Freund K, Takahashi B. Review of retinal angiomatous proliferation or type 3 neovascularization. *Retina.* 2008;28(3):375-384.
7. Kuehlewein L, Dansingani K, de Carlo T, et al. Optical coherence tomography angiography of type 3 neovascularization secondary to age-related macular degeneration. *Retina.* 2015;35(11):2229-2235.
8. Querques G, Miere A, Souied EH. Optical coherence tomography angiography features of type 3 neovascularization in age-related macular degeneration. *Dev Ophthalmol.* 2016;56:57-61.
9. Tan AC, Dansingani KK, Yannuzzi LA, Sarraf D, Freund KB. Type 3 neovascularization imaged with cross-sectional and en face optical coherence tomography angiography. *Retina.* 2017;37(2):234-246.
10. Phasukkijwatana N, Tan ACS, Chen X, Freund KB, Sarraf D. Optical coherence tomography angiography of type 3 neovascularisation in age-related macular degeneration after antiangiogenic therapy. *Br J Ophthalmol.* 2017;101(5):597-602.
11. Chen X, Al-Sheikh M, Chan CK, et al. Type 1 versus type 3 neovascularization in pigment epithelial detachments associated with age-related macular degeneration after anti-vascular endothelial growth factor therapy: a prospective study. *Retina.* 2016;36(suppl 1):S50-S64.
12. Arias L, Cervera E, Vilimelis JC, Escobar JJ, Escobar AG, Zapata MÁ. Efficacy and safety of a treat-and-extend regimen with aflibercept in treatment-naïve patients with type 3 neovascularization: a 52-week, single-arm, multicenter trial. *Retina.* 2020;40(7):1234-1244.
13. Gross N, Aizman A, Brucker A, Klancnik J, Yannuzzi L. Nature and risk of neovascularization in the fellow eye of patients with unilateral retinal angiomatous proliferation. *Retina.* 2005;25(6):713-718.

CHAPTER 16

Bilateral Macular and Peripheral Drusen in a Young Man

George Skopis ▦ William F. Mieler

History of Present Illness

A 22-year-old male patient presents to the retina clinic referred by a comprehensive ophthalmologist for a baseline retina examination and evaluation of macular deposits in both eyes. The patient is asymptomatic and denies blurry vision, floaters, flashes, nyctalopia, or metamorphopsia. He denies any past history or any ocular conditions or ocular surgeries. The patient also denies any known medical history. Of note, his paternal grandfather had polycystic kidney disease for which he had a nephrectomy 40 years ago.

OCULAR EXAMINATION FINDINGS

Best corrected visual acuity was 20/20 in both eyes. Intraocular pressure was normal. Anterior segment examination was normal in both eyes. On dilated fundus examination there were bilateral, symmetrical yellowish deposits in the macula and in the retinal periphery. The rest of the posterior segment was unremarkable.

IMAGING

Fundus photographs show drusen in the fovea extending inferiorly and temporally in both eyes (Fig. 16.1). Fluorescein angiography (FA) (both at 9 minutes) shows well-demarcated areas of hyperfluorescence in the macula of both eyes, indicating staining of drusen, and shows no signs of leakage that would indicate a choroidal neovascular membrane (Fig. 16.2).

Questions to Ask

- Does the patient have any known family history of ocular conditions? A family history could be critical in the diagnosis of inherited diseases, such as autosomal dominant familial drusen or inherited macular dystrophies.
- Has the patient had a recent upper respiratory tract infection? Some white dot syndromes are preceded by a viral prodrome and can appear similar to drusen on physical examination.
- What medications does the patient take, if any? Some medications such as pentosan polysulfate can cause deep, subretinal yellowish deposits in the macula. Although classically chloroquine/hydroxychloroquine has a bull's eye appearance in the macula, it may also present as yellowish subretinal deposits.
- Does the patient smoke or partake in illicit drug use? Although highly unlikely, as this patient is not in the correct age demographic for age-related macular degeneration (AMD), a strong social history may influence your differential diagnosis.

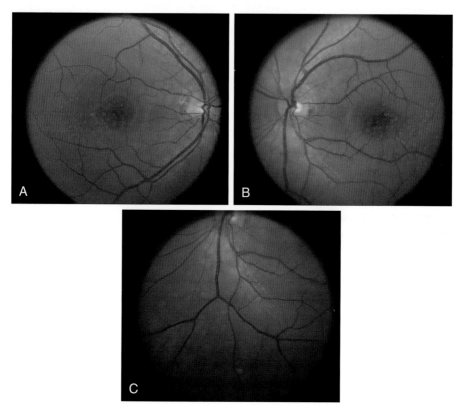

Fig. 16.1 Fundus photographs of the right and left eye. (A) The right eye showing yellowish subretinal deposits surrounding the fovea and inferior macula. (B) The left eye showing yellowish subretinal deposits surrounding the fovea and inferior macula. (C) The left eye showing more peripheral yellowish subretinal deposits.

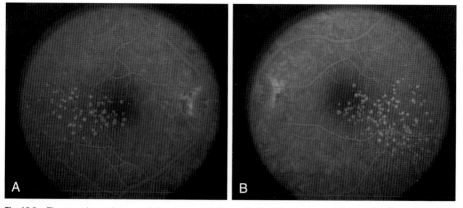

Fig. 16.2 Fluorescein angiogram of the right and left eye, both at 9 minutes. (A) Areas of well-circumscribed hyperfluorescence in the macula indicating staining of drusen of the right eye. (B) Areas of well-circumscribed hyperfluorescence in the macula indicating staining of drusen of the left eye.

Assessment

- This patient is a 22-year-old male patient presenting with no visual reports and denying any past ocular history, family history of eye disease, or any known medical issues. The patient is found to have bilateral, symmetrical drusen in the macula.

Differential Diagnosis

- Stargardt disease
- Pattern dystrophy
- AMD
- Autosomal dominant familial drusen
- Cuticular drusen
- Medication toxicity (pentosan polysulfate/hydroxychloroquine)
- White dot syndrome (multiple evanescent white dot syndrome, acute posterior multifocal placoid pigment epitheliopathy)
- Membranoproliferative glomerulonephritis type II (MPGN, dense deposit disease, C3 glomerulopathy)

Working Diagnosis

- MPGN type II (dense deposit disease)
  - The patient was sent to a primary care physician for basic lab work, including complete blood count and basic metabolic panel.
    - Basic metabolic panel shows abnormal kidney function. Urinalysis shows proteinuria.
    - Further workup and renal biopsy confirms histopathologic diagnosis of MPGN type II.

Multimodal Testing and Results

- Fundus photographs
  - On fundus examination, patients can show drusen in the macula[1] and peripheral retina[2], but drusen may not be present in all patients.[1] Patients may also have findings of retinal pigment epithelium atrophy.[3]
- Optical coherence tomography (OCT)
  - OCT findings include thickening of the Bruch membrane and drusen. Some patients may also display subretinal fluid and retinal pigment epithelial detachment.[4]
- FA
  - Unless there is development of choroidal neovascular membrane that would show early hyperfluorescence and later leakage, FA shows staining of the drusen.
- Fundus autofluorescence (FAF)
  - FAF can show patchy areas of mixed hyperautofluorescence and hypoautofluorescence.[4]

Management

- The patient presented in this case was 20/20 in both eyes and was asymptomatic, so the patient was observed.
- Patients are typically observed, as there is usually good visual acuity unless other sequelae such as a central serous retinopathy-like reaction or choroidal neovascular membrane formation (CNVM).

- Ranibizumab has been used with good results in patients who develop CNVM with improvement of visual acuity and resolution of neovascular activity.[5]
- Some reports show development of central serous chorioretinopathy (CSR) in patients with MPGN type II;[4,6] however, many of these patients are subjected to chronic oral steroid use to combat kidney transplant rejection, so it is unclear if this is a sequelae of MPGN or due to their chronic steroid use. CSR can be treated in the typical fashion of photodynamic therapy (PDT) or subthreshold laser (STL).

Follow-up Care

- There are no clear or established follow-up guidelines for office visit frequency.
- Most patients have good visual acuity, and it is reasonable to follow up every 6 to 12 months.
- Patients with CSR, choroidal neovascular membrane, or visual acuity decline require more frequent follow-up. Sequelae of disease can be treated with anti–vascular endothelial growth factor injections, PDT, or STL.

Algorithm 16.1: Algorithm for Differential Diagnosis of Yellowish Macular Deposits/Lesions

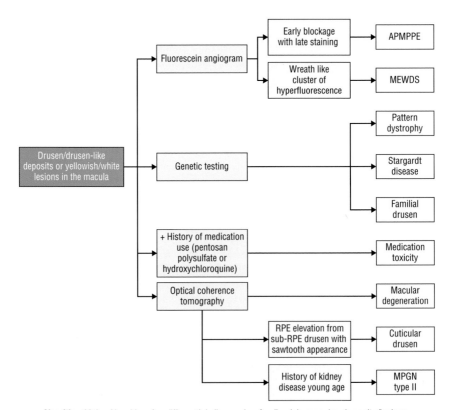

Algorithm 16.1   Algorithm for differential diagnosis of yellowish macular deposits/lesions.

Key Points

- Consider MPGN type II in all young patients with bilateral drusen, and ask about any history of kidney disease.
- Patients usually have good visual acuity and are diagnosed at a young age.
- Patients may develop vision-threatening sequelae, such as CSR or CNVM.
- Performing a detailed medical, social, and family history, as well as asking about medications, can help narrow the differential diagnosis.

References

1. Appel GB, Cook HT, Hageman G, et al. Membranoproliferative glomerulonephritis type II (dense deposit disease): an update. *J Am Soc Nephrol*. 2005;16(5):1392-1403.
2. Huang SJ, Costa DL, Gross NE, Yannuzzi LA. Peripheral drusen in membranoproliferative glomerulonephritis type II. *Retina*. 2003;23(3):429-431.
3. Kim DD, Mieler WF, Wolf MD. Posterior segment changes in membranoproliferative glomerulonephritis. *Am J Ophthalmol*. 1992;114(5):593-599.
4. Mansour AM, Lima LH, Arevalo JF, et al. Retinal findings in membranoproliferative glomerulonephritis. *Am J Ophthalmol Case Rep*. 2017;7:83-90.
5. McCullagh D, Silvestri G, Maxwell AP. Treatment of choroidal neovascularisation secondary to membranoproliferative glomerulonephritis type II with intravitreal ranibizumab. *BMJ Case Rep*. 2014;2014: bcr2013010247.
6. Ulbig MR, Riordan-Eva P, Holz FG, Rees HC, Hamilton PA. Membranoproliferative glomerulonephritis type II associated with central serous retinopathy. *Am J Ophthalmol*. 1993;116(4):410-413.

CHAPTER 17

Long-Standing Macular Scars

Daniel F. Kiernan ▨ Kent W. Small

History of Present Illness

A 60-year-old White male patient (proband case I-1) presented with blurred vision in both eyes, the right having begun to blur 30 years earlier, and the left having begun to blur more recently, impairing his ability to drive or work.

OCULAR EXAMINATION FINDINGS

On examination, his visual acuity was 20/400 in the right eye and 20/100 in the left eye. Dilated fundus examination showed a central area of excavation with atrophy surrounded by irregular hyperpigmentation and subretinal fibrosis in each eye (Fig. 17.1). Nasal to the area of atrophy in the left eye was a small subretinal hemorrhage (Fig. 17.1A and B).

IMAGING

Questions to Ask

- What was the age of onset of vision loss in one or both eyes?
- What is the extent of vision loss (e.g., driving or work impairment)?
- Is there a family history of eye disease or vision loss/functional restriction at an early age?
- Is there a history of nyctalopia?
- Is there a history of color vision abnormality/loss?

Assessment

A 60-year-old male patient reports with decreasing vision in the left eye and persistently deceased central vision in the right eye.

Differential Diagnosis and Associated Confirmatory Tests

- Toxoplasmosis: serum antibodies
- Best macular dystrophy: DNA sequencing, electroretinogram (ERG), electrooculogram (EOG)
- Cone dystrophy: ERG, DNA sequencing
- Age-related macular degeneration (AMD): optical coherence tomography (OCT), fluorescein (FA), indocyanine green angiography (ICG)
- Myopic macular degeneration with staphyloma and choroidal neovascularization (CNV): OCT, FA

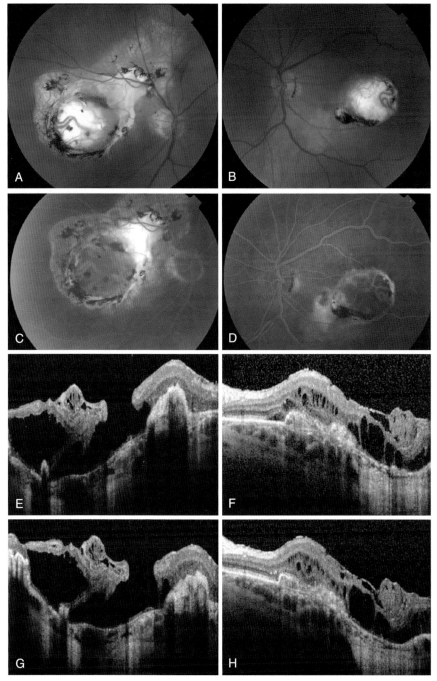

Fig. 17.1 Retinal images of Case I-1. Fundus photographs of the right (A) and the left (B) eyes of the proband show a central atrophic area with surrounding hyperpigmentation and fibrosis with subretinal hemorrhage nasal to the atrophy. Late frames of fluorescein angiogram of the right (C) and the left (D) eye show late hyperfluorescence but no obvious choroidal neovascularization. Optical coherence tomography of the right eye before (E) and after (G) and the left eye before (F) and after (H) three monthly intravitreal injections with 1.25-mg bevacizumab. The intraretinal and subretinal cystic fluid in the left nasal macula (F) was reduced after three injections (H).

- North Carolina macular dystrophy (NCMD): DNA sequencing, ERG, EOG
- CNV secondary to AMD: OCT, FA, ICG

Working Diagnosis

- CNV secondary to NCMD.

Multimodal Testing and Results

- Fundus imaging, FA, OCT, and genetic testing were obtained.
- OCT showed intraretinal and subretinal fluid consistent with CNV.
- OCT images showed central excavated atrophy with overlying central intraretinal and subretinal fluid along with intrachoroidal lacunae in both eyes. There was the appearance of macular pseudohole in the right eye, and the left eye exhibited mild subretinal fluid nasal to the excavation (Fig. 17.1E and F).
- FA showed late staining but no definite CNV in either eye (Fig. 17.1C and D).
- Genetic testing molecular analysis of the MCDR1 locus revealed a pathogenic heterozygous point mutation in the noncoding region of the DNASE1 hypersensitivity site "V1 variant," chr6:100040906 G>T (hg19) upstream of PRDM13 consistent with a diagnosis of NCMD.1.

Management

- The CNV was treated with an intravitreal anti–vascular endothelial growth factor (VEGF) agent (1.25 mg/0.05 mL bevacizumab) according to a treat-and-extend protocol.
- After five monthly injections in the right eye and eight in the left eye, visual acuity improved to 20/50 and 20/150, respectively. OCT was stable for the right eye and showed decreased intraretinal and subretinal fluid nasal of the excavation for the left eye (Fig. 17.1G and H). Family members indicated in the pedigree (Fig. 17.2) were also examined, with select notable findings as follows.

Case II-2

The patient's 40-year-old son had drusen in the central macula with subretinal deposits on OCT examination (Fig. 17.3A–D) and normal visual acuity.

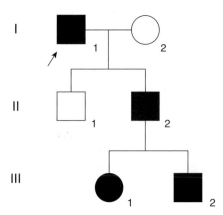

Fig. 17.2 Pedigree of family with North Carolina macular dystrophy. Four family members had macular findings (I-1, II-2, III-1, and III-2). Molecular analysis for the proband only, Case I-1 (indicated with *arrow*) revealed a heterozygous variant in a DNase-sensitive site upstream of the PRDM13 gene.

Case III-1

A 9-year-old female patient had visual acuity 20/30 in the right eye and 20/50 in the left eye. The fundus examination showed a stable central macular subretinal yellowish deposit in each eye with surrounding hypopigmentation in the left eye. OCT exhibited a central subretinal density without adjacent subretinal fluid (Fig. 17.3E–H).

Case III-2

A 7-year-old male patient had visual acuity 20/40 in the right eye and 20/60 in the left eye. In the central macula, there was a cluster of drusen. OCT showed choroidal thinning with a shallow staphyloma-like depression and subretinal densities in each eye (Fig. 17.3I–L).

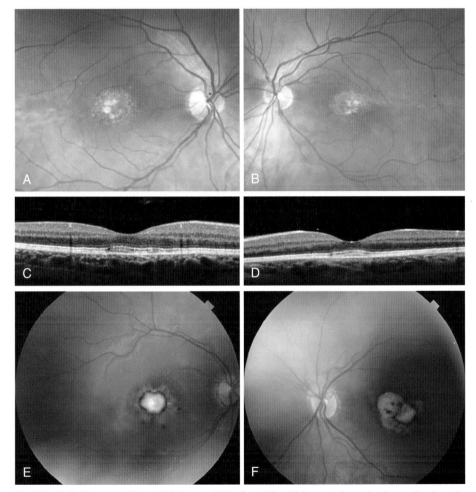

Fig. 17.3 Retinal images of Cases II-2, III-1, and III-2. Case II-2 exhibits central macular drusen-like deposits (A and B) with subretinal densities on optical coherence tomography (OCT) in each eye (C and D). Fundus photographs of Case III-1 show central subretinal fibrosis surrounded by hypopigmentation (E and F), and

Continued

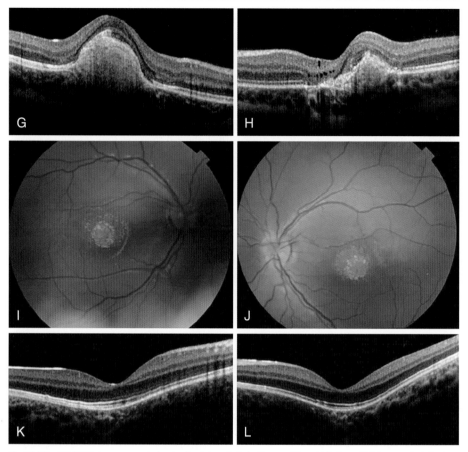

Fig. 17.3 Cont'd OCT shows a central subretinal density in both eyes (G and H). Case III-2 has central drusen-like deposits in the central macula (I and J) with subretinal deposits and a shallow staphyloma-like appearance with bilateral central choroidal thinning on OCT (K and L).

Clinical Pearls

- Recognize bilateral, often symmetrical macular lesions as a potentially inherited retinal disease rather than an acquired entity.
- Recognize that the patient may have relatively mild, if any, visual impairment despite a notable, often dramatic fundus appearance in the absence of CNV.

Recognize the Grades of NCMD

- Grade 1: Drusen centrally with normal vision
- Grade 2: Confluent drusen, absence of retinal pigment epithelium, or a disciform scar with mild to moderate visual impairment
- Grade 3: Severe-appearing coloboma-like defect in the central maculae with or without surrounding fibrosis, yet may have surprisingly mild visual impairment

Algorithm 17.1: Algorithm Showing Steps Involved in Diagnosing and Managing North Carolina Macular Dystrophy

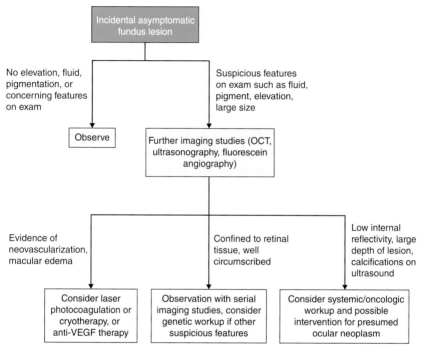

Algorithm 17.1 Algorithm showing steps involved in diagnosing and managing North Carolina macular dystrophy. Primary decision-making should be based on examination and testing demonstrating vision threatening scenarios especially choroidal neovascularization. *OCT,* Optical coherence tomography; *VEGF,* vascular endothelial growth factor.

Acknowledgements

Text and images reprinted with permission from Wolters Kluwer Health, Inc.: Bakall B, Bryan JS 3rd, Stone EM, Small KW. Choroidal neovascularization in North Carolina macular dystrophy responsive to anti-vascular endothelial growth factor therapy. *Retin Cases Brief Rep.* 2021;15(5):509-513.

Key Points

Choroidal neovascularization has been associated with NCMD, with involution and development of submacular fibrosis.[1-3] The combination of decreased visual acuity and subretinal and intraretinal fluid on OCT prompted a trial of intravitreal anti-VEGF injection to both eyes, which resulted in decreased retinal fluid and improved vision. The treatment was stopped after stability in the examination and visual acuity after a treat-and-extend protocol. The history for Case I-1 with sudden decreased central vision for the left eye at age 30 and for the right eye at age 50 was likely caused by development of CNV in the nasal macular area.

Case III-1 exhibited a central macular fibrotic lesion in each eye with a subretinal density on OCT that may correspond to early-onset involuted CNV (Fig. 17.3E–H). Early-onset CNV has also been observed in Best vitelliform macular dystrophy, with formation of central macular subretinal fibrosis.[4]

The initial genetic locus for NCMD was linked to chromosome 6q16.2 by Small et al. (1992) and was termed *MCDR1*, the first genetic locus identified for any inherited macular diseases.[5] The mutations were found by Small et al. in 2016 in 12 NCMD families. Three were point mutations in a noncoding region in a DNASE1 site 12 kb upstream from the retinal transcription factor PRDM13. The *PRDM13* gene encodes a retinal transcription factor likely important in developing a normal primate macula.[1] Although the pathogenic variant is identical in affected family members, great variability was observed in disease severity and visual acuity in this reported family. In cases of CNV complicating this rare inherited macular disease, a prompt diagnosis will lead to optimal treatment and visual outcome of affected patients. Widely available commercial genetic testing may also facilitate diagnostic confirmation of this and other suspected inherited retinal diseases.

References

1. Small KW, DeLuca AP, Whitmore SS, et al. North Carolina macular dystrophy is caused by dysregulation of the retinal transcription factor PRDM13. *Ophthalmology*. 2016;123:9-18.
2. Rhee DY, Reichel E, Rogers A, Strominger M. Subfoveal choroidal neovascularization in a 3-year-old child with North Carolina macular dystrophy. *J AAPOS*. 2007;11:614-615.
3. Small KW. North Carolina macular dystrophy: clinical features, genealogy, and genetic linkage analysis. *Trans Am Ophthalmol Soc*. 1998;96:925-961.
4. Iannaccone A, Kerr NC, Kinnick TR, et al. Autosomal recessive best vitelliform macular dystrophy: report of a family and management of early-onset neovascular complications. *Arch Ophthalmol*. 2011;129: 211-217.
5. Small KW, Weber JL, Roses A, et al. North Carolina macular dystrophy is assigned to chromosome 6. *Genomics*. 1992;13:681-685.

CHAPTER 18

Bilateral Presentation of Bull's Eye Maculopathy

Mina M. Naguib ▦ Yasha Modi ▦ Christina Y. Weng

History of Present Illness

We present a case of a 60-year-old healthy female patient with an unremarkable past ocular history referred for evaluation of fundus abnormalities in both eyes. She reports that her vision has been stable for several years and denies blurry vision, scotomata, floaters, photopsias, metamorphopsia, dyschromatopsia, or nyctalopia. Her family history was unremarkable for any ophthalmic conditions. She has no history of substance use and takes no medications.

OCULAR EXAMINATION FINDINGS

Visual acuity with correction was 20/20 in the right eye and 20/25 in the left eye. Intraocular pressure was normal. Her pupils were briskly reactive to light, equal, and without relative afferent pupillary defect. Extraocular motility and visual fields with confrontation were full. Slit lamp examination was only significant for early nuclear sclerotic cataract and mild asteroid hyalosis in both eyes. Dilated fundus examination revealed bilateral parafoveal concentric atrophy.

IMAGING

Fundus photography of both eyes illustrated symmetrical parafoveal atrophy in a bull's eye pattern (Fig. 18.1). Optical coherence tomography (OCT) of both eyes showed preserved foveal contour;

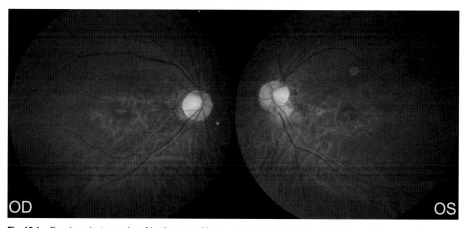

Fig. 18.1 Fundus photography of both eyes with symmetrical parafoveal atrophy in a bull's eye pattern.

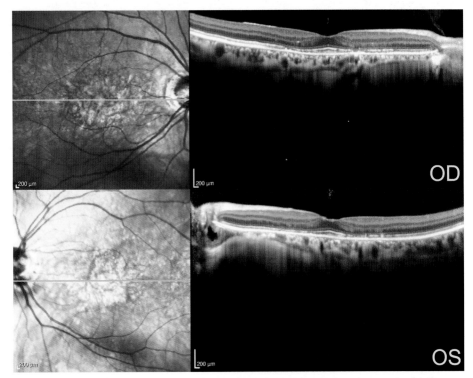

Fig. 18.2 Optical coherence tomography of both eyes demonstrating parafoveal attenuation of the outer retina and ellipsoid zone with focal thickening of the retinal pigment epithelium.

parafoveal attenuation of the outer retina and shoddy loss and attenuation of the ellipsoid zone (EZ). There is focal and irregular parafoveal thickening of the retinal pigment epithelium (RPE) (Fig. 18.2). Fundus autofluorescence (FAF) of both eyes demonstrated parafoveal patchy areas of hypo- and hyperautofluorescence (Fig. 18.3).

Questions to Ask

- Does the patient have a family history of vision problems? This symmetrical pattern of atrophy can be seen in several inherited macular dystrophies such as Stargardt disease, central areolar choroidal dystrophy (CACD), benign concentric annular macular dystrophy, and cone dystrophy.
  - Patient reports no known family history of eye conditions.
- What medications is the patient currently taking or has used in the past? Parafoveal outer retinal atrophy can be seen in chloroquine and hydroxychloroquine toxicity.
  - Patient denies current or past use of medications associated with retinal toxicity.

Assessment

- This is a case of a 60-year-old woman with no visual symptoms, no past ocular history, and a negative family history who presents with incidental findings of bilateral, symmetrical parafoveal outer retinal atrophy noted on fundus examination, OCT, and FAF.

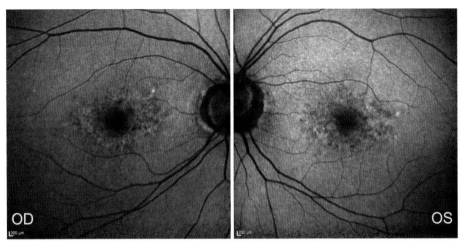

Fig. 18.3 Fundus autofluorescence of both eyes with parafoveal patchy areas of hypoautofluorescence and hyperautofluorescence.

Differential Diagnosis

- Central areolar choroidal dystrophy (CACD)
- Stargardt disease
- Medication-associated toxicity (e.g., chloroquine, hydroxychloroquine, pentosan polysulfate)
- Benign concentric annular macular dystrophy
- Cone or cone-rod dystrophy
- North Carolina macular dystrophy (NCMD)
- Pattern dystrophy of the retinal pigment epithelium
- Best disease (vitelliform macular dystrophy)

Working Diagnosis

- CACD
  - Clinical diagnosis was made based on fundus findings of well-demarcated, concentric area of parafoveal atrophy in the absence of other history, examination, or imaging findings that would be characteristic of other etiologies.
  - However, given the phenotypic variation of this entity and overlapping features with other conditions on the differential diagnosis, genetic testing was performed for diagnostic confirmation.

Multimodal Testing and Results

- Fundus photography
  - The macula reveals a bilateral, symmetrical, well-circumscribed area of parafoveal atrophy with visualization of underlying choroidal vessels and sclera in advanced cases.[1,2]
- OCT
  - As noted in our patient, OCT changes of the outer retina predominate and progress in four stages.[3]
    - Stage 1 is characterized by focal parafoveal areas of disruption of RPE and EZ anatomy.

- Stage 2 progresses to outer nuclear layer thinning with early external limiting membrane irregularity. Additionally, focal elongation of the photoreceptor outer segments can be observed.
- Stage 3 progresses to complete absence of outer retinal layers and RPE atrophy correlating to hypoautofluorescence on FAF.
- Stage 4 is characterized by progression of total outer retinal layer and RPE loss involving the fovea. Outer retinal tubulations extending from the photoreceptor layer can be seen at the borders of atrophy in the majority of cases.
- FAF
  - FAF changes also progress in four stages.[3]
    - Stage 1 shows focal areas of hyperautofluorescence.
    - Stage 2 shows speckled or patchy areas of hyper- and hypoautofluorescence as noted in our patient (Fig. 18.3).
    - Stages 3 and 4 reveal more confluent areas of RPE and outer retinal atrophy that are non-foveal-involving and foveal-involving, respectively.
- Fluorescein angiography (FA)
  - FA may show early-phase hyperfluorescence corresponding to a window defect. If RPE atrophy is incomplete, a speckled pattern of hyperfluorescence can be visualized. In late-phase images, discrete areas of hyperfluorescence may be seen at the edge of the central lesion corresponding to incomplete choriocapillaris atrophy.[1,4]
- Indocyanine green angiography
  - Two distinct phenotypes have been described.[4] The first demonstrates hyperfluorescence in the early phase and normofluorescence in the late phase. The second phenotype shows hypofluorescence in the early phase and normofluorescence with pinpoint areas of leakage within the atrophic lesion in the late phase.
- Electroretinography (ERG)
  - In full-field ERG, mildly decreased cone b-wave amplitude and prolonged b-wave implicit time are the main abnormalities observed; these may extend beyond the area of central atrophy.
  - Of note, multifocal ERG can be helpful in detecting macular dysfunction in cases of CACD that only involve a small central area,[5] and will typically show lower $P1/N1$ amplitudes and delayed $P1/N1$ implicit times.[6]
- OCT angiography
  - An increase in the avascular zone can be seen at the superficial capillary plexus (SCP) and deep capillary plexus. Microaneurysms, vascular loops, and intraretinal microvascular abnormalities, especially in the SCP, can be seen in earlier disease stages. Widespread impaired vascular perfusion may be seen in later disease stages.[7]
- Genetic testing
  - Our patient carried a p.Arg142Trp mutation in the *PRPH2* or *peripherin/RDS* gene, which leads to a CACD phenotype.
  - In most cases, CACD is inherited in an autosomal dominant fashion.[8]
  - Five identified *PRPH2* mutations can cause autosomal dominant CACD, although significant intrafamilial variation in penetrance and expressivity has been observed.[9] Macular changes typically begin in early adulthood and may progress in the fourth or fifth decade of life. This feature is highlighted by our patient, who presents with no vision symptoms, excellent visual acuity, and relatively mild disease despite her older age.
- Miscellaneous
  - Visual field testing: central scotoma corresponding to areas of atrophy; normal peripheral field.[10]
  - Color vision: Farnsworth Panel–D15 testing with disturbances affecting the blue axis.[11]

Management

- At this time there is no treatment for CACD, thus our patient was observed.
- After genetic testing, it is important to counsel the patient on the autosomal dominant inheritance pattern of this disease for the purposes of family planning. Screening of other family members should also be considered, especially because of phenotypic heterogeneity.

Follow-up Care

- Patients can be followed annually once diagnosis is confirmed

Algorithm 18.1: Algorithm for Differential Diagnosis for Bull's Eye Maculopathy

This algorithm (Algorithm 18.1) highlights the most common genetic defects and characteristic clinical or imaging findings.

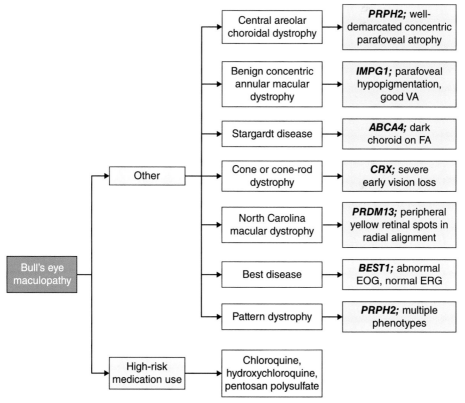

Algorithm 18.1   Algorithm for differential diagnosis for bull's eye maculopathy. *EOG,* Electrooculography; *ERG,* electroretinography; *FA,* fluorescein angiography; *VA,* visual acuity.

Key Points

- CACD should be included on the differential diagnosis for bilateral, symmetrical bull's eye maculopathy, even in the absence of family history.
- Dilated fundus examination and ancillary imaging can help differentiate CACD from other conditions with similar features.
- Genetic testing is critical in confirming the diagnosis of CACD and ruling out other inherited retinal dystrophies.
- No treatment exists for CACD, and patients can be followed annually.

References

1. Noble KG. Central areolar choroidal dystrophy. *Am J Ophthalmol.* 1977;84(3):310-318.
2. Ferry AP, Llovera I, Shafer DM. Central areolar choroidal dystrophy. *Arch Ophthalmol.* 1972;88(1):39-43.
3. Smailhodzic D, Fleckenstein M, Theelen T, et al. Central areolar choroidal dystrophy (CACD) and age-related macular degeneration (AMD): differentiating characteristics in multimodal imaging. *Invest Ophthalmol Vis Sci.* 2011;52(12):8908-8918.
4. Guigui B, Semoun O, Querques G, Coscas G, Soubrane G, Souied EH. Indocyanine green angiography features of central areolar choroidal dystrophy. *Retin Cases Brief Rep.* 2009;3(4):434-437.
5. Ponjavic V, Andréasson S, Ehinger B Full-field electroretinograms in patients with central areolar choroidal dystrophy. *Acta Ophthalmol (Copenh).* 1994;72(5):537–544.
6. Gundogan FC, Dinç UA, Erdem U, Ozge G, Sobaci G. Multifocal electroretinogram and central visual field testing in central areolar choroidal dystrophy. *Eur J Ophthalmol.* 2010;20(5):919-924.
7. Albertos-Arranz H, Sánchez-Sáez X, Martínez-Gil N, et al. Phenotypic differences in a PRPH2 mutation in members of the same family assessed with OCT and OCTA. *Diagnostics (Basel).* 2021;11(5):777.-
8. Iannaccone A. Genotype-phenotype correlations and differential diagnosis in autosomal dominant macular disease. *Doc Ophthalmol.* 2001;102(3):197-236.
9. Boon CJ, Klevering BJ, Cremers FP, et al. Central areolar choroidal dystrophy. *Ophthalmology.* 2009;116(4):771-782, 782.e1.
10. Ponjavic V, Andréasson S, Ehinger B. Full-field electroretinograms in patients with central areolar choroidal dystrophy. *Acta Ophthalmol (Copenh).* 1994;72(5):537-544.
11. Keilhauer CN, Meigen T, Weber BH. Clinical findings in a multigeneration family with autosomal dominant central areolar choroidal dystrophy associated with an Arg195Leu mutation in the peripherin/RDS gene. *Arch Ophthalmol.* 2006;124(7):1020-1027.

CHAPTER 19

Late-Onset Nyctalopia and Widespread Geographical Atrophy

Rose A. Moore ▪ Shannon A. Donley ▪ Anita Agarwal

History of Present Illness

A 59-year-old White woman of German descent presented with progressive visual difficulty in the dark for 5 years. The right eye was amblyopic secondary to anisometropia. She was otherwise healthy.

OCULAR EXAMINATION FINDINGS

Her best corrected visual acuities were 20/400 in the right eye and 20/50 in the left eye. Anterior segment examination was normal in both eyes. Fundus examination showed multiple islands of geographical atrophy (GA) involving most of the posterior pole and temporal retina in each eye. There were yellow drusen-like flecks in the nasal retina, without islands of atrophy.

IMAGING

Fundus photograph of the right eye showed multiple islands of GA involving the posterior pole (Figs. 19.1 and 19.2) and temporal retina (Figs. 19.3 and 19.4). Many of the patches of atrophy abutted neighboring patches leaving scalloped areas of preserved retina between them. Fine yellow drusen-like flecks were seen in the nasal retina, without islands of atrophy (Fig. 19.5). The fluorescein angiogram showed window defects corresponding to the GA (Fig. 19.6), and the

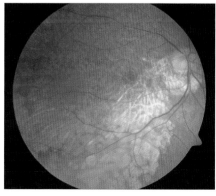

Fig. 19.1 Right fundus with multiple islands of geographical atrophy.

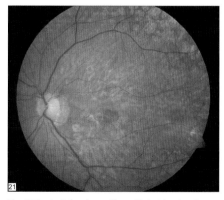

Fig. 19.2 Left fundus with multiple islands of geographical atrophy.

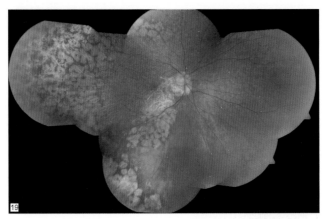

Fig. 19.3   Right eye. The islands of geographical atrophy extend to the temporal periphery. Many abut the neighboring patches leaving intervening retinal pigment epithelium in a scalloped pattern.

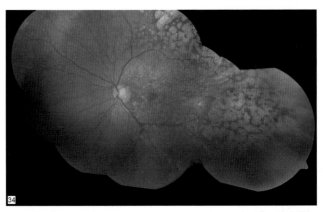

Fig. 19.4   Left eye. The islands of geographical atrophy extend to the temporal periphery with intervening preserved retinal pigment epithelium.

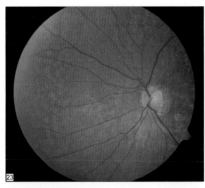

Fig. 19.5   Fine yellow drusen-like flecks in the nasal retina of the left eye.

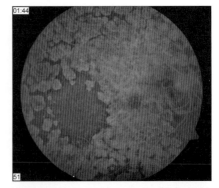

Fig. 19.6   Fluorescein angiogram shows transmission hyperfluorescence corresponding to the atrophic patches.

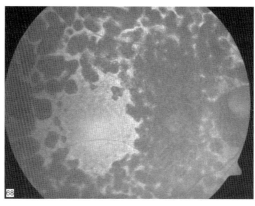

Fig. 19.7   Hypoautofluorescence corresponding to the patches of geographical atrophy.

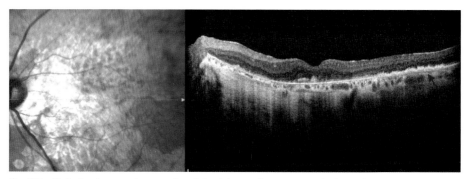

Fig. 19.8   Optical coherence tomography of the left eye shows outer retinal atrophy and retinal pigment epithelium (RPE) loss corresponding to the geographical atrophy and irregularly elevated RPE with sub-RPE material in areas of preserved retina.

corresponding atrophic areas showed reduced autofluorescence (Fig. 19.7). Optical coherence tomography revealed outer retinal atrophy corresponding to the GA but sub–retinal pigment epithelium (RPE) thickening/deposits in the intact areas (Fig. 19.8).[1-3]

Questions to Ask

- Is there a family history of similar symptoms? If there is a family history suggestive of autosomal dominant inheritance, one should consider Sorsby fundus dystrophy, peripherin/RDS dystrophy, and late-onset retinal macular degeneration (LORMD). Lack of family history suggests an autosomal recessive inheritance condition such as Gyrate atrophy or sporadic extensive macular atrophy with pseudodrusen.
  - Yes. Father was adopted and had poor vision late in life.
- Is there a history of long-term use of certain medications? Thioridazine (Mellaril), used in treatment of psychosis, and didanosine, previously used in treatment of HIV, can cause widespread chorioretinal atrophy resembling LORMD.
  - The patient has no history of long-term use of medications.

Thioridazine accumulates in the melanin granules of the RPE and uveal melanocytes and affects rhodopsin synthesis resulting in disintegration of rod outer segments. Beginning as a coarse granular salt-and-pepper pigmentary retinopathy in the periphery, the lesions progress as nummular areas of GA of the RPE and choriocapillaris that can eventually enlarge and become confluent, involving the entire fundus.

Didanosine is a nucleoside reverse transcriptase inhibitor postulated to deplete mitochondrial DNA. The clinical features begin with coarse pigment speckling in the midperipheral and peripheral fundus and progress to well-circumscribed round areas of RPE and choriocapillaris atrophy that are sharply demarcated from the posterior pole. These enlarge over time despite discontinuation of the drug, with only a few scalloped ares of remaining RPE. Patients can report nyctalopia.

Assessment

- This 59-year-old woman reports with a history of visual loss and nyctalopia of 5 years' duration and a similar history in her father. The patient demonstrates punctate drusen in the nasal retina and extensive GA in the macula and temporal retina.

Differential Diagnosis

- Sorsby fundus dystrophy
- LORMD
- Peripherin/RDS retinal dystrophy
- Extensive macular atrophy with pseudodrusen
- Gyrate atrophy
- Thioridazine toxicity
- Didanosine toxicity

Working Diagnosis

- Sorsby fundus dystrophy

Nyctalopia is a late feature of Sorsby fundus dystrophy. The macula would show extensive drusen and RPE changes along with gradually increased drusen and pseudodrusen from the posterior pole toward the periphery. Choroidal neovascularization is much more common, and an autosomal dominant family history of "early-onset wet age-related macular degeneration" is often elicitable.

- LORMD

Early findings are drusen-like flecks in asymptomatic patients. Nyctalopia begins after age 50 and worsens rapidly over 4 to 5 years. The widespread islands of GA are seen in the macula, midperiphery, and periphery. The peripheral lesions may not be uniformly distributed, with some areas, especially the nasal area, being spared until very late. Choroidal neovascularization is uncommon. It is dominantly inherited and was first described in people of Scottish descent.

- Extensive macular atrophy with pseudodrusen

This condition is generally sporadic, with no known family history. The islands of GA arise in the central macula and are limited to the posterior pole, but the pseudodrusen are extensive and found up to the equator and beyond.

Other Features

Patients with LORMD can have long zonules attached to the anterior surface of the lens, which this patient did not have.

Multimodal Testing and Results

- Goldmann visual field
  - Central scotoma and marked constriction on the right and moderate constriction on the left (Figs. 19.9 and 19.10)

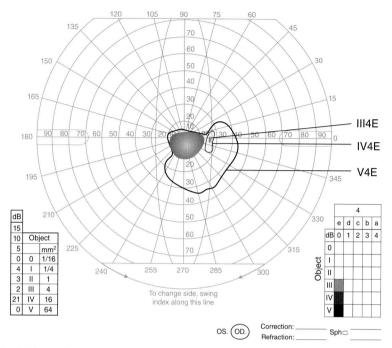

Fig. 19.9 Goldmann visual field demonstrates peripheral constriction and central scotoma in the right eye.

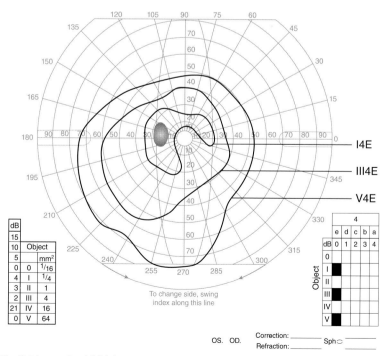

Fig. 19.10 Goldmann visual field demonstrates peripheral constriction and central scotoma in the left eye.

- Electroretinogram (ERG)
  - ERG showed markedly decreased rod and cone function in both eyes.
- Laboratory testing
  - Amino acid testing revealed the following (all in mmol/L). All values are within the normal ranges, thus ruling out gyrate atrophy.
    - Ornithine, 102 (range, 48–195)
    - Glutamine, 652 (range, 206–756)
    - Glutamic acid, 35 (range, 10–131)
    - Glycine, 186 (range, 151–490)
    - Citrulline, 46 (range, 12–55)
    - Arginine, 53 (range, 15–128)
- Genetic testing
  - The *C1QTNF5* gene is responsible for autosomal dominant LORMD. Genetic testing was not available at the time of diagnosis.[4,5]

Management and Follow-up

- The patient's family history was further investigated for evidence of similar retinal findings. Her relatives were notified as to her diagnosis of LORMD. It is important to notify a patiet's family members of the genetic diagnosis so that appropriate testing can be performed and family members can be diagnosed, treated, and/or followed for development of the disease. The patient has a younger brother and sister who are asymptomatic and who live in Germany. She has two sons, aged 32 and 34 years, who so far have no visual deficits.
- Management of LORMD is supportive with low-vision counseling and low-vision aides. There is no treatment at this time. The areas of GA progressed over the next 10 years, and the patient's night vision worsened. She could still ambulate, and her visual acuity was 20/400 in both eyes 13 years from presentation.

Algorithm 19.1: Late-onset Retinal Macular Degeneration *(LORMD)* Flowchart

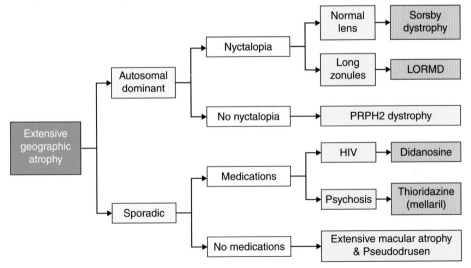

Algorithm 19.1 Late-onset retinal macular degeneration *(LORMD)* flowchart.

Key Points

- Consider LORMD when patients have drusen and widespread GA.
- Onset of night blindness is usually after age 50.
- The disease is inherited in an autosomal dominant manner.
- Look for long anterior insertion of zonules.
- Choroidal neovascular membranes can occur occasionally.[6]
- Consider genetic testing to confirm the diagnosis.

References

1. Milam AH, Curcio CA, Cideciyan AV, et al. Dominant late-onset retinal degeneration with regional variation of sub-retinal pigment epithelium deposits, retinal function, and photoreceptor degeneration. *Ophthalmology*. 2000;107(12):2256-2266.
2. Jacobson SG, Cideciyan AV, Wright E, Wright AF. Phenotypic marker for early disease detection in dominant late-onset retinal degeneration. *Invest Ophthalmol Vis Sci*. 2001;42(8):1882-1890.
3. Agarwal A, Law JC, Tarantola RM. Late-onset retinal macular degeneration: an entity not to be overlooked. *Retin Cases Brief Rep*. 2010;4(3):257-261.
4. Vanderford EK, De Silva T, Noriega D, Arango M, Cunningham D, Cukras CA. Quantitative analysis of longitudinal changes in multimodal imaging of late-onset retinal degeneration. *Retina*. 2021;41(8):1701-1708.
5. Jacobson SG, Cideciyan AV, Sumaroka A, Roman AJ, Wright AF. Late-onset retinal degeneration caused by C1QTNF5 mutation: sub-retinal pigment epithelium deposits and visual consequences. *JAMA Ophthalmol*. 2014;132(10):1252-1255.
6. Ramtohul P, Gascon P, Matonti F. Choroidal neovascularization in late-onset retinal macular degeneration. *Ophthalmol Retina*. 2019;3(2):153.

CHAPTER 20

Bilateral Gradual Visual Decline With Subtle Parafoveal Graying and Refractile Foci

Geoffrey K. Broadhead ▪ Sanjeeb Bhandari ▪ Henry E. Wiley ▪ Emily Y. Chew

History of Present Illness

A 53-year-old female patient presented with a 3-month history of gradually worsening vision in both eyes, particularly affecting reading text. She denied metamorphopsia, floaters, or scotoma. Her past ocular history was unremarkable, though past medical history included type 2 diabetes mellitus (DM).

OCULAR EXAMINATION

Corrected visual acuity was 20/50 in each eye and improved to 20/40 in each eye with a low myopic manifest refraction. Intraocular pressures were normal, and anterior segment examination was unremarkable bilaterally. Dilated fundus examination demonstrated a blunted foveal reflex with subtle graying of the parafoveal region bilaterally, subtle hyperpigmentation temporal to the fovea on the right, and sparse punctate refractile foci parafoveally in both eyes, more pronounced on the left (Fig. 20.1).

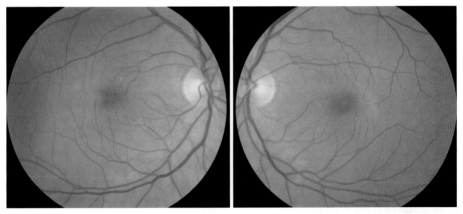

Fig. 20.1 Color fundus photographs of the right and left eyes, showing graying of the parafoveal region and refractile foci.

IMAGING

Optical coherence tomography (OCT) showed foveal intraretinal cavitations in both eyes and bilateral loss of the ellipsoid zone (EZ) layer juxtafoveally, involving the fovea on the right. Alterations of the right fovea also included disruption of the interdigitation layer, subtle irregularity of the retinal pigment epithelium/Bruch membrane layer, and retinal thinning (Fig. 20.2). Red-free (RF) photographs (Fig. 20.3) and confocal blue light reflectance (CBR) imaging (Fig. 20.4) highlighted the presence of crystalline deposits in the parafoveal regions bilaterally. Fluorescein angiography (FA) demonstrated right-angled venules temporal to the fovea with telangiectasis of juxtafoveal capillaries (more pronounced temporally) in early frames and leakage (temporally more than nasally) in late frames (Fig. 20.5).

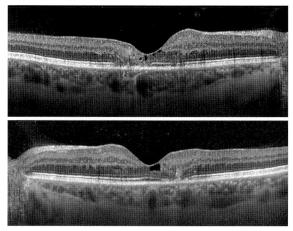

Fig. 20.2 Optical coherence tomography images of the right *(top)* and left *(bottom)* eyes, showing focal ellipsoid zone loss and intraretinal cavitations.

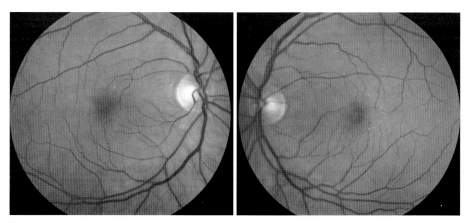

Fig. 20.3 Red-free photographs of the right and left eyes, showing parafoveal refractile foci and capillary dilation.

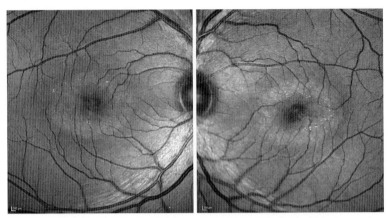

Fig. 20.4 Blue-reflectance images of the right and left eyes demonstrating a bright parafoveal halo, refractile foci, and capillary dilation.

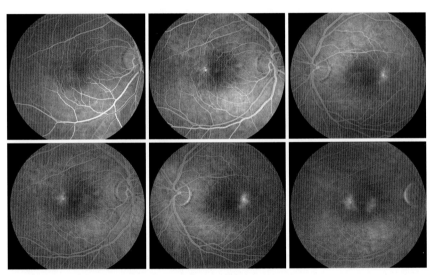

Fig. 20.5 Fluorescein angiogram images showing parafoveal capillary dilation and leakage.

Questions to Ask

- How long ago was DM diagnosed, has hyperglycemia been well controlled, and does the patient have other vascular disease? Diabetic macular edema (DME) or past retinal vein occlusion (RVO) can cause macular microvascular alterations with a variable degree of retinal thickening (macular edema [ME]).[1]
- What medications has the patient used? Certain medications (e.g., niacin, latanoprost) can cause cystoid macula edema (CME). Others (e.g., tamoxifen) can cause intraretinal cavitations and/or refractile retinal deposits.[2]
- Is there any family history of ocular diseases? Certain inherited diseases have been reported to demonstrate similar cavitations, including retinitis pigmentosa and cone dystrophies. Other inherited dystrophies can cause crystalline retinal deposits.[1]

Assessment

- This is a case of a 53-year-old female patient with DM who manifests decreased visual acuity in both eyes, bilateral parafoveal graying with refractile foci, bilateral cavitations and EZ loss without retinal thickening on OCT, and parafoveal microvascular changes with leakage on FA in both eyes.

Differential Diagnosis

- Branch or central RVO
- Diabetic retinopathy
- Cone dystrophy
- Pseudophakic CME (subclinical)
- Idiopathic macular telangiectasia (MacTel) (type II)
- Idiopathic MacTel (type III)

Working Diagnosis

- Idiopathic MacTel type II

Multimodal Testing and Results

- Fundus photos
  - Fundus examination classically shows graying of the parafoveal region, with refractile foci (Fig. 20.1). Dilated capillaries may or may not be visible. With progression, pigmentary deposition may appear temporal to the fovea.
- Fundus autofluorescence
  - Autofluorescence imaging often demonstrates mild to moderate hyperautofluorescence of the fovea and/or temporal parafovea in early MacTel, which can progress to a mixed hyper- and hypoautofluorescence pattern as pigment deposition and atrophy develop (Fig. 20.6).[3]

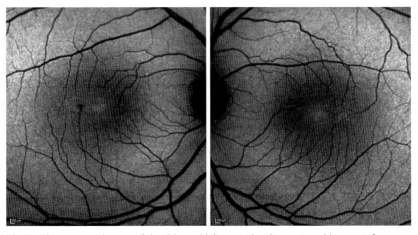

Fig. 20.6 Autofluorescence images of the right and left eyes, showing scattered hyperautofluorescence in both eyes and focal parafoveal hypoautofluorescence in the right eye.

- RF imaging
  - RF images highlight the presence of refractile foci, dilated capillaries, and/or pigment deposition (Fig. 20.3).
- CBR imaging
  - CBR can show a bright halo in the parafovea (Fig. 20.4).
- OCT
  - Classic findings on OCT include a variable degree of central or juxtafoveal EZ loss and variable intraretinal cavitation formation (Fig. 20.2). Cavitations often have a more rectangular appearance than the rounded cystic lesions seen in DME or RVO-related ME and can occur in the absence of retinal thickening.[4] As disease progresses, hyperreflective foci representing intraretinal pigmentary alterations and a potential precursor to intraretinal neovascularization can become visible.
  - In occasional more advanced cases, evidence of macular neovascularization (MNV) can be seen, with findings including ME, subretinal fluid, lipid exudates, and/or subretinal hyperreflective material (Fig. 20.7).
- FA
  - Except in very early cases where it may not yet be present, FA usually shows a variable degree of juxtafoveal and parafoveal capillary telangiectasia in early frames and leakage in late frames (Fig. 20.5).

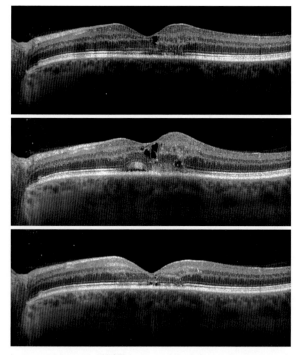

Fig. 20.7 Optical coherence tomography (OCT) images of the left eye showing macular neovascularization (MNV) development in another individual. *Top:* OCT scan 1 month before MNV development. *Middle:* OCT scan at the time of subretinal neovascularization development, showing new subretinal fluid, increased intraretinal cystic changes, and retinal thickening. *Bottom:* OCT scan 1 month after receiving the third dose of monthly intravitreal anti–vascular endothelial growth factor agent therapy, showing marked improvement in retinal thickening and resolution of exudative features.

Management

- There is currently no approved therapy for the treatment of MacTel. Management involves surveillance for possible vision-threatening complications, such as progression to proliferative MacTel with associated MNV.
- Surveillance usually consists of symptom monitoring and periodic examination. Employment of monocular monitoring techniques, such as an Amsler grid, may be used to aid early identification of new symptoms warranting evaluation.
- Use of intravitreal injection of anti–vascular endothelial growth factor (VEGF) agents to treat MacTel has been studied without demonstrating visual improvement.[5] It is therefore not recommended in the absence of MNV.
- Similarly, laser therapy to the areas of leakage and capillary abnormality also has not been shown to be effective in altering disease course or preserving vision and is not recommended.[6]
- In cases of MNV, treatment with intravitreal anti-VEGF therapy is indicated and is effective at minimizing vision loss.[5]

Follow-up Care

- There are no formal guidelines for follow-up in the absence of MNV.
- Our patient uses an Amsler grid for symptom monitoring and seeks a retinal examination every 6 to 12 months.
- In the presence of MNV, the follow-up and treatment schedule is guided by the activity of the MNV.

Algorithm 20.1: Algorithm for Retinal Cysts/Cavitations

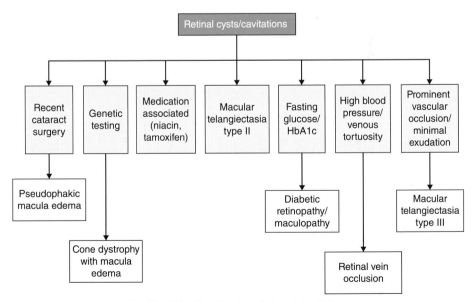

Algorithm 20.1   Algorithm for retinal cysts/cavitations.

Key Points

■ MacTel has prototypical features that help distinguish it from other entities on ophthalmoscopy and on multimodal imaging, and unlike conditions manifesting ME, it typically presents without retinal thickening.

■ Clinical signs can be subtle in the early stages and require careful evaluation to detect. The characteristic appearance of foveal intraretinal cavitations and/or patchy juxtafoveal EZ loss on OCT can be an important clue to the diagnosis, and FA is often helpful for confirmation. In later stages, the presence of temporal parafoveal pigment deposition is a helpful clinical sign. The CBR demonstrates bright hyperfluorescence that persists consistently in the early stages and throughout the course of the disease.[7]

■ Visual decline is generally gradual in nature, and rapid changes in symptoms should prompt expeditious evaluation for possible MNV.

■ No approved therapy exists for the treatment of MacTel, and neither anti-VEGF therapy nor laser has been shown to be effective as therapy for MacTel. However, in the case of concurrent MNV, anti-VEGF therapy is effective in preserving vision.

■ There are Phase III clinical trials investigating the possible role of ciliary neurotrophic growth factor in treating MacTel.[8]

References

1. Charbel Issa P, Gillies MC, Chew EY, et al. Macular telangiectasia type 2. *Prog Retin Eye Res*. 2013;34: 49-77.
2. Khan MJ, Papakostas T, Kovacs K, Gupta MP. Drug-induced maculopathy. *Curr Opin Ophthalmol*. 2020;31:563-571.
3. Wong WT, Forooghian F, Majumdar Z, Bonner RF, Cunningham D, Chew EY. Fundus autofluorescence in type 2 idiopathic macular telangiectasia: correlation with optical coherence tomography and microperimetry. *Am J Ophthalmol*. 2009;148:573-583.
4. Oh JH, Oh J, Togloom A, Kim SW, Huh K. Characteristics of cystoid spaces in type 2 idiopathic macular telangiectasia on spectral domain optical coherence tomography images. *Retina*. 2014;34:1123-1131.
5. Roller AB, Folk JC, Patel NM, et al. Intravitreal bevacizumab for treatment of proliferative and nonproliferative type 2 idiopathic macular telangiectasia. *Retina*. 2011;31:1848-1855.
6. Park DW, Schatz H, McDonald HR, Johnson RN. Grid laser photocoagulation for macular edema in bilateral juxtafoveal telangiectasis. *Ophthalmology*. 1997;104:1838-1846.
7. Sallo FB, Leung I, Zeimer M, et al. Abnormal retinal reflectivity to short-wavelength light in type 2 idiopathic macular telangiectasia. *Retina*. 2018;38(suppl 1):S79-S88.
8. Chew EY, Clemons TE, Jaffe GJ, et al. Effect of ciliary neurotrophic factor on retinal neurodegeneration in patients with macular telangiectasia type 2: a randomized clinical trial. *Ophthalmology*. 2019; 126:540-549.

CHAPTER 21

Transient Peripheral White Retinal Lesions

Daniel W. Wang ■ William F. Mieler

History of Present Illness

A 57-year-old male patient presents with progressive blurry vision in both eyes (OU). The onset of his symptoms was gradual, and he mentions that vision was particularly poor during low light conditions, and that this has prevented him from driving at night. The patient reports no difficulty with color vision and endorses no notable personal history of ocular disease.

Ocular Examination Findings

Visual acuity without correction was 20/20 OU. Intraocular pressure was 17 OU by applanation. Pupils were round, equal, and reactive without a relative afferent pupillary defect in each eye. External and anterior segment examination was unremarkable with trace nuclear sclerotic cataracts. On dilated fundus examination, both optic nerves appeared normal without pallor. The macula was flat without mottling or edema. The vessels appeared normal without attenuation (Fig. 21.1). The retinal periphery showed numerous scattered white spots but no pigmentary alteration (Fig. 21.2).

Questions to Ask

- Is there any family history of known retinal dystrophies or ocular disease? Conditions such as ocular albinism, gyrate atrophy, or retinitis pigmentosa often have genetic associations and may commonly be seen in other family members.
  - No
- What systemic medications is the patient taking? Certain medications, such as phenothiazines and oral isotretinoin, have been associated with nyctalopia.
  - Patient is taking only lisinopril for hypertension.
- What were the onset and duration of the patient's symptoms? Conditions such as cataracts and glaucoma typically have a slow progression and evolve over several years.
  - Patient endorses that symptoms were gradually worsening over the past 6 months.
- Does the patient have a history of bariatric surgery, or does the patient have major dietary restrictions?
  - Yes, the patient underwent uncomplicated bariatric surgery for obesity 5 years before presentation.

Assessment

- This is a 57-year-old male patient with no previous ocular disease, though with a history of bariatric surgery presenting with progressive nyctalopia.

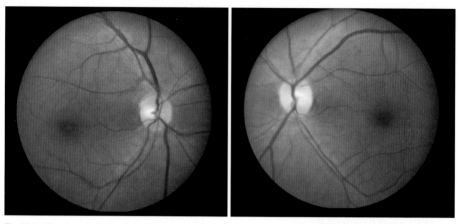

Fig. 21.1 Fundus photographs of both eyes demonstrating a grossly normal appearance of the posterior pole. The media is clear. There is no pallor or glaucomatous changes of the optic nerve. The retinal vessels are of normal course and caliber. The macula is normal and without mottling or pigmentary changes.

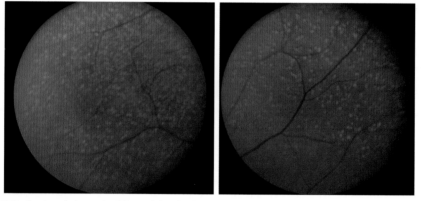

Fig. 21.2 Fundus photograph of the peripheral retina of both eyes demonstrating uniformly scattered, deep whitish-yellow dots.

Differential Diagnosis

- Retinitis pigmentosa
- Vitamin A deficiency
- Zinc deficiency
- Cataract
- Albinism
- Gyrate atrophy
- Oguchi disease
- Optic atrophy

Working Diagnosis

- Vitamin A deficiency

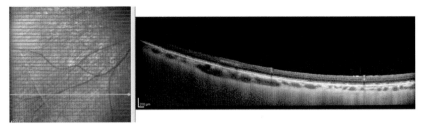

Fig. 21.3 Ocular coherence tomography of the right eye demonstrating focal hyporeflective excrescences below the ellipsoid zone corresponding to the whitish dots seen on fundus examination.

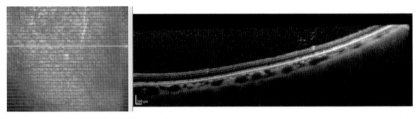

Fig. 21.4 Ocular coherence tomography of the right eye again demonstrates hyperreflective material accumulating beneath the focal disrupted ellipsoid zone.

Multimodal Testing and Results

■ Fundus photos
  ■ Color fundus photos show a grossly normal fundus appearance in the posterior pole, but numerous whitish-yellow dots are visualized in the retinal periphery[1] (Fig. 21.2).
■ Optical coherence tomography (OCT)
  ■ Normal appearance with intact layers and normal contour through the fovea of both eyes; subretinal hyperreflective material along with an irregular appearance of the interdigitating zone and the ellipsoid zone as is appreciated in the retina periphery where whitish dots are most prominent[2] (Figs. 21.3 and 21.4).

Electroretinogram

■ Electroretinogram (ERG) demonstrating a depressed scotopic response with depressed amplitude combined response in both eyes

Management

Vitamin A is an essential nutrient that is acquired through a diet with animal-derived products, leafy green and yellow vegetables, or synthetic vitamin A analogs. Vitamin A deficiency has been well documented in patients who have undergone bariatric surgery and individuals with vegan-based diets.[3,4] In adult patients, treatment typically consists of 200,000 IU given orally for 2 days, with a third dose provided at least 2 weeks later.[5] However, studies have shown that lower doses are sufficient for visual recovery.[6] Intramuscular therapy is thought to lead to faster recovery and may be employed when corneal involvement with impending perforation is a concern or when severe gastrointestinal malabsorption is present.[7] Sublingual vitamin A preparations have also been described.[8] Patients with concomitant zinc deficiency should also undergo zinc supplementation. Topical lubrication has utility in the treatment of concomitant ocular surface disease.

Follow-up Care

The patient should be carefully monitored for other ocular sequelae of xerophthalmia. Monitoring of vitamin A levels during active vitamin supplementation is conducted with serial serum testing. Retinal response to treatment may be followed with ERG and other ancillary testing such as OCT. Providers should work closely with the patient's primary care physician and/or dietitian as patient education is critical to ensure well-balanced, nutrient-rich diets. After the patient was administered vitamin A supplementation, the peripheral white spots disappeared.

Algorithm 21.1: Differential Diagnosis and Algorithm for Nyctalopia

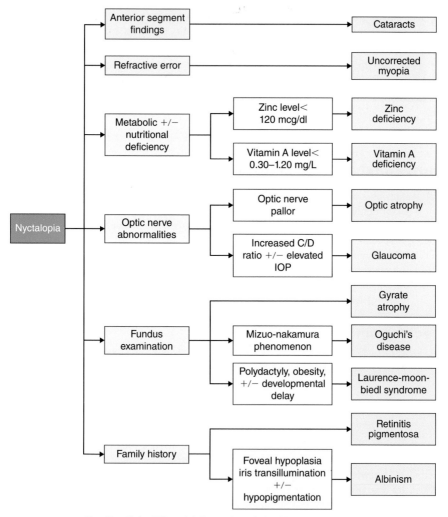

Algorithm 21.1   Differential diagnosis and algorithm for nyctalopia.

References

1. Aleman TS, Garrity ST, Brucker AJ. Retinal structure in vitamin A deficiency as explored with multimodal imaging. *Doc Ophthalmol*. 2013;127:239-243.
2. Berkenstock MK, Castoro CJ, Carey AR. Outer retina changes on optical coherence tomography in vitamin A deficiency. *Int J Retina Vitreous*. 2020;6:23.
3. Zalesin KC, Miller WM, Franklin B, et al. Vitamin A deficiency after gastric bypass surgery: an underreported postoperative complication. *J Obes*. 2011;2011:760695.
4. Hovinen T, Korkalo L, Freese R, et al. Vegan diet in young children remodels metabolism and challenges the statuses of essential nutrients. *EMBO Mol Med*. 2021;13(2):e13492.
5. World Health Organization. Initial treatment. In: *Management of Severe Malnutrition: A Manual for Physicians and Other Senior Health Workers*. Geneva, Switzerland: World Health Organization; 1999:17-18.
6. Chae T, Foroozan R. Vitamin A deficiency in patients with a remote history of intestinal surgery. *Br J Ophthalmol*. 2006;90:955-956.
7. Gilbert C. How to manage children with the eye signs of vitamin A deficiency. *Community Eye Health*. 2013;26(84):68.
8. Singer JR, Bakall B, Gordon GM, Reddy RK. Treatment of vitamin A deficiency retinopathy with sublingual vitamin A palmitate. *Doc Ophthalmol*. 2016;132:137-145.

CHAPTER 22

Bilateral Atypical Drusen and Slow Dark Adaptation in a Woman

Eleni K. Konstantinou   ▓   Tiarnán D. L. Keenan

History of Present Illness

A 63-year-old female patient was referred for evaluation of atypical drusen in both eyes. She reported normal central vision in both eyes. Her past medical history included hypothyroidism, hypertension, and hypercholesterolemia.

OPHTHALMIC EXAMINATION FINDINGS

Visual acuity was 20/16 without correction in each eye. Intraocular pressures were normal. External and anterior segment examination showed mild nuclear sclerotic cataracts. Dilated fundus examination demonstrated an extensive interlacing network of yellowish deposits, including some punctate lesions, involving the maculae (with relative sparing nasally) and extending beyond the arcades (particularly temporally and superotemporally) in both eyes, as well as large, soft drusen in the temporal macula of the left eye (Figs. 22.1 and 22.2).

IMAGING

Optical coherence tomography (OCT) showed that the interlacing network in both eyes consisted of multiple lesions of hyperreflective material above the retinal pigment epithelium (RPE) (Fig. 22.3). Some lesions comprised mounds of hyperreflective material that altered the ellipsoid zone (EZ), whereas others were conical and broke through the EZ. Soft drusen were also observed in some B-scans, comprising nonconical lesions of hyperreflective material below the RPE layer. Fundus autofluorescence (FAF) imaging revealed an extensive interlacing network (i.e., a reticular appearance) in both eyes comprising hypoautofluorescent lesions surrounded by areas of hyperautofluorescence (Fig. 22.4). A similar appearance was observed on near-infrared reflectance (NIR) imaging (Fig. 22.5).

Questions to Ask

- Does the patient have slow dark adaptation? Reticular pseudodrusen (RPD) are typically accompanied by prolonged dark adaptation.[1]
  - Dark adaptation was highly prolonged. The patient admitted to her vision taking many minutes to adapt to the low light conditions of a movie theatre and described the phenomenon of afterimages of bright lights persisting sometimes for several hours.

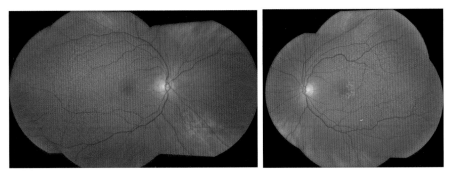

Fig. 22.1 Montage of color fundus photography of both eyes, demonstrating an extensive interlacing (i.e., reticular) network of yellowish deposits, including some punctate lesions (i.e., both ribbons and dots), involving the maculae and extending beyond the arcades. Large, soft drusen are also observed temporal to the fovea macula in the left eye.

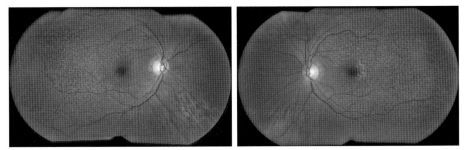

Fig. 22.2 Montage of red-free fundus photography of both eyes, showing extensive reticular pseudodrusen involving the maculae and extending beyond the arcades.

- Is the patient known to have age-related macular degeneration (AMD)? RPD are observed most commonly in AMD.
  - Yes
- Is there a family history of inherited retinal disease (particularly Sorsby fundus dystrophy, late-onset retinal degeneration, fundus albipunctatus, or retinitis punctata albescens)? RPD can be observed in these conditions.[2]
  - No
- Does the patient have systemic features of pseudoxanthoma elasticum (e.g., characteristic skin lesions, intermittent claudication, coronary artery disease, or gastrointestinal bleeding)? RPD can also be observed in this condition.[2]
  - No
- Could the patient have vitamin A deficiency (e.g., from dietary deprivation, gastrointestinal conditions, or liver disease), which has been linked to RPD?[2]
  - No
- Related to AMD, questions on smoking history and oral supplement use are appropriate.
  - The patient had never smoked cigarettes and took Age Related Eye Disease Study (AREDS2) supplements.

Assessment

- This 63-year-old female patient had extensive RPD in both eyes and no apparent monogenic retinal disease or systemic condition as a potential cause. Other findings of AMD were present.

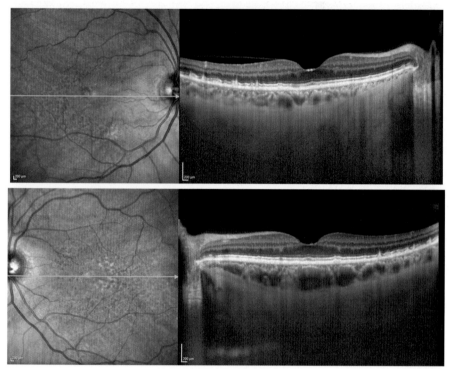

Fig. 22.3 Spectral-domain optical coherence tomography of both eyes, showing multiple lesions of hyper-reflective material above the retinal pigment epithelium (RPE) (i.e., subretinal location), predominantly in the temporal macula. Some lesions are observed as mounds of hyperreflective material that alter the ellipsoid zone (EZ) (i.e., stage 2 reticular pseudodrusen), whereas others are conical and break through the EZ (i.e., stage 3 reticular pseudodrusen). Temporal to the fovea, particularly in the left eye, soft drusen are also observed, comprising nonconical lesions of hyperreflective material below the RPE.

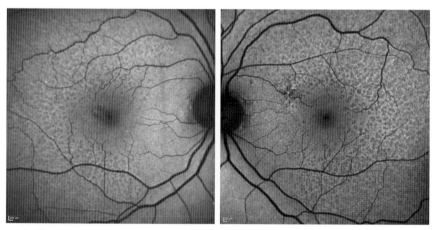

Fig. 22.4 Blue-light fundus autofluorescence imaging of both eyes, showing an extensive interlacing (i.e., reticular) network comprising hypoautofluorescent lesions surrounded by areas of hyperautofluorescence. Some hypoautofluorescent lesions have a "target" appearance, with a central area of isoautofluorescence surrounded by a halo of hypoautofluorescence.

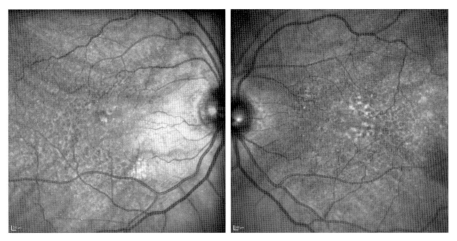

Fig. 22.5 Near-infrared reflectance imaging of both eyes, showing an extensive interlacing (i.e., reticular) network comprising lesions with low signal surrounded by areas of high signal. Some lesions have a "target" appearance, with a central area of higher signal surrounded by a halo of low signal.

Differential Diagnosis

- RPD should be distinguished from other retinal deposits, including soft drusen, cuticular drusen, RPE pigmentary abnormalities, and flecks[3]
- AMD is the most common cause of RPD
- RPD can also be seen in some monogenic retinal diseases:
  - Sorsby fundus dystrophy (*TIMP3* mutations)
  - Late-onset retinal degeneration (LOLD) (*CTRP5* mutations)
  - Fundus albipunctatus (*RDH5* mutations)
  - Retinitis punctata albescens (*RLBP1* or *RDH5* mutations)
- Pseudoxanthoma elasticum
- Vitamin A deficiency
- Extensive macular atrophy with pseudodrusen
- Otherwise normal retina (i.e., with RPD as either an aging phenomenon or an isolated feature in atypical AMD)

Working Diagnosis

- Intermediate AMD with extensive RPD in both eyes

Multimodal Testing and Results

- Color fundus photography (CFP) (Fig. 22.1)
  - Often poorly visualized. If apparent, typically observed as (1) a network of faint interlacing ribbons, (2) more discrete dot-like deposits, and/or (3) moderately confluent globules in the midperiphery.[4]
- OCT (Fig. 22.3)
  - Lesions of hyperreflective material above the RPE layer.
  - Often considered in three or four stages: stage 1, diffuse granular hyperreflective material; stage 2, mounds of hyperreflective material that alter the EZ; stage 3, conical lesions of

hyperreflective material that break through the EZ[5]; and stage 4, hyperreflective lesions fading into the inner retinal layers.[6]
- Proposed as the base modality for defining RPD, given high sensitivity and specificity, and ability to determine their subretinal location.[2]
- FAF (Fig. 22.4)
  - Interlacing network comprising hypoautofluorescent lesions, sometimes with a "target" appearance (i.e., a central area of isoautofluorescence encased by a halo of hypoautofluorescence), surrounded by areas of hyperautofluorescence
- NIR (Fig. 22.5)
  - Similar appearance to FAF
  - High sensitivity and specificity for detecting RPD
- Deep learning algorithms have been trained to detect RPD presence automatically from FAF and/or CFP images[7,8]
- Dark adaptation
  - RPD presence in AMD is strongly associated with very slow dark adaptation[1]
- Genetic testing
  - RPD presence in AMD is strongly associated with a high AMD polygenic risk score and is preferentially associated with risk variants at *ARMS2/HTRA1* rather than *CFH*[9]

Management

- The management of a patient with RPD is guided by the parent condition.
- In this case of a patient with intermediate AMD, management comprised recommendations for daily AREDS2 oral supplement use, home monitoring for symptoms of progression (using an Amsler grid or other home monitoring program), avoidance of smoking, and a healthy diet (Mediterranean pattern).[10]
- RPD presence in AMD might make eyes inappropriate for subthreshold nanosecond laser (SNL) treatment. In post hoc analyses of one randomized controlled trial of SNL for eyes with intermediate AMD, RPD presence appeared to be a strong factor in predicting a negative response (i.e., increased risk of progression to late AMD or nascent geographical atrophy).[11]

Follow-up Care

- Follow-up is guided by the parent condition. For AMD, this is determined by the disease stage; for example, every 6 to 24 months for early AMD and every 6 to 18 months for intermediate disease.[10]
- However, RPD presence in AMD is associated with increased risk of progression to late disease, particularly geographical atrophy, type 3 neovascular AMD, and isolated outer retinal atrophy.[2,9] Therefore our patient was recommended for repeat evaluation and multimodal imaging at least every 6 months. As always, prompt evaluation is required for any new symptoms.

Algorithm 22.1: Algorithm for Workup of Reticular Pseudodrusen: Staging and Differential Diagnosis of their Parent Condition

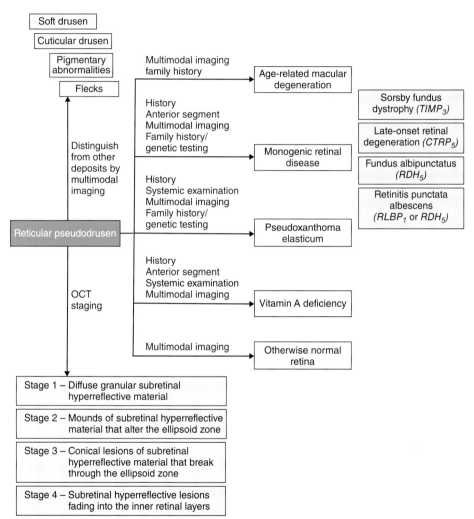

Algorithm 22.1 Algorithm for workup of reticular pseudodrusen: staging and differential diagnosis of their parent condition.

Key Points

■ RPD are often poorly visualized on fundus examination or CFP but are typically highly apparent on OCT, NIR, and FAF imaging. On OCT they are distinguished by their sub-retinal location.

■ RPD are commonly observed in AMD; the phenotype comprises RPD, a thin choroid, and slow dark adaptation.

■ These eyes are at higher risk of progression to late AMD and preferentially to particular subtypes: geographical atrophy, type 3 neovascular AMD, and isolated outer retinal atrophy.

■ However, RPD may be a manifestation of other conditions, including monogenic retinal diseases. They may be seen in pseudoxanthoma elasticum, which has important systemic implications, and in vitamin A deficiency, which is treatable.

References

1. Flamendorf J, Agrón E, Wong WT, et al. Impairments in dark adaptation are associated with age-related macular degeneration severity and reticular pseudodrusen. *Ophthalmology*. 2015;122(10):2053-2062.
2. Wu Z, Fletcher EL, Kumar H, Greferath U, Guymer RH. Reticular pseudodrusen: A critical phenotype in age-related macular degeneration. *Prog Retin Eye Res*. 2022;88:101017. doi: 10.1016/j.preteyeres.2021.101017.
3. Khan KN, Mahroo OA, Khan RS, et al. Differentiating drusen: drusen and drusen-like appearances associated with ageing, age-related macular degeneration, inherited eye disease and other pathological processes. *Prog Retin Eye Res*. 2016;53:70-106.
4. Suzuki M, Sato T, Spaide RF. Pseudodrusen subtypes as delineated by multimodal imaging of the fundus. *Am J Ophthalmol*. 2014;157(5):1005-1012.
5. Zweifel SA, Spaide RF, Curcio CA, Malek G, Imamura Y. Reticular pseudodrusen are subretinal drusenoid deposits. *Ophthalmology*. 2010;117(2):303-312.e1.
6. Querques G, Canouï-Poitrine F, Coscas F, et al. Analysis of progression of reticular pseudodrusen by spectral domain: optical coherence tomography. *Invest Ophthalmol Vis Sci*. 2012;53:1264-1270.
7. Keenan TDL, Chen Q, Peng Y, et al. Deep learning automated detection of reticular pseudodrusen from fundus autofluorescence images or color fundus photographs in AREDS2. *Ophthalmology*. 2020; 127(12):1674-1687.
8. Chen Q, Keenan TDL, Allot A, et al. Multimodal, multitask, multiattention (M3) deep learning detection of reticular pseudodrusen: toward automated and accessible classification of age-related macular degeneration. *J Am Med Inform Assoc*. 2021;28(6):1135-1148.
9. Domalpally A, Agrón E, Pak JW, et al. Prevalence, risk, and genetic association of reticular pseudodrusen in age-related macular degeneration: Age-Related Eye Disease Study 2 report 21. *Ophthalmology*. 2019;126(12):1659-1666.
10. American Academy of Ophthalmology. *Preferred Practice Pattern 2019*. American Academy of Ophthalmology; 2019. Available at: https://www.aao.org/preferred-practice-pattern/age-related-macular-degeneration-ppp. Accessed May 2, 2023.
11. Guymer RH, Wu Z, Hodgson LAB, et al. Subthreshold nanosecond laser intervention in age-related macular degeneration: the LEAD randomized controlled clinical trial. *Ophthalmology*. 2019;126(6):829-838.

CHAPTER 23

Bilateral Diffuse Macular and Peripheral Yellow spots

Katherine A. Joltikov ▪ Jennifer I. Lim

History of Present Illness

We present a case of a 58-year-old man with a past medical history of gout on allopurinol, and past ocular history of myopia and age-related macular degeneration (AMD), referred for further AMD management. He was diagnosed with AMD 3 years ago, and he reports worsening vision in both eyes (right eye more than the left eye) since the time of diagnosis. He denies floaters, photopsias or flashes, or nyctalopia. He denies any history of trauma or ocular surgeries.

OCULAR EXAMINATION FINDINGS

Visual acuities with correction were 20/400 in the right eye and 20/60 in the left eye. His spectacle lenses measured $-3.00 + 0.75 \times 160$ (right eye) and $-3.50 + 0.50 \times 170$ (left eye), and there was no improvement in vision with manifest refraction. Intraocular pressures were normal. External and anterior segment examinations showed mild nuclear sclerotic cataracts but were otherwise unremarkable. Dilated fundus examination revealed multiple small, discrete, round drusen throughout the macular regions and extending into the periphery of both eyes. Retinal pigment epithelium (RPE) atrophy was present in the macula of the right eye, and a vitelliform-like, subfoveal lesion was present in the left eye (Fig. 23.1). The vitelliform lesion was not associated with hemorrhage, hard exudates, or subretinal fluid.

IMAGING

Optical coherence tomography (OCT) showed the presence of multiple drusen in a sawtooth pattern in both eyes. In the right eye, there was RPE atrophy with loss of the ellipsoid zone and external limiting membrane layer subfoveally. In the left eye, OCT showed subfoveal hyperreflective material (Fig. 23.2) in a mound of elevated RPE.

Optical coherence tomography angiography (OCTA) did not show any neovascular membranes in either eye.

Questions to Ask

- Is there a pattern to the drusen distribution?
  - AMD typically shows scattered drusen of various sizes in the macular area. There may be associated RPE mottling, hyperpigmentation, or hypopigmentation due to RPE atrophy. AMD eyes may have intermediate and soft drusen, as well as reticular pseudodrusen

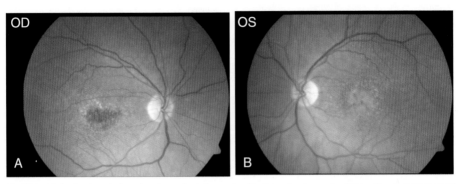

Fig. 23.1 Color fundus photos showing retinal pigment epithelium atrophy and cuticular drusen in both eyes. (B) In the left eye there is vitelliform subfoveal lesion without hemorrhage, hard exudates, or subretinal fluid.

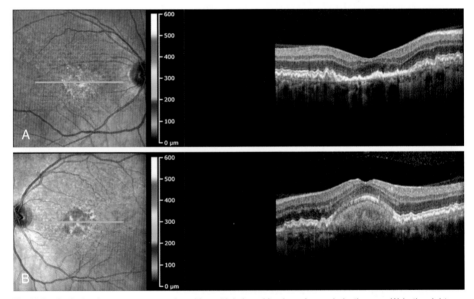

Fig. 23.2 Optical coherence tomography with multiple basal laminar drusen in both eyes. (A) In the right eye the sawtooth drusen pattern is seen, as well as retinal pigment epithelium (RPE) atrophy with loss of the ellipsoid zone and external limiting membrane layer subfoveally. There are also shallow elevations of RPE. (B) In the left eye the sawtooth pattern of drusen is still visible, although there is also a mound-shaped elevation of the RPE with subfoveal hyperreflective material.

and cuticular drusen. Exudative neovascular AMD may show turbid fluid similar to the exudation seen with pattern dystrophy.

- Autosomal dominant malattia leventinese show drusen in a radial pattern in the macula and peripapillary, sometimes described as a honeycomb pattern. In later stages, drusen can become large and confluent and appear similar to AMD.
- Cuticular or basal laminar drusen are dispersed throughout the macular area and beyond in a "milky way" or "starry night" pattern. This pattern is best seen with fluorescein angiography (FA).

- Pattern dystrophy lesions range from a circular yellow foveal spot with or without a hyperpigmented spot centrally (foveomacular dystrophy) to an X-shaped configuration (butterfly pattern) or other patterns of yellowish deposits.
    - Yes. The drusen were dispersed throughout the macular areas and present in the periphery of both eyes.
- Is there any family history of AMD or drusen?
    - Patients with AMD may have affected relatives as there is a genetic component.
    - No, the patient was not aware of any family history of AMD.
- Is there any family history of Best disease or hereditary retinal condition?
    - Best disease typically has vitelliform lesions in the macular areas. These lesions may be unifocal or multifocal; they may resemble an egg yolk or pseudohypopyon or have various degrees of "scrambled egg" appearance. Best disease is typically autosomal dominant.
    - Pattern dystrophies may be dominantly inherited. Genetic testing is becoming more common. If suspected, family members should also be examined.
    - No, the patient was not aware of any family ocular history and did not have any examinations as a young adult or child.
- At what age were the drusen first noted?
    - Cuticular drusen are seen during young adulthood. They become more numerous over time and can coalesce.
    - Unknown, because the patient did not have any examination as a young adult.
- Does the patient have renal disease? Membranoproliferative glomerulonephritis type 2 is associated with cuticular drusen.
    - No
- Is the RPE detached?
    - Basal laminar drusen represent thickening of the basal lamina of the RPE, and the RPE is not detached. In contrast, typical drusen in AMD are beneath the RPE, which is detached in exudative AMD.
    - No
- At what age did the patient start to notice decrease in vision?
    - Typically, cuticular drusen patients develop the exudative form in their late 50s and beyond.
    - The patient was 55 years old.
- Is there associated hemorrhage with the lesion?
    - Hemorrhage may indicate the presence of choroidal neovascularization. FA may be indicated in those cases.
    - No

Assessment

- This is a case of a 58-year-old man previously diagnosed as having AMD who shows bilateral cuticular/basal laminal drusen and a subfoveal vitelliform lesion in the left eye.

Differential Diagnosis

- Cuticular drusen with vitelliform lesion
- AMD
- Autosomal dominant drusen (malattia leventinese)
- Patten dystrophy including adult-onset vitelliform maculopathy
- Best vitelliform macular dystrophy

Working Diagnosis

- Cuticular drusen with vitelliform lesion

Multimodal Testing and Results

- Fundus photos
  - Fundus examination will reveal numerous small yellow nodular drusen bilaterally. Geographic atrophy, choroidal neovascular membranes, or vitelliform pigment epithelial detachments may be present.
- OCT
  - OCT will show numerous basal laminar drusen, which appear different from typical drusen that do not have basal laminar thickening.[1]
  - There can be variable reflectivity of the cuticular drusen on OCT. There are three described patterns of cuticular drusen on OCT:[2]
    - Type 1: shallow elevations of RPE with difficult-to-discern contents (Fig. 23.2A)
    - Type 2: drusen in a sawtooth pattern (Fig. 23.2A and B)
    - Type 3: broad, mound-shaped elevations of RPE (Fig. 23.2B)
- OCTA
  - May show a choroidal neovascular membrane (was not seen in our patient)
- Fundus autofluorescence (FAF)
  - Demonstrates numerous hypoautofluorescent drusen with a rim of hyperautofluorescence
- FA
  - Demonstrates numerous hyperfluorescent drusen, conferring a starry-sky appearance (as seen on this representative photo in Fig. 23.3)
- Electroretinogram (ERG) and electrooculogram (EOG)
  - ERG would be expected to be normal in cuticular drusen with vitelliform lesion.
  - ERG may be abnormal in pattern dystrophy but is not typically performed.
  - EOG would be normal in cuticular drusen and abnormal in Best disease, with an Arden ratio of 1.5 or less.

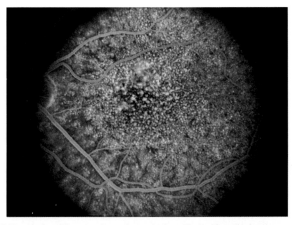

Fig. 23.3 Representative photo of fluorescein angiography in patient with cuticular drusen, showing starry-sky appearance (https://imagebank.asrs.org/file/13588/basal-laminar-drusen-cuticular). This image was originally published in the Retina Image Bank® website. David Callanan, MD. Basal Laminar Drusen / Cuticular. Retina Image Bank. 2014; Image Number # 13588 © the American Society of Retina Specialists.

- Genetic testing
  - This can be obtained to help rule out genetic disorders such pattern dystrophy, Best disease, and malattia leventinese.

Management

- Isolated cuticular drusen does not require treatment. Moreover, it is important to recognize the stage of subfoveal vitelliform lesion as not choroidal neovascularization and thus avoid unnecessary treatment.
- Patient should be monitored for development of geographic atrophy, choroidal neovascularization, and vitelliform pigment epithelium detachments.
- In cases of choroidal neovascularization (CNV), photodynamic therapy has been shown to be effective.[3]
- Vitelliform lesions may be observed and may spontaneously regress.[4] Treatment of vitelliform lesions with PDT may worsen the vitelliform lesions and is not recommended.[5]
- It is unknown if patients with cuticular drusen would benefit from AREDS vitamins.[6]

Follow-up Care

- There are no previously established guidelines for follow-up.
- Our patient is followed on an annual basis.
- If the patient is symptomatic or demonstrates progression on OCT, more frequent follow-up is indicated.

Algorithm 23.1: Differential Diagnosis for Cuticular Drusen With Vitelliform Lesion

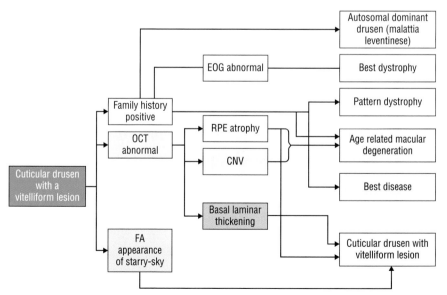

Algorithm 23.1   Differential diagnosis for cuticular drusen with vitelliform lesion. *CNV,* Choroidal neovascularization; *FA,* fluorescein angiography; *OCT,* optical coherence tomography; *RPE,* retinal pigment epithelium.

Key Points

■ Consider cuticular drusen in patients with OCT finding of basal laminar thickening, with or without a vitelliform lesion.

■ Vitelliform lesions should be observed and can regress spontaneously; no treatment is needed.

■ Patients should be monitored for development of RPE atrophy and CNV when vitelliform lesions are seen.

References

1. Gass JD, Jallow S, Davis B. Adult vitelliform macular detachment occurring in patients with basal laminar drusen. *Am J Ophthalmol*. 1985;99:445-459.
2. Balaratnasingam C, Cherepanoff S, Dolz-Marco R, et al. Cuticular drusen: clinical phenotypes and natural history defined using multimodal imaging. *Ophthalmology*. 2018;125(1):100-118.
3. Guigui B, Martinet V, Leveziel N, Coscas G, Soubrane G, Souied EH. Photodynamic therapy for choroidal neovascularisation secondary to basal laminar drusen. *Eye (Lond)*. 2009;23:2115-2118.
4. Gass JD, Jallow S, Davis B. Adult vitelliform macular detachment occurring in patients with basal laminar drusen. *Am J Ophthalmol*. 1985;99:445-459.
5. Ergun E, Costa D, Slakter J, Yannuzzi LA, Stur M. Photodynamic therapy and vitelliform lesions. *Retina*. 2004;24:399-406.
6. Age-Related Eye Disease Study Research Group. A randomized, placebo-controlled, clinical trial of high-dose supplementation with vitamins C and E, beta carotene, and zinc for age-related macular degeneration and vision loss: AREDS report no. 8. *Arch Ophthalmol*. 2001;119:1417-1436.

Inflammatory/Autoimmune Macular Diseases

CHAPTER 24

Night Blindness in a Man With a Normal Fundus Examination

Alexis Warren ▪ William F. Mieler

History of Present Illness

We present a case of a 31-year-old male patient who is HIV positive and has had nyctalopia for several years. Patient denies any flashes of light or color deficiencies.

OCULAR EXAMINATION FINDINGS

Visual acuity was 20/20 in the right eye and 20/25 in the left eye. Intraocular pressure was normal. Dilated fundus examination exhibited bilateral optic disc drusen but otherwise normal macula and peripheral retinal examination.

IMAGING

Fundus examination had no visually significant abnormalities (Fig. 24.1). Optical coherence tomography (OCT) showed normal foveal contour with mild attenuation of the ellipsoid zone (EZ) in both eyes (Figs. 24.2–24.4).

Questions to Ask

- Is the nyctalopia progressive? When was it first noticed? Patients with congenital stationary night blindness (CSNB) usually have these symptoms from birth with limited progression over time. Because of this, some patients may not be aware of their difficulty with night vision as it seems "normal" to them.
  - No
- What is the patient's refractive error? Patients with CSNB may present with minimal fundus findings, but this condition has been associated with myopia, strabismus, and even nystagmus.
  - This patient is emmetropic with normal motility.
- Does the patient have any vitamin or nutritional deficiencies? It is important to check for acquired causes of nyctalopia that can mimic nonreversible causes of night blindness. Additionally, it is important to recognize that several medications employed in the treatment of patients who are HIV positive may impair vitamin A absorption.
  - Vitamin A levels were decreased in this patient but were adequately supplemented with limited to no improvement in symptoms.

Assessment

- This is a case of a 31-year-old male patient who is HIV positive with nonprogressive nyctalopia, a normal fundus examination, and an electronegative electroretinogram (ERG).

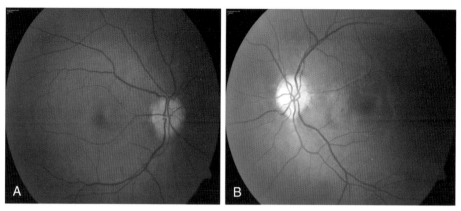

Fig. 24.1 Fundus photography of the right and left eyes with optic nerve drusen.

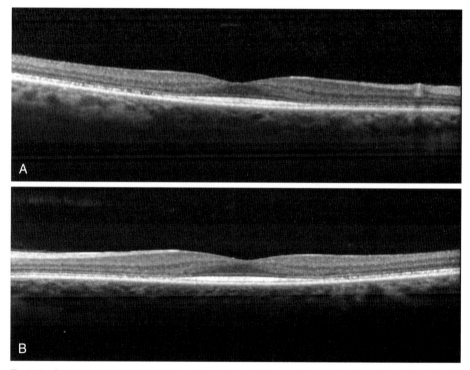

Fig. 24.2 Optical coherence tomography of the right and left eye with macular attenuation of the ellipsoid layer excluding the subfoveal area.

Differential Diagnosis

- Congenital Stationary Night blindness (CSNB)
- Retinitis pigmentosa
- Vitamin A deficiency
- Zinc deficiency

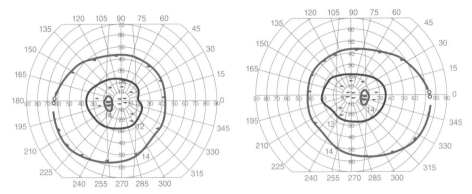

Fig. 24.3 Goldmann visual fields were normal without peripheral field defects.

- Oguchi disease
- Fundus albipunctatus
- Rod-cone dystrophy

Working Diagnosis

- CSNB

Multimodal Testing and Results

- Fundus photographs. The fundus examination in these patients is usually normal, although there are two variants with abnormal fundi.[1]
    - Fundus albipunctatus: These patients have multiple white dots throughout the fundus sparing the central fovea.[1]
    - Oguchi disease: The fundus examinations have a yellow "metallic" sheen in the light-adapted state, but with 2 to 3 hours of dark adaptation this will go away, and the fundus will appear normal.
- OCT
    - Our patient showed some attenuation diffuse attenuation of the EZ, but classically CSNB patients with normal fundi have an unremarkable OCT.[2]
    - Patients with the fundus albipunctatus variant show hyperreflective deposits at the layer of the outer retina.[3]
- Electroretinogram (ERG). The ERG findings of CSNB can be divided into several subtypes:
    - Riggs type (type I): The scotopic ERG shows no a- or b-wave with a dim flash and a decreased b:a ratio with a bright flash. The photopic response is normal.[4]
    - Schubert-Bornschein (type II): This is characterized by the electronegative ERG with a normal a-wave but reduced b-wave. This diagnosis is also further classified as complete or incomplete form.[4,5]
        - Complete (dysfunction of the ON bipolar cells): The photopic ERG shows an almost a-wave with a broadened trough and a sharply increasing b-wave with loss of oscillatory potentials.[5]
        - Incomplete (dysfunction of the ON and OFF bipolar cells): The photopic ERG is more affected, specifically the 30-Hz flicker, which is delayed and often shows a bifid peak due to some residual rod function.[4,5]

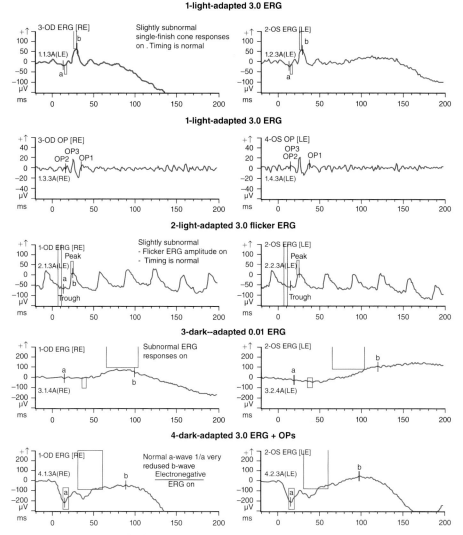

Fig. 24.4 Electroretinogram (ERG) exhibited slightly decreased photopic responses. Dark-adapted testing showed decreased rod responses with a normal a-wave and significantly reduced b-wave consistent with an electronegative ERG.

- Genetic testing A number of genetic mutations have been identified based upon the subtype and inheritance pattern of the disease (Table 24.1).

Management

- Laboratory tests for nutritional deficiencies revealed decreased serum vitamin A levels, which were appropriately supplemented.
- Given persistent lack of improvement of nyctalopia and electronegative ERG, a diagnosis of CSNB was made. Genetic testing confirmed this diagnosis with a heterozygous mutation in the *TRPM1* gene.

TABLE 24.1 ■ Genetic Mutations Identified in CSNB

Subtype	Inheritance Pattern and Gene Mutation
Incomplete Schubert-Bornschein[6]	X-linked • *CACNA1F* and *CABP4*
Complete Schubert-Bornschein[6,7]	X-linked • *NYX* Autosomal recessive • *GRM6, TRPM1, GPR179,* or *LRIT3*
Riggs type[7]	Autosomal dominant • *GNAT1* and *PDE6B* Autosomal recessive • *SCL24A1*
Fundus albipunctactus[8]	Autosomal recessive • *RDH5*
Oguchi disease[8]	Autosomal recessive • *GRK1* and *SAG*

Follow-up Care

- There are currently no approved treatments for CSNB.
- Given the good visual acuity and nonprogressive nature of this diagnosis, a favorable prognosis is expected.

Algorithm 24.1: Algorithm Showing Differential Diagnosis for Nyctalopia

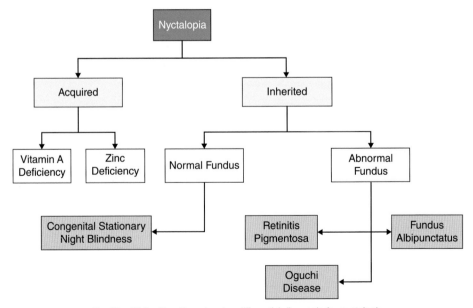

Algorithm 24.1   Algorithm showing differential diagnosis for nyctalopia.

Key Points

- CSNB is a genetic retinal condition that can inherited in an X-linked, autosomal recessive, or autosomal dominant inheritance pattern.[4]
- Fundus examination can be unremarkable but can also be pathognomonic in cases such as fundus albipunctatus or Oguchi disease.[8]
- Diagnostic testing, such as an electronegative ERG, is important and can be very helpful in diagnosing this condition.[1]
- This condition is not normally progressive, and these patients can maintain relatively good vision and high-functioning lifestyles.[1]
- There has been no change in the patient's symptoms or visual function with 3 years follow-up.

References

1. Tsang SH, Sharma T. Congenital stationary night blindness. In: Tsang SH, Sharma T, eds. *Atlas of Inherited Retinal Diseases*. Springer International Publishing; 2018:61-64.
2. Chen RW, Greenberg JP, Lazow MA, et al. Autofluorescence imaging and spectral-domain optical coherence tomography in incomplete congenital stationary night blindness and comparison with retinitis pigmentosa. *Am J Ophthalmol*. 2012;153(1):143-154.e2.
3. Wang NK, Chuang LH, Lai CC, et al. Multimodal fundus imaging in fundus albipunctatus with RDH5 mutation: a newly identified compound heterozygous mutation and review of the literature. *Doc Ophthalmol*. 2012;125(1):51-62.
4. Kim AH, Liu PK, Chang YH, et al. Congenital stationary night blindness: clinical and genetic features. *Int J Mol Sci*. 2022;23(23):14965.
5. Miyake Y, Yagasaki K, Horiguchi M, Kawase Y, Kanda T. Congenital stationary night blindness with negative electroretinogram: a new classification. *Arch Ophthalmol*. 1986;104(7):1013-1020.
6. Bijveld MM, Florijn RJ, Bergen AA, et al. Genotype and phenotype of 101 Dutch patients with congenital stationary night blindness. *Ophthalmology*. 2013;120(10):2072-2081.
7. Zeitz C, Robson AG, Audo I. Congenital stationary night blindness: an analysis and update of genotype-phenotype correlations and pathogenic mechanisms. *Prog Retin Eye Res*. 2015;45:58-110.
8. Dryja TP. Molecular genetics of Oguchi disease, fundus albipunctatus, and other forms of stationary night blindness: LVII Edward Jackson Memorial Lecture. *Am J Ophthalmol*. 2000;130(5):547-563.

CHAPTER 25

Hypopyon Uveitis

Monique Munro ▪ Pooja Bhat

History of Present Illness

A 20-year-old woman of Middle Eastern descent presented because of acute onset of floaters, decreased vision, and redness in the left eye without pain, photophobia, or other ocular symptoms. She was evaluated by her referring provider and diagnosed with uveitis with cystoid macular edema and started on topical corticosteroid. Upon completion of corticosteroid taper, the patient developed recurrent uveitis in the left eye with development of decreased vision in the right eye and was referred for assessment.

Questions to Ask

- Does the patient have an ocular history that could be associated with her symptoms? Has she been diagnosed with myopia? Are these any symptoms suggestive of prior uveitis in both eyes?
- Systemic symptoms: Does the patient have any history of recurrent oral ulcers, intermittent tinnitus, or joint pain in hands and feet?
- Family history: Is there any history of autoimmune hepatitis, psoriasis, or leukemia?
- Social and travel history: Does the patient own any cats? Is there any history of alcohol, tobacco, intravenous drug use, high-risk sexual activity, or recent travel?
  - The patient owns one cat and has experienced bites and scratches. She denies a history of alcohol, tobacco, intravenous drug use, high-risk sexual activity, or recent travel.

Ocular Exam Findings

Visual acuity was counting fingers at 2 inches in the right eye and light perception in the left eye. Intraocular pressures were normal. The external examination was normal. Anterior segment examination showed mild conjunctival injection with ciliary flush, 4+ pigmented and white blood cells with mild flare in both eyes. An inferior hypopyon was present in the right eye.

Dilated fundus examination showed 3+ vitreous cell bilaterally with 1+ haze in the right eye and 2 to 3+ haze in the left eye. The right optic nerve was hyperemic and edematous. Scattered areas of inner retinal whitening were noted in the right eye with sheathing of the arterioles and venules. Details of the optic nerve, macula, vessels, and periphery in the left eye were limited due to vitritis.

Imaging

Optos ultra–wide-field color fundus photographs (Figs. 25.1 and 25.2) were obtained. Fig. 25.1 demonstrates hyperemia with disc edema, patches of retinitis within the macula, diffuse vasculitis, and patches of retinitis in all four quadrants with a small inferotemporal

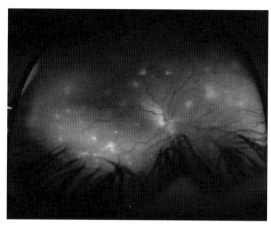

Fig. 25.1   Optos ultra–wide-field color fundus photograph of the right eye demonstrating diffuse foci of deep retinal white lesions.

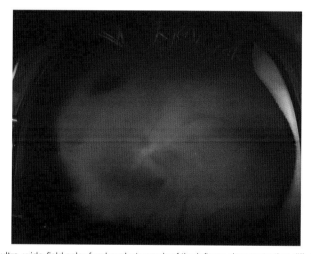

Fig. 25.2   Optos ultra–wide-field color fundus photograph of the left eye demonstrating diffuse media opacity.

hemorrhage. Fig. 25.2 demonstrates significant media opacity secondary to vitreous cells with optic nerve head edema.

Spectral domain optical coherence tomography (OCT) demonstrated macular edema bilaterally with outer retinal cysts and subretinal fluid in the right eye. Nasal retinal edema was observed in the left eye (Figs. 25.3 and 25.4).

Optos ultra–wide-field fluorescein angiogram (FA) showed arteritis and phlebitis bilaterally in the mid to late phase with disc staining. Early blockage in the areas of retinitis with late staining was observed (Figs. 25.5–25.8).

Differential Diagnosis

- Hypopyon uveitis
  - Behcet disease
  - HLA-B27 uveitis

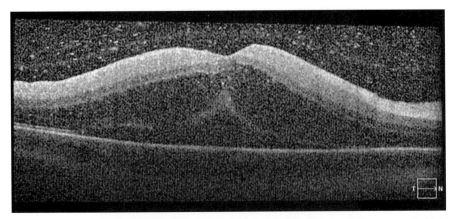

Fig. 25.3 Optical coherence tomography of the right eye demonstrating vitreous opacities, inner retinal thickening, outer retinal edema, and subretinal fluid. The choroid appears normal.

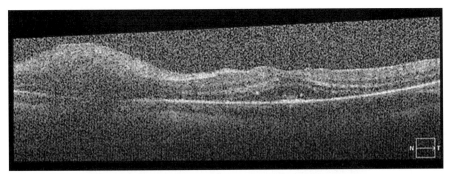

Fig. 25.4 Optical coherence tomography of the left eye demonstrating inner retinal thickening, outer retinal edema, and subretinal fluid. The choroid appears normal. More significant inner retinal edema is present adjacent to the optic nerve head.

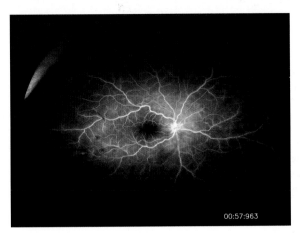

Fig. 25.5 Optos ultra–wide-field fluorescein angiogram of the right eye demonstrating diffuse capillary leakage with optic nerve head edema.

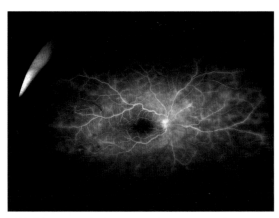

Fig. 25.6 Optos ultra–wide-field fluorescein angiogram of the right eye during recirculation phase demonstrating progressive diffuse capillary leakage with involvement of the larger arteries and veins along with optic nerve head edema.

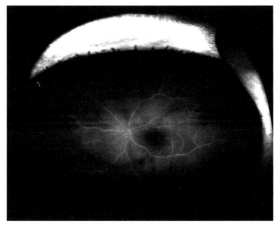

Fig. 25.7 Optos ultra–wide-field fluorescein angiogram of the left eye demonstrating diffuse capillary leakage with optic nerve head edema. There is media opacity present obscuring the view.

- Endophthalmitis: acute and chronic
- Pseudohypopyon
- Retinitis with/without occlusive vasculitis
  - Connective tissue, vasculitis, and other autoimmune disease: systemic lupus erythematosus, polyarteritis nodosa, and granulomatosis with polyangiitis, Vogt-Koyanagi-Harada disease, multiple sclerosis
  - Sarcoidosis
  - Infectious: necrotizing herpetic retinitis, cytomegalovirus, syphilis, toxoplasmosis
  - Malignancy: leukemia, lymphoma

Working Diagnosis

- Behcet disease with panuveitis bilaterally versus other occlusive vasculitis.

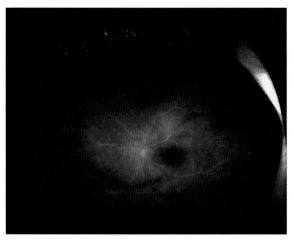

Fig. 25.8 Optos ultra–wide-field fluorescein angiogram of the left eye during recirculation phase demonstrating progressive diffuse capillary leakage with involvement of the larger arteries and veins along with optic nerve head edema.

Multimodal Testing and Results

Serology: HLA-B51 is supportive but not diagnostic of Bechet disease. An elevated white count, erythrocyte sedimentation rate, and C-reactive protein may occur.[1-3] Serology to consider to assess for additional autoimmune, infectious, or masquerade causes include complete blood count, comprehensive metabolic panel, rapid plasma reagin quantitative, FTA-ABS, HLA-B-27, angiotensin-converting enzyme, red-free, anti-nuclear antibody, anti-neutrophil cytoplasmic antibody, QuantiFERON-TB Gold, HIV, SSA/SSB, dsDNA, and Lyme disease testing.[1,2]

Neuroimaging: Magnetic resonance imaging of the brain and orbits in neuro-Behcet disease can demonstrate white matter and cortical changes that can mimic multiple sclerosis and/or stroke. Hypointense to isointense lesions may be seen on T1-weighted images and hyperintense lesions on T2-weighted and fluid-attenuated inversion recovery. Hyperintense lesions may be seen on diffusion-weighted images. Meningeal enhancement may be seen. Cerebral sinus or vein thrombosis may occur.[1-4]

- Neuroimaging was unremarkable in this patient.

Lumbar puncture may be indicated in those suspected of neuro-Bechet disease or with other neurological symptoms to differentiate between multiple sclerosis and other autoimmune or infectious entities.[1,3]

Fundus photographs: Retinal findings in Behcet disease include necrotizing retinitis, retinal vasculitis hemorrhages, edema, and media opacity from vitritis.[1]

OCT may demonstrate cystoid macular edema, as seen in this patient, and very severe cases may have serous detachments.[5]

FA: Early phase shows blockage corresponding to zones of retinitis, and late phase shows staining. The areas of leakage and staining surround retinal arteries and veins. Areas of capillary dropout with possible neovascularization may be seen in chronic cases. FA is essential to show the extent of the burden of disease.[5]

Indocyanine green angiography (ICG) is not commonly used. If performed, however, it may demonstrate areas of hyper- and hypofluorescence.[5] The findings on ICG are often nonspecific.[5]

Pathergy testing is available but not frequently used.[4]

Management

- Recommend emergent admission because of tinnitus and suspected neuro-Behcet disease
- Rheumatology consult
- Intravenous solumedrol 1 g/day for 3 days recommended if severe and/or with neurological symptoms

Follow-up Care

- Discharged on prednisone 60 mg and azathioprine 50 mg daily with anti–tumor necrosis factor approval pending
- The patient had a course of relapsing uveitis because of noncompliance with medications, but achieved stability on adalimumab with a taper of oral prednisone with resolution of retinitis (Figs. 25.9 and 25.10) and final vision of 20/50 in both eyes

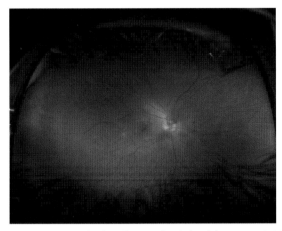

Fig. 25.9 Optos ultra–wide-field color fundus photograph of the right eye postcorticosteroid treatment demonstrating resolution of the retinal lesions.

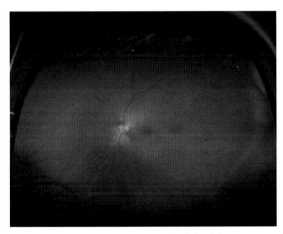

Fig. 25.10 Optos ultra–wide-field color fundus photograph of the left eye postcorticosteroid treatment demonstrating resolution of the retinal lesions.

Algorithm 25.1: Approach to Retinal Whitening

The following criteria may be used to differentiate neuro-Behcet disease from other causes of uveitis with neurological manifestations.[4]

Definite neuro-Behcet disease must meet all of the following:

1. Satisfies the International Study Group (ISG) Criteria 1990 or other accepted Behcet disease criteria guidelines
2. Neurological symptoms known to be caused by Behcet disease and supported by one of the following:
   a. Neuroimaging
   b. Cerebrospinal fluid (CSF)
3. No other cause for neurological findings

Probable neuro-Behcet:

1. Satisfies the above criteria with systemic features of Behcet disease but not meeting ISG criteria
2. Neurological syndrome not satisfying the above with Bechet disease meeting ISG criteria

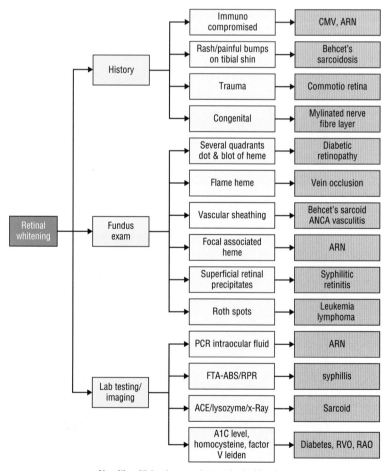

Algorithm 25.1   Approach to retinal whitening.

Key Points

■ Behcet disease is a chronic multisystem inflammatory disease that is characterized by mucosal ulcerations, skin lesions, and ocular inflammation.

■ Uveitis with hypopyon is the most common ocular finding.

■ HLA-B51 is not diagnostic but supportive.

■ Neuro-Bechet disease occurs in 5% to 10% of patients.

■ A thorough history with review of systems, ophthalmic examination, and multimodal ophthalmic imaging, along with systemic workup, neuroimaging, and CSF studies, as indicated, can differentiate neuro-Behcet disease from other causes of uveitis with neurological symptoms.

■ Acute presentations should be treated with systemic corticosteroids. Chronic inflammation and relapses of ocular inflammation are controlled with immunomodulatory therapy, with the goal of steroid-free remission.

References

1. Caruso P, Moretti R. Focus on neuro-Behçet's disease: a review. *Neurol India*. 2018;66(6):1619-1628.
2. Saip S, Akman-Demir G, Siva A. Neuro-Behçet syndrome. *Handb Clin Neurol*. 2014;121:1703-1723.
3. Borhani-Haghighi A, Kardeh B, Banerjee S, et al. Neuro-Behcet's disease: an update on diagnosis, differential diagnoses, and treatment. *Mult Scler Relat Disord*. 2020;39:101906.
4. Kalra S, Silman A, Akman-Demir G, et al. Diagnosis and management of Neuro-Behçet's disease: international consensus recommendations. *J Neurol*. 2014;261(9):1662-1676.
5. Tugal-Tutkun I, Ozdal PC, Oray M, Onal S. Review for diagnostics of the year: multimodal imaging in Behçet uveitis. *Ocul Immunol Inflamm*. 2017;25(1):7-19.

CHAPTER 26

Treatment-Resistant Bilateral Neurosensory Macular Detachment

Stephen J. Smith ▦ Mark W. Johnson

History of Present Illness

We present a case of a 77-year-old man referred for evaluation of nonresolving submacular fluid after 18 months of frequent anti–vascular endothelial growth factor (VEGF) injections (aflibercept and ranibizumab) for presumed exudative age-related macular degeneration (AMD). The past ocular history was notable for a diagnosis of possible idiopathic central serous chorioretinopathy (ICSC) 10 years earlier, with associated retinal pigment epithelium (RPE) changes but normal visual acuity. He had undergone bilateral photodynamic therapy (PDT) without resolution of the macular fluid. His chief report was persistently blurred vision with metamorphopsia in both eyes unresponsive to PDT and anti-VEGF therapy.

His past medical history was significant for a diagnosis of monoclonal gammopathy of undetermined significance (MGUS).

OCULAR EXAMINATION FINDINGS

The best corrected visual acuities were 20/50 in the right eye and 20/63 in the left eye. Intraocular pressures were normal. Anterior segment examination was unremarkable, including clear corneas with no crystalline deposits. Dilated fundus examination was notable for RPE atrophy inferonasal to the fovea in the right eye and submacular fluid with scattered subretinal vitelliform deposits and mild choroidal folds in both eyes (Fig. 26.1A and B). There were no typical or basal laminar drusen in either eye.

IMAGING

Optical coherence tomography (OCT) imaging of the right eye showed RPE atrophy, a thick choroid, and a macular neurosensory retinal detachment with mild intraretinal fluid (Fig. 26.1C). OCT imaging of the left eye demonstrated a thick choroid and submacular fluid (Fig. 26.1D). Fundus autofluorescence (FAF) photography showed scattered hyperautofluorescence corresponding to subretinal vitelliform material, most prominent inferiorly in the left eye (Fig. 26.1E and F). Fluorescein angiography (FA) revealed scattered transmission defects in each eye with mild late staining but without definite leakage in either eye (Fig. 26.1G and H). Of particular note was the absence of evidence for choroidal neovascularization in either eye by any imaging modality.

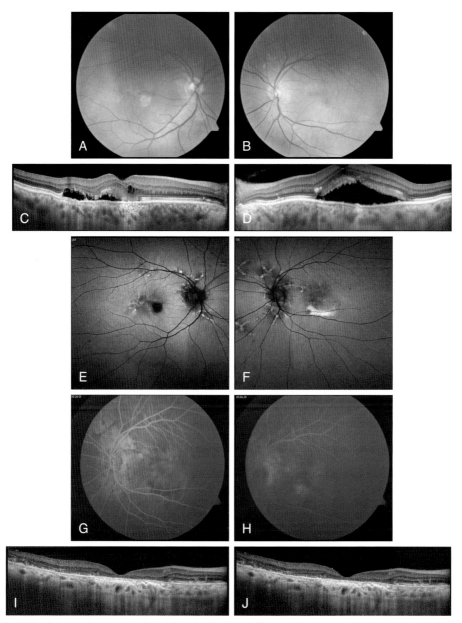

Fig. 26.1 Color fundus photographs of the right (A) and left (B) eyes demonstrate retinal pigment epithelium (RPE) atrophy inferior to the fovea in the right eye and scattered vitelliform deposits and mild choroidal folds in both eyes. Horizontal optical coherence tomography (OCT) image of the right eye (C) shows RPE atrophy, a thick choroid, and subretinal and mild intraretinal fluid. Horizontal OCT image of the left eye (D) shows a thick choroid and submacular fluid. Fundus autofluorescence photographs of both eyes (E and F) demonstrate scattered hyperautofluorescence corresponding to subretinal vitelliform material., Early (G) and late (H) fluorescein angiography images of the left eye show scattered transmission defects with mild late staining but without definite leakage. After ibrutinib therapy, horizontal OCT images show resolution of subretinal fluid in the right (I) and left (J) eyes with a significant reduction in choroidal thickness in both eyes.

Questions to Ask

- Does the patient have a history of steroid use? ICSC should be high on the differential diagnosis of treatment-resistant submacular fluid, particularly in a patient with RPE atrophy.
  - The patient denied any history of previous or current steroid use.
- What medications does the patient take? Medications such as mitogen-activated protein kinase (MEK) inhibitors can cause subretinal fluid.
  - The patient denied use of MEK inhibitors.
- Is there a history of uncontrolled hypertension? Hypertensive choroidopathy can result in serous macular detachments.
  - The patient did not have untreated hypertension.
- Does the patient have a family history of AMD, basal laminar drusen, pattern macular dystrophy, or polypoidal choroidal vasculopathy (PCV)? These are common causes of submacular fluid.
  - The patient denied a family history of these conditions, and his examination and imaging findings were not suggestive of these diagnoses.
- Is there a history of bone pain, neurological symptoms, or symptoms related to anemia? These symptoms can be seen with multiple myeloma, Waldenström macroglobulinemia, and primary amyloidosis, which are rare causes of treatment-resistant neurosensory macular detachment typically associated with clinical signs of hyperviscosity retinopathy.[1]
  - No. However, the patient did have a diagnosis of MGUS and was being monitored by his hematologist.
- Is there any previous diagnosis of an optic pit? Cavitary optic disc anomalies such as optic disc pit and coloboma can result in treatment-resistant neurosensory macular detachment.
  - The patient had no history of cavitary optic disc anomalies and no evidence for these on examination.

Assessment

- This is a case of a 77-year-old man with a past ocular history of possible ICSC presenting with bilateral, treatment-resistant, and angiographically silent macular detachment.

Differential Diagnosis

- ICSC
- Exudative AMD
- PCV
- Vitelliform macular detachment associated with basal laminar drusen
- Adult vitelliform pattern dystrophy
- Immunogammopathy maculopathy or monoclonal gammopathy of macular significance (MGMS)
- Optic pit maculopathy
- Hypertensive choroidopathy
- Medication-associated subretinal fluid (e.g., MEK inhibitor maculopathy)

Working Diagnosis

- MGMS
- MGMS has recently been described in patients with MGUS. These patients present with submacular fluid and variable subretinal vitelliform material without signs of hyperviscosity retinopathy. The findings may be bilateral or unilateral.[2,3]

Multimodal Testing and Results

- Fundus photos
  - On fundus examination, the patient will typically *not* demonstrate signs of hyperviscosity retinopathy. By definition, MGUS does not achieve sufficiently high serum protein levels to cause hyperviscosity. Hyperviscosity retinopathy, including dilated, tortuous vessels and retinal hemorrhages, is typically seen if the disease transforms to a malignant condition such as multiple myeloma or Waldenström macroglobulinemia.
- OCT
  - As mentioned, our patient's OCT showed bilateral choroidal thickening with neurosensory macular detachment.
  - Treatment-resistant macular detachment with variable accumulation of vitelliform material is the classic finding seen in MGMS.[3]
- FA
  - FA in both eyes was notable for the lack of leakage.
  - MGMS is characterized by angiographically silent macular neurosensory detachments. These detachments are hypothesized to be due to a transudative process driven by higher-than-normal circulating levels of protein in the serum.
- FAF
  - As in our patient, FAF shows variable hyperautofluorescence corresponding to subretinal vitelliform accumulations.[2,3]
- Laboratory testing
  - Idiopathic and refractory neurosensory macular detachment may be a sign of underlying malignancy or indicate a premalignant condition. Total serum protein and serum protein electrophoresis should be obtained in such patients.

Management

- This patient underwent malignant transformation to immunoglobulin (Ig)G-κ lymphoplasmacytic lymphoma, an IgG variant of Waldenström macroglobulinemia. He was treated with Bruton tyrosine kinase (BTK) inhibitor, with gradual resolution of submacular fluid and reduction in choroidal thickening (Fig. 26.1I and J). Trace submacular fluid recurred when the BTK inhibitor dose was reduced but remained stable through 6 months of follow-up.
- General management for MGMS is observation with close follow-up by hematology/oncology specialists. Systemic therapy is indicated in the event of malignant transformation, and this frequently results in resolution of submacular fluid.[3]

Follow-up Care

- There are no previously established guidelines for follow-up, but we have followed our patients every 3 to 6 months with dilated fundus examination and imaging.
- If the patient demonstrates progression on OCT, more frequent follow-up may be indicated.

Algorithm 26.1: Algorithm Representing Macular Subretinal Fluid in Eyes Without Inflammation

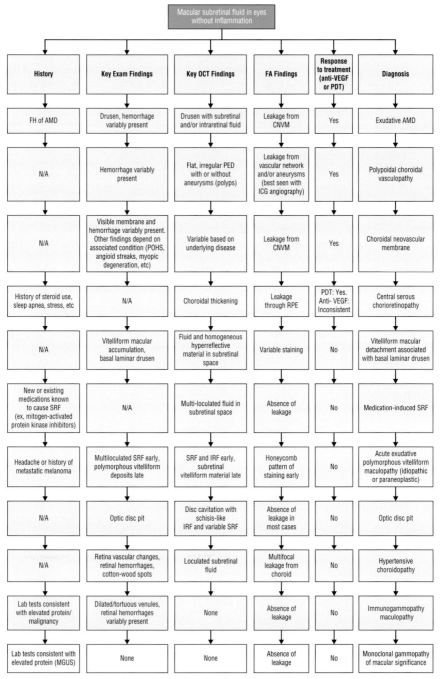

Algorithm 26.1 Algorithm representing macular subretinal fluid in eyes without inflammation. *AMD*, Age-related macular degeneration; *CNVM*, choroidal neovascular membrane; *FA*, fluorescein angiography; *FH*, ; *ICG*, indocyanine green angiography; *IRF*, ; *MGUS*, monoclonal gammopathy of undetermined significance; *N/A*, not applicable; *OCT*, optical coherence tomography; *PDT*, photodynamic therapy; *PED*, pigment epithelial detachment; *POHS*, presumed ocular histoplasmosis syndrome; *RPE*, retinal pigment epithelium; *SRF*, subretinal fluid; *VEGF*, vascular endothelial growth factor.

Key Points

- Consider MGMS in patients with angiographically silent, treatment-resistant neurosensory macular detachment.
- Laboratory evaluation, including total serum protein and serum protein electrophoresis, should be obtained in these patients.
- A diagnosis of MGMS may be a harbinger of malignant transformation, and these patients should be referred to a hematologist/oncologist for evaluation and periodic monitoring.

References

1. Ho AC, Benson WE, Wong J. Unusual immunogammopathy maculopathy. *Ophthalmology*. 2000;107:1099-1103.
2. Rusu IM, Mrejen S, Engelbert M, et al. Immunogammopathies and acquired vitelliform detachments: a report of four cases. *Am J Ophthalmol*. 2014;157:648-657.e1.
3. Smith SJ, Johnson MW, Ober MD, et al. Maculopathy in patients with monoclonal gammopathy of undetermined significance. *Ophthalmol Retina*. 2020;4(3):300-309.

CHAPTER 27

Malignant Photopsias

Monique Munro ▪ Jennifer I. Lim ▪ Pooja Bhat

History of Present Illness

A 65-year-old White man presented in 2015 with bilateral light sensitivity and 4 months of mobile, white spots in his vision that persisted when his eyes were closed. He also reported difficulty reading, as well as symptoms suggesting peripheral visual field constriction, such as difficulties with navigating.

Questions to Ask

- Additional ocular symptoms
  - No additional visual symptoms
- Medical history
  - Testicular cancer (seminoma) in 1982, treated with chemotherapy and pelvic radiation. In 2013, he was found to recurrent seminoma. He had since been on surveillance with testing every 6 months (computed tomography scans, colonoscopies, and repeat routine blood work) revealing no evidence of metastasis or other cancers.
- Family history
  - Strong family history of cancer: renal cell cancer (father), breast cancer (mother), colon cancer (brother)
- History of photopsias: autoimmune retinopathy patients describe shimmering or twinkling lights.
  - This patient described moving white spots.
- Impaired dark adaptation due to progressive damage to rods when suspicious of autoimmune retinopathies
  - This patient did not describe classic nyctalopia but did report constriction of visual fields, which could imply rod dysfunction.
- Social history: assess for possible social and travel risk factors for infectious causes, such as syphilis, human immunodeficiency virus, and tuberculosis.
  - Negative
- Medications: assess for medications known to cause pigmentary retinopathy, such as phenothiazine, antipsychotics, chlorpromazine, and thioridazine.
  - Noncontributory
- Review of symptoms: to assess for symptoms associated with causes of uveitis, white dot syndromes, infectious signs, and undiagnosed malignancy.
  - No additional systemic symptoms in this patient

Ocular Examination Findings

Visual acuity was 20/20 in the right eye and 20/15 in the left eye. Intraocular pressures were normal. Anterior segment examination was unremarkable bilaterally. Fundus examination

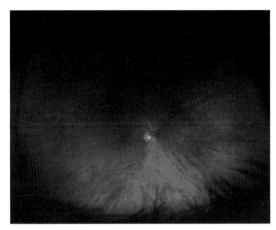

Fig. 27.1 Optos ultrawide field color fundus photograph of the right eye demonstrating mild optic nerve pallor, attenuated arterioles, and retinal pigmentary changes.

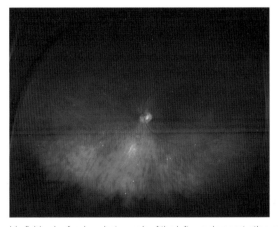

Fig. 27.2 Optos ultrawide field color fundus photograph of the left eye demonstrating mild optic nerve pallor, attenuated arterioles, and retinal pigmentary changes.

demonstrated optic nerve pallor and attenuated arterioles with retinal pigmentary changes in both eyes (Figs. 27.1 and 27.2).

Goldmann visual field testing demonstrated bilateral superior arcuate visual field defects, respecting the horizontal meridian.

Optical coherence tomography (OCT) demonstrated sparring of the outer retina at the fovea in both eyes with outer retinal loss involving the photoreceptors, ellipsoid zone, and external limiting membrane parafoveally in both eyes (Figs. 27.3 and 27.4).

Fundus autofluorescence showed hypoautofluorescence along the superior temporal regions in both eyes with diffuse stippled hyperautofluorescence in the remainder of the fundus in both eyes (Figs. 27.5 and 27.6).

Fluorescein angiogram demonstrated stippled staining of the retina bilaterally with no abnormalities of the optic nerve heads or vessels in both eyes (Figs. 27.7 and 27.8).

Full field electroretinogram demonstrated markedly reduced cone and rod functions bilaterally (Fig. 27.9).

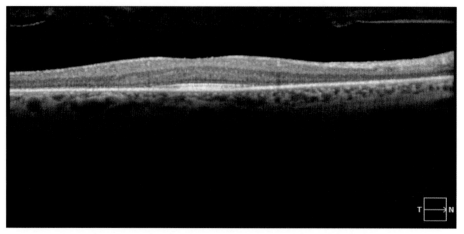

Fig. 27.3 Optical coherence tomography of the right eye demonstrating outer retinal loss involving the photoreceptors, ellipsoid zone, and external limiting membrane parafoveally.

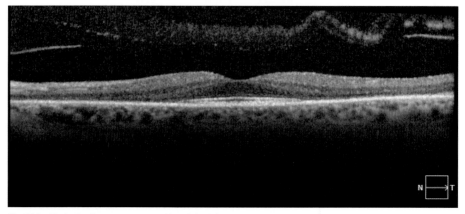

Fig. 27.4 Optical coherence tomography of the left eye demonstrating outer retinal loss involving the photoreceptors, ellipsoid zone, and external limiting membrane parafoveally.

Differential Diagnosis

- Melanoma-associated retinopathy
- Nonneoplastic autoimmune retinopathy
- Retinal dystrophies/degenerations (e.g., retinitis pigmentosa, cone dystrophy)
- Toxic, nutritional, or medication-related retinopathy/optic neuropathy
- Uveitis and white dot syndromes (e.g., acute zonal occult outer retinopathy, multiple evanescent white dot syndrome, birdshot retinopathy)
- Infection: syphilis
- Masquerades (e.g., intraocular foreign body)

Working Diagnosis

- Cancer-associated retinopathy (CAR) versus nonneoplastic autoimmune retinopathy spectrum

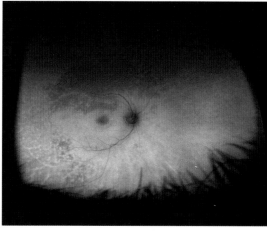

Fig. 27.5   Optos ultrawide field fundus autofluorescence of the right eye demonstrating hypoautofluorescence along the superior temporal regions with diffuse stippled hyperautofluorescence in the remainder of the fundus.

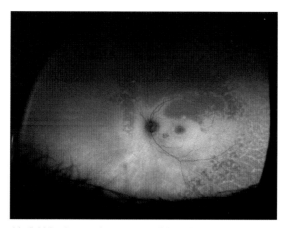

Fig. 27.6   Optos ultrawide field fundus autofluorescence of the left eye demonstrating hypoautofluorescence along the superior temporal regions with diffuse stippled hyperautofluorescence in the remainder of the fundus.

Multimodal Testing and Results

- Visual field testing: may demonstrate central, paracentral, or ring scotomas.[1-3]
- OCT: irregular/loss of outer retinal layers has been documented histologically[2] (photoreceptors, ellipsoid zone, external limiting membrane) and is observed on OCT.[4]
- Electroretinogram (ERG): with progressive damage, decreased and delayed rod and cone amplitudes may occur with a negative waveform. Multifocal ERG may be useful in cases where cones are predominantly involved.[1-3,5]
- Antiretinal antibody testing: Western blot, enzyme-linked immunosorbent assay, and immunohistochemistry testing is available at select laboratories. False-negative results are not uncommon.[1,2,6]
    - Positive autoantibodies against alpha enolase (46 kDa), carbonic anhydrase II (30 kDa), and glyceraldehyde 3-phosphate dehydrogenase (36 kDa), as well as autoantibodies against 56 kDa and 70 kDa proteins, obtained in this patient.

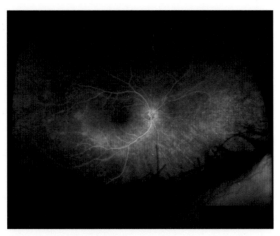

Fig. 27.7 Optos ultrawide field fluorescein angiogram of the right eye demonstrating stippled staining of the retina with no abnormalities of the optic nerve heads or vessels.

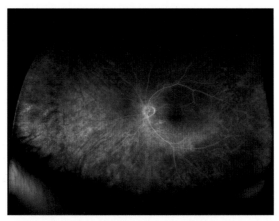

Fig. 27.8 Optos ultrawide field fluorescein angiogram of the left eye demonstrating stippled staining of the retina with no abnormalities of the optic nerve heads or vessels.

- Systemic workup for underlying malignancy in conjunction with a primary care provider or internist.[1-3]
  - No recurrence of new primary malignancies found in this patient.

Management

- Treatment of the underlying malignancy.[1-3]
- Treatment to stabilize vision is controversial. Immunomodulating therapy has been used and should be pursued with oncology guidance to prevent interference with treatment of the underlying malignancy or recurrence/metastasis.[1-3]
  - A trial of oral prednisone was commenced at 60 mg daily. It was gradually tapered over 6 weeks. Given the risk profile of immunomodulating medications and the patient's history of cancer and strong family history of cancer, the decision was made in conjunction with oncology to not pursue systemic immunomodulating therapy.

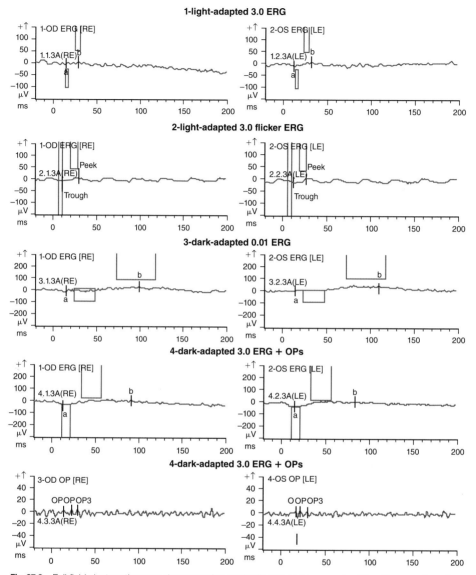

Fig. 27.9 Full field electroretinogram demonstrating markedly reduced cone and rod functions on all modes.

■ The patient was temporized with serial subtenon triamcinolone acetonide 40 mg/mL injections with approval request for intravitreal dexamethasone implant. The patient declined further treatment and was followed for 6 months total, then subsequently lost to follow-up.

Follow-up Care

The visual prognosis is often poor, and long-term prognosis can be challenging given mortality associated with the primary malignancy.[1-3]

Algorithm 27.1: Approach to Photopsias

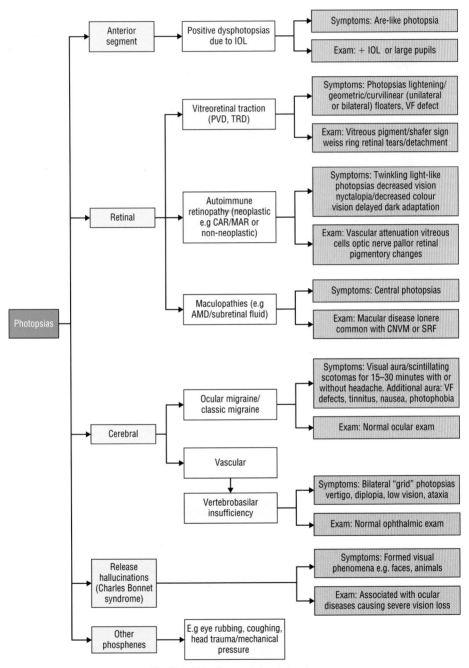

Algorithm 27.1 Approach to photopsias.

Key Points

- Patients with CAR and autoimmune retinopathy present with subacute visual decline. Depending on whether rods or cones are predominantly involved, symptoms may include positive visual phenomena, decreased vision and/or nyctalopia, peripheral visual field loss, and prolonged dark adaptation. The symptoms and findings tend to be bilateral but can be asymmetrical.[1-3]
- CAR is an uncommon paraneoplastic process where autoantibodies develop against the retina with resultant degeneration.[1-3]
- Early in the disease the fundus examination is normal. As the process progresses, arteriolar attenuation, mottled pigmentary retinal changes, and optic disc pallor result. Vitreous cell and low-grade anterior chamber cell may be present. Cystoid macular edema may occur.[1,6]
- The most common antigen in CAR is recoverin, a protein found in rods and cones. Additional autoantibodies include transducin-beta, carbonic anhydrase, alpha-enolase, arrestin, and heat-shock protein 70.[1-3,6]
- Common associated malignancies include small cell lung cancer (most common), non–small cell lung cancer, ovarian/endometrial/uterine carcinoma, breast carcinoma, and prostate carcinoma.[1-3,7]

References

1. Hecklenlively JR, Ferreyra HA. Autoimmune retinopathy: a review and summary. *Semin Immunopathol.* 2008;30:127-134.
2. Chan JW. Paraneoplastic retinopathies and optic neuropathies. *Surv Ophthalmol.* 2003;48(1):12-38.
3. Khan N, Huang JJ, Foster CS. Cancer associated retinopathy (CAR): an autoimmune-mediated paraneoplastic syndrome. *Semin Ophthalmol.* 2006;21:135-141.
4. Neena R, Jain A, Anantharaman G, Antony MA. Carcinoma-associated retinopathy (CAR): role of electroretinography (ERG) and optical coherence tomography (OCT) in diagnosis and predicting treatment outcome. *Am J Ophthalmol Case Rep.* 2021;21:101008.
5. Ferreyra HA, Jayasundera T, Kahn NW, et al. Management of autoimmune retinopathies with immunosuppression. *Arch Ophthalmol.* 2009;127(4):390-397.
6. Adamus G, Ren G, Weleber RG. Autoantibodies against retinal proteins in paraneoplastic and autoimmune retinopathy. *BMC Ophthalmol.* 2004;4:5.
7. Mohamed Q, Harper CA. Acute optical coherence tomographic findings in cancer-associated retinopathy. *Arch Ophthalmol.* 2007;125(8):1132-1133.

CHAPTER 28

Unilateral Paracentral Scotoma and Photopsia in a Young Woman With Myopia

Arthi D. Bharadwaj ▦ Maura Di Nicola ▦ Ann-Marie Lobo

History of Present Illness

We present a case of a 39-year-old woman with a past medical history of high myopia referred for evaluation of bilateral chorioretinitis. She reports symptoms of a paracentral scotoma and photopsias in the left eye. These symptoms had initially improved upon administration of oral prednisone. However, the patient experienced recurrent symptoms 5 months after initial treatment, and repeat oral steroids demonstrated limited efficacy. She denies any history of ocular surgeries.

OCULAR EXAMINATION FINDINGS

Best corrected visual acuity was 20/20 in both eyes. Intraocular pressure was within normal limits. External examination and slit lamp examination were unremarkable. Dilated fundus examination showed two hypopigmented, circumscribed lesions nasally in the right eye. Multiple well-defined, hypopigmented, round lesions nasal to the disc were noted in the left eye, with one lesion demonstrating blurred margins.

IMAGING

Fundus photographs captured ophthalmoscopic findings of hypopigmented, round lesions bilaterally, with blurred margins in one of the lesions in the left eye (Fig. 28.1A, B). Fundus autofluorescence demonstrated hypoautofluorescent, round lesions (Fig. 28.1C). Fluorescein angiography (FA) of the right eye was unremarkable. The left eye demonstrated multiple hypofluorescent lesions nasally with late staining (Fig. 28.1D, E). One lesion demonstrated early hyperfluorescence with mild late leakage. There was no evidence of choroidal neovascularization (CNV) on optical coherence tomography (OCT) or FA. Indocyanine green angiography (ICGA) of the right eye was unremarkable. In the left eye, multiple hypocyanescent lesions were seen nasally (Fig. 28.1F, G). OCT revealed normal foveal contour bilaterally (Fig. 28.1H, I). OCT over the hypopigmented lesions demonstrated chorioretinal nodules and atrophy of the outer retina (Fig. 28.1J, K).

Questions to Ask

- What is the patient's gender and refractive error? Punctate inner choroidopathy (PIC) affects individuals in all demographics but commonly presents in young women with myopia.[1,2]
  - Female
    - $-13.00 + 1.50 \times 78$ in the right eye and $-13.00 + 2.00 \times 100$ in the left eye

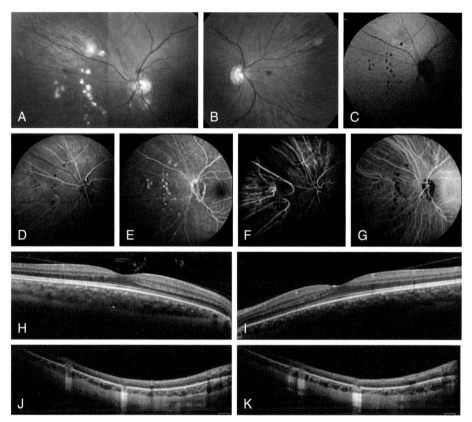

Fig. 28.1 Fundus photography shows hypopigmented, round lesions bilaterally (A–B). The lesions appear hypoautofluorescent on fundus autofluorescence (C), hypofluorescent with late staining on fluorescein angiography (D–E), and hypocyanescent on indocyanine green angiography (F–G). Optical coherence tomography demonstrates normal foveal contour bilaterally (H–I) with chorioretinal nodules and atrophy of the outer retina corresponding to the lesions (J–K).

- Does the patient have a recent history of infection or a family history of autoimmune disease? Similar to other white dot syndromes, PIC is theorized to be an autoimmune disease of genetic predisposition triggered by environmental stressors.[1]
  - There is no recent infection or family history of autoimmune disease.
  - QuantiFERON-TB Gold, *Treponema pallidum* antibodies, and rapid plasma reagin are negative, and angiotensin converting enzyme and lysozyme are normal.
- Are symptoms unilateral or bilateral? In PIC, symptoms typically present unilaterally despite it being a bilateral disease.[1,3]
  - Unilateral symptoms, bilateral disease
- Where is the inflammation located? In PIC, lesions are most often localized to the posterior pole without inflammation, as opposed to multifocal choroiditis (MFC), which can present with varying degrees of anterior chamber and vitreous inflammation and often has more peripherally located lesions.[1,2]
  - Peripapillary chorioretinal lesions without anterior chamber or vitreous inflammation
- Is CNV present? CNV represents a complication of PIC seen in 20% to 60% of cases, producing clinical symptoms of vision loss or metamorphopsia.[1,3,4]
  - No CNV is present.

Assessment

- This is a case of a 39-year-old woman with past ocular history significant for high myopia demonstrating bilateral PIC without CNV.

Differential Diagnosis

- MFC and panuveitis
- Presumed ocular histoplasmosis syndrome
- Sarcoidosis
- Birdshot chorioretinopathy
- Tuberculosis
- Progressive subretinal fibrosis and uveitis syndrome
- Acute posterior multifocal placoid pigment epitheliopathy
- Myopic degeneration
- Multiple evanescent white dot syndrome
- Serpiginous choroiditis

Working Diagnosis

- PIC (alternative names: punctate inner choroiditis, multifocal inner choroiditis)

Multimodal Testing and Results

- Fundus photographs
  - Fundus photography in patients with PIC shows multiple small, yellow-white lesions. In the acute phase, these lesions appear yellow or white with indistinct borders, whereas in the chronic phase, these areas become well defined and atrophic with variable pigmentation.[4]
- Fundus autofluorescence
  - Active lesions demonstrate slight hyperautofluorescence, whereas inactive, atrophic lesions appear hypoautofluorescent.[5]
  - Reactivation of a previously inactive lesion may present with a ring of hyperautofluorescence surrounding an area of hypoautofluorescence.[1]
- OCT
  - OCT can identify the structure of lesions, detect disease recurrence before clinical presentation, and help assess disease stage.
  - In the acute phase, OCT demonstrates the accumulation of inflammatory material between the Bruch membrane and the retinal pigment epithelium, with subsequent involvement of the subretinal space and outer retina.[5]
  - When the atrophic, punched-out lesions develop, outer retina atrophy and increased signal transmission are demonstrated on OCT.
  - The presence of CNV can be detected on OCT with the presence of subretinal hyperreflective material and subretinal and intraretinal fluid.
- Optical coherence tomography angiography (OCTA)
  - Consider OCTA to distinguish inflammatory infiltrate from CNV, as the treatment for each varies. OCTA has been shown to detect the presence of CNV in patients with inconclusive multimodal imaging.[1]
- FA
  - In the acute phase, PIC lesions usually appear hyperfluorescent in the early phase with staining or leakage in the late phase. Occasionally, they may display blocked fluorescence early.[1,2]

- In the chronic phase of the disease, the circular lesions become atrophic and demonstrate window defects on FA.
- CNV on PIC is often classic (type 2) and exhibits a lacy pattern of early hyperfluorescence with late leakage unless blocked by the presence of subretinal hemorrhage.[6]
- ICGA
  - ICGA shows hypocyanescent circular spots that can be more numerous than seen clinically.[7]
  - Hypocyanescence in the early and late phases suggests choroidal hypoperfusion. Hypercyanescent spots on choroidal vessels may indicate a vasculitic process.[1,2]

Management

- Presentation of a new or active PIC lesion, especially if it threatens vision or with secondary CNV, warrants interventions such as systemic or local corticosteroids, corticosteroid-sparing immunosuppressive therapy, anti–vascular endothelial growth factor (VEGF) intravitreal therapy, or photodynamic therapy.[1]
  - Our patient presented with mild, residual inflammation in the left eye and elected to undergo one more course of systemic steroids with slow taper. For a subsequent flare that presented with a new macular lesion showing hyperautofluorescence on fundus autofluorescence and visible as an outer retinal nodule with shadowing into the choroid on OCT (Fig. 28.2A-C), she had a periocular steroid injection to avoid side effects of systemic corticosteroids. The lesion resolved after treatment (Fig. 28.2D).
- Cases of PIC without active or vision-threatening lesions and without CNV can be observed.[1,2]
- Steroid treatment, either systemic or local, is often used as first-line therapy in the acute phase of the disease.[1]
- Local treatment with intravitreal or periocular corticosteroids can be a viable option for patients with contraindications to systemic treatment or pregnant patients.
- Consider corticosteroid-sparing immunomodulatory therapy (IMT) for patients with contraindications to corticosteroids or requiring maintenance therapy for frequent recurrence.[1,4]
- Multiple studies report efficacy of anti-VEGF intravitreal injections for PIC complicated by CNV.[1,2]

Follow-up Care

- There is no standardized treatment or follow-up protocol for PIC.
- Follow-up care varies based on the patient's symptoms and treatment course (local or systemic corticosteroids, IMT, anti-VEGF).
- Patients on high-dose systemic steroids need close follow-up to monitor response to and possible side effects from treatment. The goal should be to taper and discontinue corticosteroids.

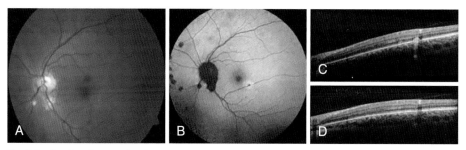

Fig. 28.2 Fundus photography demonstrating a new, active macular lesion (A). The lesion is hyperautofluorescent on fundus autofluorescence and is visible as an outer retinal nodule on optical coherence tomography (OCT) (B–C). OCT demonstrates complete resolution of the nodule after periocular steroid injection (D).

- Patients on IMT (e.g., methotrexate, mycophenolate mofetil) require close follow-up and laboratory monitoring (every 6–12 weeks) for potential side effects.
- Anti-VEGF injections are initially administered every 4 weeks for CNV. The treatment interval is then adjusted based on the response of the lesion to the medication, as monitored by OCT.
- Our patient was initially followed every 6 to 8 weeks, with a progressive increase in the follow-up interval.

Algorithm 28.1 Algorithm Representing Differential Diagnosis for Punctate Inner Choroidopathy (PIC)

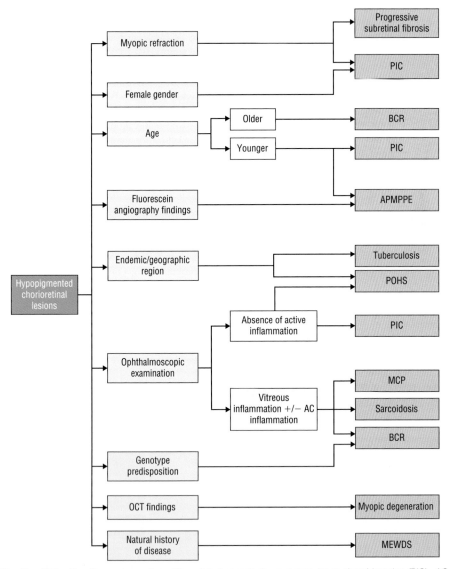

Algorithm 28.1   Algorithm representing differential diagnosis for punctate inner choroidopathy *(PIC)*. *AC,* Anterior chamber; *APMPPE,* acute posterior multifocal placoid pigment epitheliopathy; *BCR,* birdshot chorioretinopathy; *MCP,* multifocal choroiditis and panuveitis; *MEWDS,* multiple evanescent white dot syndrome; *OCT,* optical coherence tomography; *POHS,* presumed ocular histoplasmosis syndrome.

Key Points

- Although PIC commonly presents in young women with myopia, the disease is rare and may be underdiagnosed in other demographics.[1,4]
- When complicated by CNV, PIC may resolve spontaneously or rapidly progress to severe vision loss. Thus the disease requires early detection and frequent monitoring by OCT and autofluorescence imaging.[1,3]
- Treat new or active vision-threatening PIC lesions with oral or local corticosteroids; IMT can be used for long-term management.[1,2]
- Consider local treatment (intravitreal or periocular steroids) if there are contraindications to systemic therapy.
- Consider anti-VEGF therapy for CNV secondary to PIC.[1,2]

References

1. Ahnood D, Madhusudhan S, Tsaloumas MD, et al. Punctate inner choroidopathy: a review. *Surv Ophthalmol*. 2017;62(2):113-126.
2. Campos J, Campos A, Mendes S, et al. Punctate inner choroidopathy: a systematic review. *Med Hypothesis Discov Innov Ophthalmol*. 2014;3(3):76-82.
3. Baxter SL, Pistilli M, Pujari SS, et al. Risk of choroidal neovascularization among the uveitidies. *Am J Ophthalmol*. 2013;156(3):468-477.
4. Mount GR, Kaufman EJ. White dot syndromes. In: *StatPearls*. StatPearls Publishing. Updated March 13, 2023. Accessed May 10, 2023. Available at: https://www.ncbi.nlm.nih.gov/books/NBK557854/.
5. Spaide RF, Goldberg N, Freund KB. Redefining multifocal choroiditis and panuveitis and punctate inner choroidopathy through multimodal imaging. *Retina*. 2013;33(7):1315-1324.
6. Olsen TW, Capone A, Sternberg P, et al. Subfoveal choroidal neovascularization in punctate inner choroidopathy. *Ophthalmology*. 1996;103(12):2061-2069.
7. Raven ML, Ringeisen AL, Yonekawa Y, et al. Multi-modal imaging and anatomic classification of the white dot syndromes. *Int J Retina Vitreous*. 2017;3:12.

CHAPTER 29

Persistent Bilateral Flashes With Vitreous Cell and Haze

Karl N. Becker ■ Pooja Bhat

History of Present Illness

A 69-year-old White woman with no significant past medical history was referred by an outside ophthalmologist for evaluation and management of bilateral photopsias of 3 months' duration. She reported mild blurring of her vision that had not resolved after obtaining new eyeglasses. She noted no floaters, pain, or photophobia and had no history of ocular surgery or procedures. She denied nyctalopia. Her family history was remarkable for an aunt with age-related macular degeneration.

OCULAR EXAMINATION FINDINGS

Visual acuity with correction was 20/25 in both eyes, pupils were reactive without afferent pupillary defect, but confrontation visual fields were constricted. Intraocular pressures were 9 in the right eye (OD) and 12 in the left eye (OS). There was no evidence of inflammation in the anterior segment of either eye, although trace nuclear sclerosis was noted in both eyes (OU). Dilated examination showed bilateral 2+ anterior and posterior vitreous cells and 2+ central vitreous haze. Fundus examination showed several small drusen along the arcades OU, few intermediate-sized drusen OU, and a large druse OD. The remainder of her examination, including that of optic discs, vasculature, macula, and periphery, was otherwise unremarkable (Fig. 29.1, color fundus photographs). No tears, holes, or breaks were identified in either eye.

IMAGING

Fluorescein angiography (FA) showed bilateral late staining of the discs and staining with leakage of the retinal venules, which was greater in the right eye. Indocyanine green angiography (ICGA) was performed showing numerous scattered nummular hypocyanescent lesions nasal to the disc OU as well as within the periphery.

Optical coherence tomography (OCT) of each eye showed a few drusen and no cystoid macular edema (CME).

Questions to Ask

■ Does the patient have a history of systemic inflammatory disease, including sarcoidosis, or other systemic diseases, such as central nervous system lymphoma, that may be related to intraocular disease? Does the patient have a history of symptoms consistent with any of these diseases, including shortness of breath, cough, rashes, or joint pain and swelling?
  ■ No

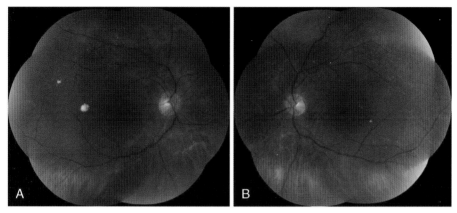

Fig. 29.1 Color montage images of the right (A) and left (B) eyes. (A) shows vitreous haze, several small drusen along the arcades, few intermediate drusen, and a large druse. (B) shows clear vitreous, as well as few small and intermediate drusen.

- Does the patient have family history of systemic inflammatory disease?
  - No
- Does the patient have a history of systemic infection, including tuberculosis (TB) or syphilis? Does the patient have risks for exposure to these infections, including being from an endemic area (another country for TB), or high-risk sexual behavior? Does the patient have a history of symptoms consistent with these infections?
  - No

Assessment

- A 69-year-old woman with no past medical history presents with mild blurred vision and persistent photopsias. Clinical findings include vitreous haze with inflammation, FA with optic nerve staining and vascular leakage, and ICGA with numerous hypocyanescent lesions nasal to the disc OU and within the periphery.

Differential Diagnosis

- Birdshot chorioretinopathy (BSCR)
- Ocular sarcoidosis
- TB choroiditis
- Primary vitreoretinal lymphoma

Working Diagnosis

- Birdshot chorioretinopathy

Multimodal Testing and Results

- Fundus photographs
  - Classically seen "birdshot lesions" of hypopigmented lesions surrounding and nasal to the optic disc were not seen in this patient. There was no evidence of retinal vasculitis on fundus examination.

- OCT
  - This patient's OCT showed no CME, a common complication of BSCR seen in 84% of patients.[1]
- Fundus autofluorescence (FAF)
  - FAF imaging obtained at patient presentation showed no abnormalities outside the hyperautofluorescence of the drusen in the right eye (Figs. 29.2 and 29.3). FAF findings in other patients may include hypoautofluorescence of the birdshot lesions.
- FA
  - FA for our patient showed typical signs of posterior segment inflammation, including disc hyperfluorescence and perivenular leakage.[2]

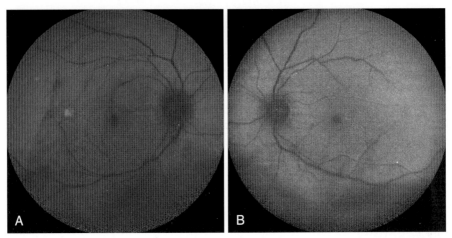

Fig. 29.2 Fundus autofluorescence images of the right (A) and left (B) eyes. (A) shows hyperautofluorescence of the temporal druse. (B) shows normal fundus autofluorescence with no remarkable findings.

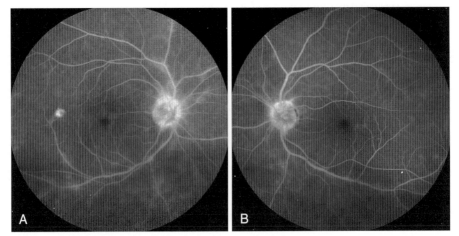

Fig. 29.3 Late fundus fluorescein angiogram images of the right (A) and left (B) eyes. (A) shows staining of the temporal large druse, staining of the nerve, and leakage of the larger venules. (B) shows staining of the nerve, and leakage of the larger venules.

- ICGA
    - ICGA was revealing of the diagnosis for our patient, displaying characteristic hypocyanescent birdshot lesions surrounding and nasal to the disc and within the periphery. ICGA can often show more numerous lesions than seen on clinical examination.[3] In the case of our patient, no birdshot lesions were seen on fundus examination, but ICGA was diagnostic of the condition (Fig. 29.4).
- Optical coherence tomography angiography (OCTA)
    - OCTA was not performed initially for this patient, but typical findings can include capillary loops and telangiectatic vessels in the superficial capillary plexus and deep capillary plexus.[4] On later imaging for this patient, increased intercapillary spaces and flow voids in the choriocapillaris were observed.[4,5]

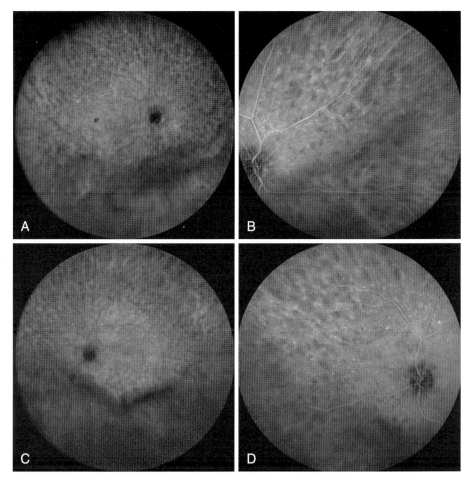

Fig. 29.4   Late indocyanine green angiography images of both eyes showing characteristic hypocyanescent birdshot lesions surrounding and nasal to the disc. Shown are right eye wide field (A) and higher-magnification (B) images, as well as left eye wide field (C) and high-magnification (D) images.

- Electroretinogram (ERG)
  - Testing revealed much-reduced rod B wave amplitudes and cone B wave amplitudes in the lower limit of normal in each eye, with slightly reduced 30-Hz implicit times observed, all of which can be typical changes.
- Visual field testing
  - Baseline Goldman visual field testing showed a full field OD and slight inferonasal constriction OS.

Management

- Patient had testing that showed HLA-A29 positivity, as well as negative infectious markers for syphilis and TB.
- The patient was started on systemic corticosteroids on her initial visit. At the next visit, she noted decreased photopsias.
- Patient was started on mycophenolate mofetil and increased to 1.5 g twice daily. With tapering of her oral steroids, increased photopsias were noted, and local steroid injection was pursued with posterior subtenon triamcinolone acetonide.
- The patient was eventually started on infliximab and the dose was increased to 10 mg/kg every 4 weeks.

Follow-up Care

- Patient has continued to follow up every 1 to 3 months depending on disease activity, with FAs performed to evaluate for retinal vasculitis. ERG and visual fields are performed annually.

Key Points

- Birdshot chorioretinopathy lesions may be undetectable on fundus examination, FA, and FAF. ICGA may be necessary to visualize birdshot lesions.
- Birdshot chorioretinopathy should be considered in patients with persistent photopsias and evidence of inflammation, especially older White women.
- Patients should be followed on a regular basis and at shorter intervals based on clinical findings, along with yearly ERG and visual field testing.

Algorithm 29.1: Algorithm for Photopsias

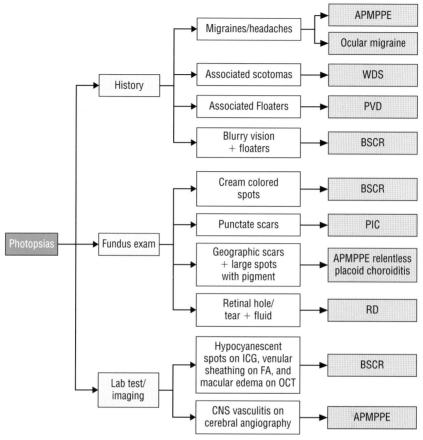

Algorithm 29.1   Algorithm for photopsias.

References

1. Rothova A, Berendschot TT, Probst K, van Kooij B, Baarsma GS. Birdshot chorioretinopathy: long-term manifestations and visual prognosis. *Ophthalmology*. 2004;111(5):954-959.
2. Priem HA, Oosterhuis JA. Birdshot chorioretinopathy: clinical characteristics and evolution. *Br J Ophthalmol*. 1988;72(9):646-659.
3. Herbort CP, Mantovani A, Papadia M. Use of indocyanine green angiography in uveitis. *Int Ophthalmol Clin*. 2012;52(4):13-31.
4. Pohlmann D, Macedo S, Stübiger N, Pleyer U, Joussen AM, Winterhalter S. Multimodal imaging in birdshot retinochoroiditis. *Ocul Immunol Inflamm*. 2017;25(5):621-632.
5. de Carlo TE, Bonini Filho MA, Adhi M, Duker JS. Retinal and choroidal vasculature in birdshot chorioretinopathy analyzed using spectral domain optical coherence tomography angiography. *Retina*. 2015;35(11):2392-2399.

CHAPTER 30

Sudden-Onset Bilateral Scotomas With Punched-Out, Pigmented Lesions

Pooja Bhat   ■   Ricky Z. Cui

History of Present Illness

We present a case of a 38-year-old Parisian man with an unremarkable past medical history referred for management of multifocal choroiditis (MFC). While in Paris in 2011, he experienced sudden-onset scotomas bilaterally with a prodrome of headaches without neck pain. He denied fevers, redness, pain, photophobia, photopsia, metamorphopsia, or floaters. He underwent two oral steroid tapers and was transitioned to azathioprine, which was stopped because of drug-induced pancreatitis. Our patient was then started on mycophenolate mofetil.

OCULAR EXAMINATION FINDINGS

Visual acuity without correction was 20/20 in both eyes. Intraocular pressure was normal. External and anterior segment examination was unremarkable. Dilated fundus examination showed bilateral peripapillary atrophy with punctate scars surrounding the optic disc; pigmented, punched-out confluent scars within the macula but sparing the fovea; and prominent choroidal pattern, MFC-type scars in the posterior pole and midperiphery without vitreous cell or haze (Fig. 30.1A and B).

PREVIOUS TESTING

Our patient had elevated angiotensin-converting enzyme levels with no hilar lymphadenopathy noted on computed tomography of the lung. Biopsy of the accessory salivary gland was normal. Other normal/negative tests include lumbar puncture, antineutrophilic cytoplasmic antibody, antinuclear antibodies, and extensive infectious disease workup.

Questions to Ask

- Is the patient from a region endemic to histoplasmosis, or has he had exposure to bats (e.g., while spelunking)? The lesions in MFC can resemble presumed ocular histoplasmosis syndrome. In fact, the term MFC was initially used to describe eyes with presumed ocular histoplasmosis syndrome (POHS).[1]
  - No

- Are the fundus lesions confined to the posterior pole? It can be difficult to distinguish punctate inner choroidopathy (PIC) and MFC, but patients with PIC are typically myopic women with smaller lesions confined to the posterior pole without associated intraocular inflammation.[2]
    - No, the lesions are large, confluent, and present in the posterior pole as well as the mid-periphery without intraocular inflammation.
- Did the patient have any recent travel history before the onset of symptoms? This information is helpful for an infectious workup, including tuberculosis (TB), toxoplasmosis, and West Nile virus.
    - The patient traveled to Vietnam shortly before the onset of his symptoms, but extensive infectious disease workup, including purified protein derivative skin testing and QuantiFERON-TB Gold, was negative.
- Does the patient have a history of cancer? Malignancies have been reported as masquerade syndromes of MFC.[3]
    - No

Assessment

- This is a case of a 38-year-old man with no past medical history demonstrating bilateral idiopathic MFC.

Differential Diagnosis

- Infectious
    - TB
    - POHS
    - Syphilis
    - Pneumocystis choroiditis
    - West Nile virus
    - Recurrent toxoplasmosis
- Noninfectious
    - Sarcoidosis
    - Birdshot chorioretinopathy (can resemble active MFC)
    - Acute posterior multifocal placoid pigment epitheliopathy with progression to relentless placoid chorioretinopathy
    - PIC
- Malignant
    - Lymphoma
    - Metastasis

Working Diagnosis

- Idiopathic MFC

Multimodal Testing and Results

- Fundus photographs
    - Fundus examination showed bilateral peripapillary atrophy with adjacent scarring, punched-out pigmented scars within the macula (following blood vessels) with sparring of the fovea, and prominent choroidal pattern, MFC-type scars of varying sizes in the posterior pole and midperiphery (Fig. 30.1A, B).

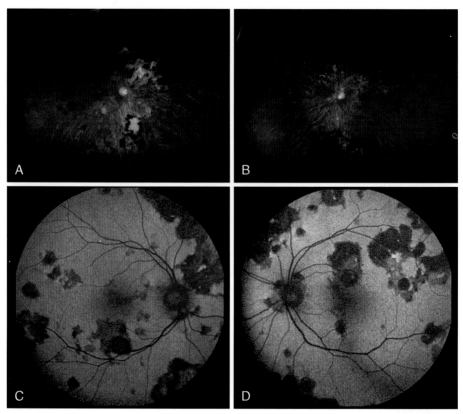

Fig. 30.1 Fundus and fundus autofluorescence photographs from the initial encounter. (A) Right eye demonstrates peripapillary atrophy with punctate scars around the optic disc. The macula has pigmented, punched-out, occasionally confluent scars with sparing of the fovea. Prominent choroidal pattern, multifocal choroiditis–type scars are seen in the posterior pole and midperiphery, following blood vessels, without evidence of sheathing, snowballs, or active granulomas. (B) Left eye has large confluent scars superonasal and inferior to the optic disc with prominent choroidal pattern, punctate scars temporally following the blood vessels, without evidence of sheathing or granulomas. (C) Right eye demonstrates no area of hyperautofluorescence. (D) Left eye did not demonstrate hyperautofluorescence within the fovea but shows hyperautofluorescence within a scar at the termination of the superotemporal arcade.

- Active lesions are typically yellow-white because of choroidal lesions with blurred margins due to overlying retinal edema, whereas inactive lesions are gray with more defined borders. Punctate hemorrhages can occasionally be visualized.[4]
- Fundus autofluorescence
  - Left eye showed an area of hyperautofluorescence within a scar at the termination of the superotemporal arcade; right eye did not show hyperautofluorescence within the fovea (Fig. 30.1C, D).
  - In active disease, diffuse hyperautofluorescent lesions can be seen in the peripapillary region and posterior pole with late staining of the optic nerve. As the inflammation subsides, the lesions become atrophic and hypoautofluorescent.[5]
- Optical coherence tomography (OCT)
  - OCT showed foveal sparing scars with focal loss of outer retina in the right eye and foveal sparing scars with focal loss of outer and inner retina in the left eye (Fig. 30.2).

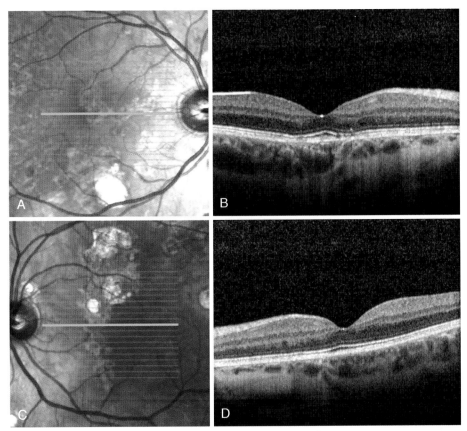

Fig. 30.2 Optical coherence tomography (OCT) macula from the initial encounter. (A) Infrared image of the right eye corresponding to the findings on OCT macula. (B) Right eye demonstrates focal loss of outer retina at the level of the scar with sparing of the fovea. (C) Infrared image of the left eye corresponding to the findings on OCT macula. (D) Left eye demonstrates multiple foveal-sparing scars within the macula with punched-out loss of the outer retina, as well as several areas with inner retina involvement.

- In active lesions, retinal pigment epithelium (RPE) elevation can be seen because of deposition of material in the sub-RPE space. Subretinal or sub-RPE material with associated fluid is suggestive of choroidal neovascular membrane (CNVM).[6]
- Fluorescein angiography (FA)
  - FA demonstrated staining of the multifocal scars bilaterally without any leakage (Fig. 30.3).
  - Acute inflammatory lesions typically have minimal early hyperfluorescence but display late staining, which may be indicative of active CNVM.[7]
- Indocyanine green angiography (ICG)
  - Lesions in both eyes were hypocyanescent in the early and late phase (Fig. 30.4).
  - Active CNVM typically presents with late hypercyanescence.[8]
- Electroretinogram (ERG)
  - Our patient did not undergo ERG testing. Patients with MFC may have normal, moderately reduced, or severely reduced ERGs.[9]

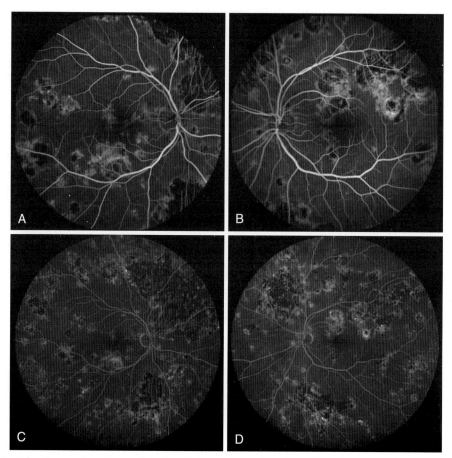

Fig. 30.3 Fluorescein angiogram from the initial encounter, early and late phase. (A) Right eye demonstrates early staining of the multifocal scars. (B) Left eye also demonstrates early staining. (C) The multifocal scars in the right eye did not demonstrate leakage of fluorescein dye. (D) Leakage was not noted in the left eye.

- Goldmann visual field (GVF)
  - GVF revealed existing blind spots without expansion and no new blind spots (Fig. 30.5).
  - Visual fields are important to track disease progression and monitor for development of optic neuropathy, which is an uncommon complication of MFC.[10]

Management

- The patient was on oral mycophenolate mofetil 1 gram two times daily, oral prednisone 10 mg, and oral potassium on presentation.
- Given continued disease inactivity, our goal was to achieve steroid-free disease remission while on systemic immunomodulatory therapy.
- Oral mycophenolate mofetil was increased to the full dose of 1.5 gram two times daily, and oral prednisone was tapered slowly because the patient had flared in the past with taper of oral steroid.

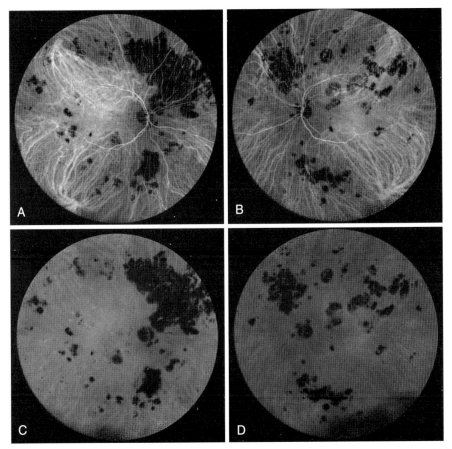

Fig. 30.4   Indocyanine green angiography (ICG) from the initial encounter. (A) ICG of the right eye shows multiple hypocyanescent lesions. (B) Left eye also demonstrates multiple hypocyanescent lesions. (C) Right eye lesions are hypocyanescent in the late phase. (D) Left eye lesions are also hypocyanescent in the late phase.

- Oral corticosteroids are the first line for treatment. Periocular or intraocular corticosteroid injections or implants can be used as local anti-inflammatory therapy.[6]
- Immunomodulator therapy should be considered for steroid-dependent, severe, or refractory cases.[11]
- Intravitreal anti–vascular endothelial growth factor therapy is used for treatment of choroidal neovascularization and macular edema.[12]

Follow-up Care

- Our patient was followed closely every 3 months with dilated fundus examination, fundus autofluorescence, and OCT macula.
- We obtained FA + ICG yearly (or sooner if we were suspected a flare of the disease) and GVF tests.
- Because the patient is treated with mycophenolate mofetil, high-risk monitoring labs (complete blood count, comprehensive metabolic panel) every 8 to 12 weeks were obtained.

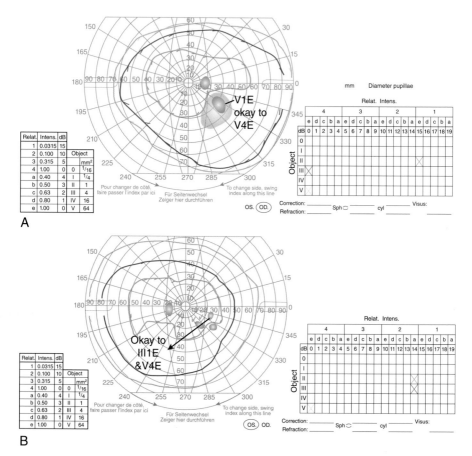

Fig. 30.5 Goldmann visual field test. (A) Right eye demonstrates an inferotemporal relative scotoma that does not show expansion compared with previous studies. No new scotomas were detected. (B) Left eye demonstrates stable inferonasal relative scotomas without new blind spots.

Algorithm 30.1: Differential Diagnosis for Multifocal Choroiditis

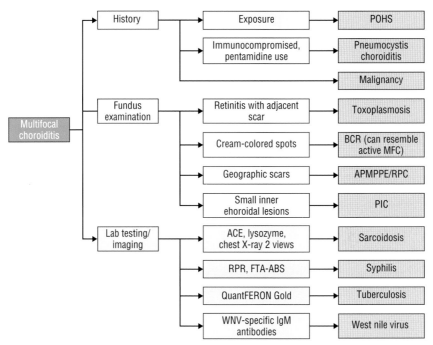

Algorithm 30.1 Differential diagnosis for multifocal choroiditis. *ACE,* angiotensin-converting enzyme; *APMPPE,* acute posterior multifocal placoid pigment epitheliopathy; *BSCR,* birdshot chorioretinopathy; *FTA-ABS,* fluorescent treponemal antibody absorption; *IgM,* immunoglobulin M; *MFC,* multifocal choroiditis; *PIC,* punctate inner choroidopathy; *POHS,* presumed ocular histoplasmosis syndrome; *RPC,* relentless placoid chorioretinitis; *RPR,* rapid plasma reagin; *WNV,* West Nile virus.

Key Points

- MFC is a phenotypic description and is distinct from PIC with larger size of lesions seen in MFC, distributed within the posterior pole and periphery, and associated intraocular inflammation.
- It is important to rule out infectious, inflammatory, and malignant processes in patients with suspected MFC because it is a diagnosis of exclusion.
- Immunomodulatory therapy is important for steroid-free disease remission in severe or refractory cases.
- In the absence of CNVM and scarring, patients may have a good visual prognosis.
- Patients should be followed on a regular basis with dilated fundus examinations and multimodal testing to monitor for disease progression.

References

1. Essex RW, Wong J, Jampol LM, Dowler J, Bird AC. Idiopathic multifocal choroiditis: a comment on present and past nomenclature. *Retina.* 2013;33(1):1-4.
2. Gilbert RM, Niederer RL, Kramer M, et al. Differentiating multifocal choroiditis and punctate inner choroidopathy: a cluster analysis approach. *Am J Ophthalmol.* 2020;213:244-251.
3. Browning DJ, Fraser CM. Primary intraocular lymphoma mimicking multifocal choroiditis and panuveitis. *Eye.* 2007;21(6):880-881.
4. Li J, Li Y, Li H, Zhang L. Imageology features of different types of multifocal choroiditis. *BMC Ophthalmol.* 2019;19(1):39.
5. Kramer M, Priel E. Fundus autofluorescence imaging in multifocal choroiditis: beyond the spots. *Ocul Immunol Inflamm.* 2014;22(5):349-355.
6. Tavallali A, Yannuzzi LA. Idiopathic multifocal choroiditis. *J Ophthalmic Vis Res.* 2016;11(4):429-432.
7. Dolz-Marco R, Fine HF, Freund KB. How to differentiate myopic choroidal neovascularization, idiopathic multifocal choroiditis, and punctate inner choroidopathy using clinical and multimodal imaging findings. *Ophthalmic Surg Lasers Imaging Retina.* 2017;48(3):196-201.
8. Slakter JS, Giovannini A, Yannuzzi LA, et al. Indocyanine green angiography of multifocal choroiditis. *Ophthalmology.* 1997;104(11):1813-1819.
9. Gilbert RM, Niederer RL, Kramer M, et al. Differentiating Multifocal Choroiditis and Punctate Inner Choroidopathy: A Cluster Analysis Approach. *Am J Ophthalmol.* 2020;213:244-251.
10. Thorne JE, Wittenberg S, Kedhar SR, Dunn JP, Jabs DA. Optic neuropathy complicating multifocal choroiditis and panuveitis (MFCPU). *Am J Ophthalmol.* 2007;143(4):721-723.
11. Jabs DA, Rosenbaum JT, Foster CS, et al. Guidelines for the use of immunosuppressive drugs in patients with ocular inflammatory disorders: recommendations of an expert panel. *Am J Ophthalmol.* 2000;130:492-513.
12. Parodi MB, Iacono P, Kontadakis DS, et al. Bevacizumab vs. photodynamic therapy for choroidal neovascularization in multifocal choroiditis. *Arch Ophthalmol.* 2010;128:1100-1103.

CHAPTER 31

Bilateral Munir-Focal Serous Retinal Detachments

Daniel W. Wang ▓ William F. Mieler

History of Present Illness

A 36-year-old female patient with an unremarkable past medical history and past ocular history presents with blurry vision of both eyes. Her symptoms were acute in onset and have been progressive over the past week. She endorses generalized malaise, fatigue, mild photophobia, and worsening headaches.

OCULAR EXAMINATION FINDINGS

Visual acuity with correction was 20/200 in the right eye and 20/60 in the left eye, with no improvement with pinhole. Intraocular pressure was normal at 12 and 14, respectively. Pupils were round, equal, and reactive without a relative afferent pupillary defect. External examination was unremarkable. Anterior segment examination showed trace anterior chamber cell and flare in both eyes but otherwise was unremarkable. Dilated fundus examination showed vitreous cell in both eyes. Both optic nerves appeared hyperemic with mild blurring of the disc margins. Cystoid macular edema along with subretinal fluid was appreciated in the macula region. Vessels appeared mildly tortuous but with normal course and caliber. Shallow inferior subretinal fluid was appreciated in the periphery of both retinas.

Questions to Ask

- What is the patient's ethnic background? There is thought to be a genetic predisposition to the pathogenesis of Vogt-Koyanagi-Harada (VKH) disease. Multiple interleukin genes and human leukocyte antigens are associated with VKH in different ethnic populations, especially in Asian, Middle Eastern, Native American, and Hispanic populations.[1,2] The typical age of onset is between 20 to 50 with a woman predisposition.
  - The patient was Hispanic and in her mid-30s.
- Does the patient have prodromal symptoms? Uveitic conditions such as acute posterior multifocal placoid pigment epitheliopathy (APMPPE) may present with prodromal symptoms such as headaches, fever, nausea, tinnitus, and neck stiffness.
  - The patient reported generalized malaise, fever, and headaches 4 days before the development of ocular symptoms.
- Does the patient have a history of ocular trauma or previous surgery? History of ocular trauma or intraocular surgery should be obtained in the consideration of sympathetic ophthalmia, which may have a similar ocular presentation and shared pathophysiology to VKH.
  - None

- What medications does the patient take? High-dose steroids may precipitate subretinal fluid accumulation in the setting for central serous chorioretinopathy.
  - None
- What is the patient's refractive error? Nanophthalmic eyes are at risk for developing uveal effusion syndrome.
  - The patient had myopia, wearing −3.25 D prescription glasses.

Assessment

- This is a case of a 36-year-old Hispanic female patient with no past ocular or surgical history presenting with generalized malaise and bilateral serous retinal detachments.

Differential Diagnosis

- Vogt-Koyanagi-Harada (VKH) disease
- APMPPE
- Sympathetic ophthalmia
- Central serous chorioretinopathy
- Panuveitis secondary to infection (e.g., syphilis, tuberculosis, *Bartonella*), secondary to autoimmune conditions (sarcoidosis, systemic lupus erythematosus) or secondary to malignancy
- Posterior scleritis
- Myopic retinoschisis
- Optic pit maculopathy

Working Diagnosis

- VKH disease

Multimodal Testing and Results

- Fundus photographs
  - Color fundus photographs were taken at presentation: right eye with disk edema and hyperemia along with subretinal fluid extending from the disk temporally through the macula (Fig. 31.1). Focal serous retinal detachment was noted inferiorly as well. The left eye had disk edema, hyperemia, and an inferior serous detachment (Fig. 31.2).
- OCT
  - Right eye showing serous retinal detachment with foveal involvement with overlying intraretinal fluid. Left eye has serous subretinal fluid with foveal involvement (Fig. 31.3). In the acute uveitic phase, significant choroidal thickening and serous retinal detachments will be observed. Characteristic septations may be seen, thought to be fibrin membranes and inflammatory products, creating lobular structures.[3,4]
- Fluorescein angiography (FA)
  - Classically, multifocal choroidal hyperfluorescent dots may be visualized in the early phase followed by multiple focal hyperfluorescent areas with diffuse leakage in the late phase.[2,5] FA in the chronic-recurrent stage of VKH disease may demonstrate various nonspecific window defects secondary to choroidal neovascularization, retinal pigment epithelium atrophy, neovascularization, and subretinal fibrosis.[3,4]

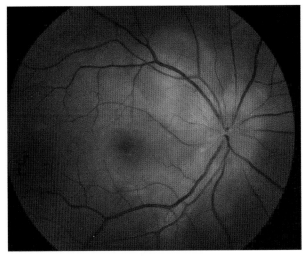

Fig. 31.1 Fundus photograph of the right eye demonstrating optic nerve head edema with hyperemia. Subretinal fluid is appreciated in the macula along with a focal serous retinal detachment along the superior vascular arcade.

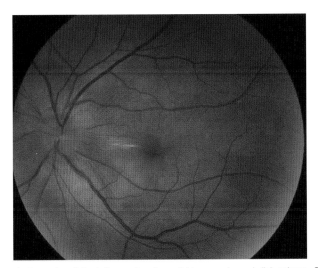

Fig. 31.2 Fundus photographs of the left eye showing mild hyperemia and disk edema. Subretinal fluid is observed extending from the disc to the macula.

Management

Workup for other causes of ocular inflammation, including infectious and autoimmune, is essential. Erythrocyte sedimentation rate, C-reactive protein, QuantiFERON-TB Gold, rapid plasma reagin, fluorescent treponemal antibody, angiotensin-converting enzyme, chest x-ray,

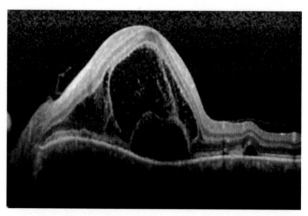

Fig. 31.3 Optical coherence tomography of the right macula demonstrating a serous retinal detachment with multiple septae of overlying intraretinal fluid and disruption of the outer retinal layers.

antinuclear antibody, and p-/c–antineutrophil cytoplasmic antibodies should be obtained. In equivocal cases, a lumbar puncture can be performed to look for lymphocytic and monocytic pleocytosis in the cerebrospinal fluid.[6]

Treatment goals in VKH revolve around early inflammation suppression and the prevention of recurrence to ward off the sequelae of secondary complications such as glaucoma, retinal detachment, and choroidal neovascularization. General management involving systemic corticosteroid treatment is preferred, particularly during the acute uveitic stage. Earlier studies have shown that the route of corticosteroid administration (oral or intravenous [IV]) does not affect final visual acuity or the recurrence of disease in the treatment of acute VKH.[7] IV methylprednisone administration for 3 days followed by high-dose oral prednisone is often given for severe disease. The steroid dose should be slowly tapered over 6 months to prevent recurrence.[8] Because of the chronicity of the disease, antimetabolites, biologics, tumor necrosis factor–alpha inhibitors, and other steroid-sparing agents may be employed early, and the patient should be carefully monitored for regular blood work in conjunction with the rheumatology department.[3] Intravitreal and subtenon injections of triamcinolone may be considered in recalcitrant disease and/or in patients who cannot undergo or tolerate systemic agents.[2,4,9] Adjunctive topical steroids and cycloplegics may decrease inflammation in the anterior chamber and decrease photophobia.

Follow-up Care

Close and frequent follow-up is required early during the acute uveitic phase to track treatment efficacy during the initiation and taper of systemic therapies. Regular blood work should be obtained during the administration of immunosuppressant agents and often is managed in conjunction with an internist to watch for potential complications or side effects from the treatment. The patient should additionally closely be monitored for ocular complications secondary to persistent or recurrent intraocular inflammation such as cataracts, secondary glaucoma, and choroidal neovascular membranes.

Algorithm 31.1: Applicable Differential Diagnosis for Serous Retinal Detachment

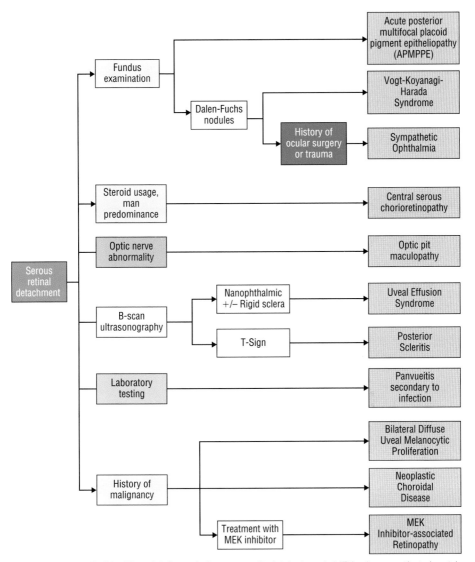

Algorithm 31.1   Applicable differential diagnosis for serous retinal detachment. *MEK,* mitogen-activated protein kinase.

Key Points

- panuveitis, serous retinal detachment, sunset glow fundus, corticosteroid.

References

1. Ng JY, Luk FO, Lai TY, Pang CP. Influence of molecular genetics in Vogt-Koyanagi-Harada disease. *J Ophthalmic Inflamm Infect.* 2014;4:20.
2. Goto H RK, Rao N. Vogt–Koyanagi–Harada disease. In: Schachat AP SS, Hinton DR, Wilkinson CP, Wiedemann, eds. *Ryan's Retina.* Elsevier; 2018:1505-1515 [chapter 78].
3. Du L, Kijlstra A, Yang P. Vogt-Koyanagi-Harada disease: novel insights into pathophysiology, diagnosis and treatment. *Prog Retin Eye Res.* 2016;52:84-111.
4. Rao N. Vogt-Koyanagi-Harada disease. In: J YMaD, ed. *Ophthalmology.* Elsevier; 2014:761-763 [chapter 7.17].
5. Yeh PT YC, Yang CH, Lin CP. Nonrhegmatogenous retinal detachment. In: Schachat AP SS, Hinton DR, Wilkinson CP, Wiedemann P, eds. *Ryan's Retina.* Elsevier; 2018:1828-1849 [chapter 99].
6. Kitaichi N, Matoba H, Ohno S. The positive role of lumbar puncture in the diagnosis of Vogt-Koyanagi-Harada disease: lymphocyte subsets in the aqueous humor and cerebrospinal fluid. *Int Ophthalmol.* 2007;27(2-3):97-103.
7. Urzua CA, Velasquez V, Sabat P, et al. Earlier immunomodulatory treatment is associated with better visual outcomes in a subset of patients with Vogt-Koyanagi-Harada disease. *Acta Ophthalmol.* 2015;93(6):e475-e480.
8. Read RW, Rechodouni A, Butani N, et al. Complications and prognostic factors in Vogt-Koyanagi-Harada disease. *Am J Ophthalmol.* 2001;131(5):599-606.
9. Rubsamen PE, Gass JD. Vogt-Koyanagi-Harada syndrome: clinical course, therapy, and long-term visual outcome. *Arch Ophthalmol.* 1991;109(5):682-687.

CHAPTER 32

Bilateral Multifocal Placoid Lesions in a Young Woman

Lucia Sobrin ▦ Ashley Li

History of Present Illness

We describe a case of a 25-year-old woman who presented with 1 week of blurred vision in both eyes, bilateral central scotomas, and intermittent headaches. She endorsed photophobia but denied floaters, flashes, and diplopia. She denied any history of ocular conditions or ocular surgeries.

OCULAR EXAMINATION FINDINGS

Visual acuity without correction was 20/60 in the right eye and 20/40 in the left eye. Intraocular pressure was normal. External and anterior segment examinations were unremarkable. Dilated fundus examination revealed multifocal placoid lesions in the macula extending through the fovea in the right eye and involving the inferior fovea in the left eye.

IMAGING

Color fundus photography of both eyes showed multifocal placoid lesions of the macula, most prominent centrally and along the superior and inferior arcades of the right eye and in the superotemporal and inferior macula of the left eye (Fig. 32.1). Autofluorescence of both eyes revealed regions of intermixed hypo- and hyperautofluorescence with surrounding rings of hyperautofluorescence (Fig. 32.2). Fluorescein angiography (FA) indicated early hypofluorescence (blockage) corresponding to the placoid lesions followed by late, irregular hyperfluorescent staining of the lesions in both eyes (Figs. 32.3 and 32.4). Optical coherence tomography (OCT) of the retina revealed disruption of the ellipsoid zone (EZ) and retinal pigment epithelium (RPE) in both eyes (Fig. 32.5).

Questions to Ask

- Does the patient have any neurological symptoms? If neurological symptoms are present, that may be concerning for central nervous system (CNS) vasculitis.
  - Patient reported intermittent headaches.
- What is the patient's recent travel history?
  - No recent travel history
- Has the patient had any tuberculosis (TB) exposure or history of TB? TB with ocular involvement can cause macular serpiginous-like choroiditis.
  - No exposure to TB or history of TB
- Are there any systemic symptoms such as rashes, joint pain, or fever? Acute posterior multifocal placoid pigment epitheliopathy (APMPPE) may be preceded by flu-like symptoms.
  - Patient reported joint pain and viral-like illness before onset of visual symptoms.

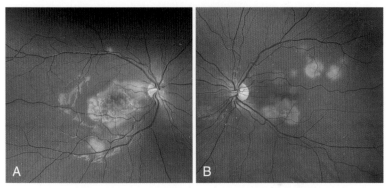

Fig. 32.1   Color fundus photographs of both eyes with multifocal placoid lesions. (A) Fundus photograph of the right eye with lesions in the central macular and along the superior and inferior arcades. (B) Fundus photograph of the left eye with lesions most prominently in the inferior and superotemporal macula.

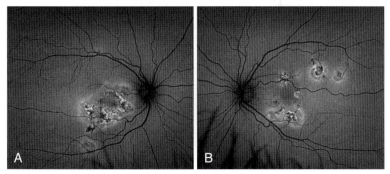

Fig. 32.2   Fundus autofluorescence (FAF) of both eyes with areas of hyper- and hypoautofluorescence. (A) FAF of the right eye shows the lesions to have mixed hyper- and hypoautofluorescence surrounded by halos of hyperautofluorescence. (B) FAF of the left eye also shows lesions to have mixed hyper- and hypo-autofluorescence surrounded by halos of hyperautofluorescence.

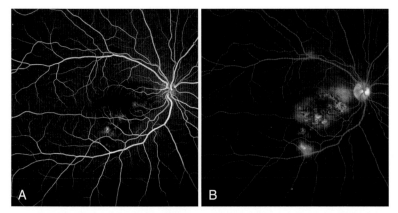

Fig. 32.3   Fluorescein angiography (FA) of the right eye. (A) In the early stage of the FA, hypofluorescence (block-age) of lesions can be observed. (B) In the late stage of FA, these lesions display hyperfluorescence (staining).

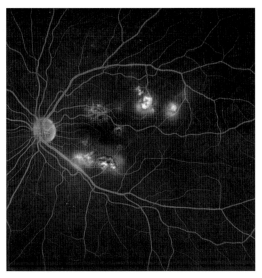

Fig. 32.4 Late-stage fluorescein angiography of the left eye displays hyperfluorescence (staining) of lesions.

- What is the patient's sexual history? Syphilis may also cause placoid retinitis.
  - No history of high-risk sexual behavior

Assessment

This is a case of a 25-year-old woman with no past ocular history demonstrating bilateral multifocal placoid lesions in the macula.

Differential Diagnosis

- APMPPE
- Serpiginous chorioretinitis
- Syphilitic posterior placoid chorioretinitis
- TB-associated serpiginous-like chorioretinitis
- Relentless placoid chorioretinitis

SEROLOGICAL TESTING

QuantiFERON-TB Gold, syphilis antibody screen, and toxoplasmosis IgG/IgM were negative.

Working Diagnosis

Acute posterior multifocal placoid pigment epitheliopathy

Multimodal Testing and Results

- Color fundus photography
  - Multiple creamy white-yellow placoid lesions, typically in the posterior pole, located at the level of the RPE and inner choroid.[1]

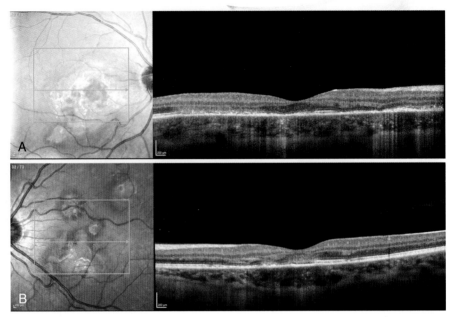

Fig. 32.5   Optical coherence tomography (OCT) of both eyes displays disruption of the ellipsoid zone (EZ) and retinal pigment epithelium (RPE) layers. (A) OCT of the right eye lesions shows disruption of the EZ and RPE in the macula and some hyperreflectivity of the outer retinal layers. (B) OCT of the left eye lesions also shows disruption of the EZ and RPE.

- OCT
  - On OCT, disruption of the EZ and RPE layers should be seen in areas with lesions. Hyperreflectivity is also observed in the outer retinal layers.[2]
- Fundus autofluorescence
  - Hypoautofluorescent lesions with an edge of relative hyperautofluorescence.[2]
- FA
  - On FA, our patient demonstrated the classic pattern of early hypofluorescence and late hyperfluorescence ("block early, stain late").[1]
- Serological testing
  - To rule out infectious etiologies such as syphilis or TB, blood work should be performed.
- Neuroimaging
  - For patients with neurological symptoms or suspected CNS involvement, further neurological testing should be pursued starting with brain magnetic resonance imaging (MRI). Lumbar puncture or magnetic resonance angiography may also be needed.[3] Our patient had a normal brain MRI.

Management

- There is no standard therapy for APMPPE. General management of APMPPE is observation as most cases are self-limiting and resolve over time, usually over 4 weeks.[4]
- Oral steroids are used in cases with subfoveal involvement and decreased vision. Oral steroids and systemic immunosuppressive therapy are indicated if there is an associated CNS vasculitis.[3]
- Patients with neurological symptoms should undergo a full neurological workup for CNS vasculitis.

Follow-up Care

- Patients should be followed weekly and then every few weeks initially. Lesions typically heal over weeks. The visual prognosis is generally good, although cases with foveal involvement tend to have worse visual outcomes.[4]
- More severe cases with lesions in the fovea or CNS vasculitis should be monitored more closely and treated with steroids and/or immunosuppressive agents. Cerebrovascular complications can occur with cerebral vasculitis in these patients.

Algorithm 32.1: Algorithm for Diagnosis of Acute Posterior Multifocal Placoid Pigment Epitheliopathy

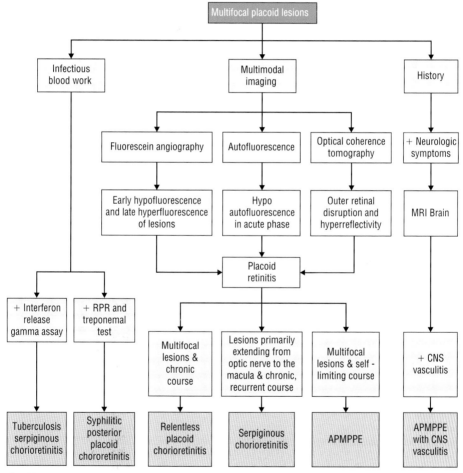

Algorithm 32.1 Algorithm for diagnosis of acute posterior multifocal placoid pigment epitheliopathy. *APMPPE,* acute posterior multifocal placoid pigment epitheliopathy; *CNS,* central nervous system; *MRI,* magnetic resonance imaging.

Key Points

- APMPPE should be considered in cases of unilateral or bilateral multifocal placoid lesions.
- A comprehensive review of systems and lab work should be performed to exclude infectious etiologies.
- If neurological symptoms are present, workup for CNS vasculitis should be performed.
- APMPPE generally self-resolves, but in more severe cases, oral steroids can be used.

References

1. Gass J. Acute posterior multifocal placoid pigment epitheliopathy. *Arch Ophthalmol*. 1968;80(2):177-185.
2. Steiner S, Goldstein D. Imaging in the diagnosis and management of APMPPE. *Int Ophthalmol Clin*. 2012;52(4):211-219.
3. O'Halloran H, Berger J, Robertson D, et al. Acute multifocal placoid pigment epitheliopathy and central nervous system involvement: nine new cases and a review of the literature. *Ophthalmology*. 2001;108(5):861-868.
4. Fiore T, Iaccheri B, Androudi S, et al. Acute posterior multifocal placoid pigment epitheliopathy: outcome and visual prognosis. *Retina*. 2009;29(7):994-1001.

CHAPTER 33

Bilateral Progressive Vision Loss in an Otherwise Healthy Man

Rukhsana G. Mirza ▪ Hassan N. Tausif ▪ Nathan C. Sklar

History of Present Illness

A 31-year-old otherwise healthy male patient with nonspecific upper respiratory illness 2 months earlier presents with blurry vision in the left eye with distortion. This has persisted for about 1 month and is associated with occasional photopsia and minimal floaters.

OCULAR EXAMINATION FINDINGS

Best-corrected visual acuity was 20/20 in the right eye and 20/40 in the left eye. Intraocular pressures were normal in both eyes, and slit-lamp biomicroscopy was notable for 2+ anterior vitreous cell in the left eye. Dilated fundus examination revealed creamy white lesions involving the fovea of the left eye at the level of the retinal pigment epithelium (Fig. 33.1). The right eye was notable for mild vitritis and inactive pigmented epithelial scars in the macula and midperiphery.

IMAGING

Optical coherence tomography (OCT) with raster through the fovea demonstrates subretinal fluid and pigment epithelial detachment. Fluorescein angiography (FA) showed early hypofluorescence and late hyperfluorescence of active lesions.

Questions to Ask

- What associated systemic medical problems does the patient have? Autoimmune diseases such as sarcoidosis can cause bilateral panuveitis with inflammatory retinal changes.
  - None
- Does the patient have history of sexually transmitted infections or exposure to tuberculosis (TB)? Infectious etiologies including syphilis and TB can cause ocular inflammation and placoid and subretinal granulomatous lesions, respectively.
  - No

Assessment

- This is a case of a 31-year-old male patient with no past ocular, medical, or surgical history with relapsing, remitting decreased vision involving both eyes with panocular inflammation and multifocal lesions deep to the retina.

207

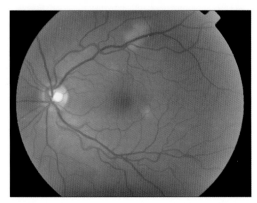

Fig. 33.1 Color fundus photograph of the left eye demonstrating clear media, sharp and healthy optic nerve, normal appearing vessels with multifocal creamy lesions deep to the retina in the macula and outside the superior arcade. (With permission from Mirza R, Jampol L. White spot syndromes and related diseases. In: Ryan SJ, Schachat AP, Sadda SR, eds. *Ryan's Retina*. Elsevier; 2018:1531.[1])

Differential Diagnosis

- Inflammatory placoid diseases
  - Acute posterior multifocal placoid pigment epitheliopathy (APMPPE)
  - Serpiginous choroiditis (SC)
  - Persistent placoid maculopathy
  - Relentless placoid chorioretinitis (RPC)
- Other inflammatory etiologies
  - Multifocal choroiditis with panuveitis (MCP)
  - Sarcoidosis
- Infectious inflammatory masqueraders
  - Tuberculosis (TB)
  - Acute syphilitic posterior placoid chorioretinopathy

Multimodal Testing and Results

- Fundus photographs
  - Fundus examination reveals multiple creamy yellow to white lesions deep to the retina in the posterior pole and midperiphery with older inactive lesions demonstrating pigmentation and scarring.[2]
- FA
  - FA shows early hypofluorescence with late hyperfluorescence of active lesions.[3] There is also staining of chorioretinal scars in the late phase with blockage from older hyperpigmented lesions.[4]
- Indocyanine green angiography (ICG)
  - ICG shows hypofluorescence in the areas corresponding to clinical lesions.[5]

Management

- Given the relatively good vision at presentation, the decision was made to observe and follow closely. At 2-month follow-up, the active lesions in the left eye began to pigment, and the fluid under the fovea resolved. However, the patient began to notice decreased vision in the right eye with best-corrected visual acuity dropping to 20/100. An active creamy lesion was noted in the fovea of the right eye with subretinal fluid.

- The patient was started on 60 mg of oral prednisone. However, the vision in the right eye continued to deteriorate and measured 20/400. Intravitreal triamcinolone acetonide was injected.[6] Oral prednisone was tapered slowly by 10 mg every month.
- Six months after starting steroids, visual acuity improved to 20/50 in the right eye and 20/20 in the left eye.
- New active lesions were seen after tapering the oral steroids. Prednisone was increased to 40 mg daily, and cyclosporine 150 mg daily was added while the steroids were tapered. The prednisone was then tapered 10 mg per month while cyclosporine was maintained (Fig. 33.2).
- The patient was monitored closely every 3 to 4 months until the lesions stabilized.
- As the patient required long-term immunosuppression, regular follow-up visits were maintained to ensure adequate treatment and monitor for disease activity.
- In total, there were between 50 and 100 healed inactive lesions in both eyes extending from the posterior pole to the equator.

Working Diagnosis

- Relentless placoid chorioretinitis
  - RPC was first described by Jones and colleagues in 2000 when they described six cases of white dot syndrome with features of both APMPPE and SC with a more atypical clinical appearance and course.[2]

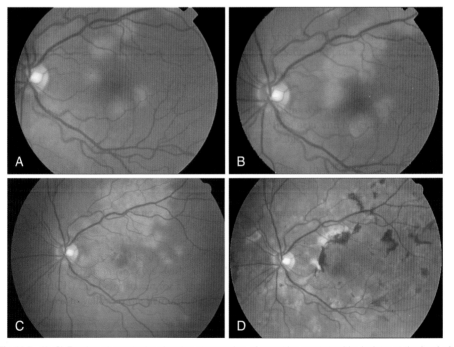

Fig. 33.2 (A–C) Fundus photographs showing progression of posterior creamy white lesions at the level of the retinal pigment epithelium over the course of 1 month. (D) Fundus photograph of the same patient 2 years later. (With permission from Mirza R, Jampol L. White spot syndromes and related diseases. In: Ryan SJ, Schachat AP, Sadda SR, eds. *Ryan's Retina*. Elsevier; 2018:1531.)

Follow-up Care

- Given the rarity of this disease entity, guidelines for follow-up care have not been well established.
- As with most chronic vision-threatening conditions, the frequency of follow-up correlates with disease activity. Patients with active lesions should be monitored monthly. As the lesions begin to pigment and no new lesions are apparent, follow-up intervals can be extended to 2, 3, and 6 months as determined clinically appropriate. Patients who require long-term immunosuppression will need to be followed more closely.

COMPARISON OF PLACOID RETINOPATHIES

Algorithm 33.1: Algorithm for Relentless Placoid Chorioretinitis

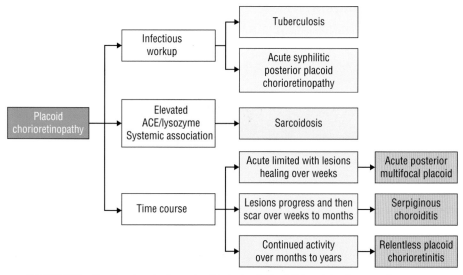

Algorithm 33.1   Algorithm for relentless placoid chorioretinitis. *ACE,* angiotensin-converting enzyme.

Key Points

- RPC must be on the differential when considering APMPPE and SC.
- Lesions extend beyond the posterior pole.
- Multimodal imaging can supplement clinical examination to aid in arriving at the correct diagnosis.[4]
- The differentiating factors include progression without treatment and relapsing remitting clinical course.
- Treatment includes high-dose systemic steroids with supplementation of periocular and intraocular steroids.[6] Steroid-sparing immunomodulatory therapy including cyclosporine[2] or adalimumab[7] may be required to minimize new activity while tapering prednisone.
- Infectious etiologies such as TB and syphilis must be excluded before initiating high-dose systemic steroids.[2]

References

1. Mirza R, Jampol L. White spot syndromes and related diseases. In: Schachat AP, Sadda SR, eds. *Ryan's Retina*. Elsevier; 2018:1531.
2. Raven ML, Ringeisen AL, Yonekawa Y, et al. Multi-modal imaging and anatomic classification of the white dot syndromes. *Int J Retina Vitreous*. 2017;3:12.
3. Jones BE, Jampol L, Yannuzzi L, et al. Relentless placoid chorioretinitis. *Arch Ophthalmol*. 2000;118: 931-938.
4. Mirza RG, Jampol LM. Relentless placoid chorioretinitis. *Int Ophthalmol Clin*. 2012;52(4):237-242.
5. Amer R., Floresu T. Optical coherence tomography in relentless placoid chorioretinitis. *Clin Exp Ophthalmol*. 2008;36(4):388-390.
6. Roth DB, Ballintine S, Mantopoulos D, Prenner J, Fine HF. Relentless placoid chorioretinitis: successful long-term treatment with intravitreal triamcinolone. *Retin Cases Brief Rep*. 2019;13(2):150-153.
7. Asano S, Tanaka R, Kawashima H, Kaburaki T. Relentless placoid chorioretinitis: a case series of successful tapering of systemic immunosuppressants achieved with adalimumab. *Case Rep Ophthalmol*. 2019; 10:145-152.

CHAPTER 34

Flashes and Floaters With a Well-Demarcated Peripapillary Lesion of the Right Eye

Aliaa Abdelhakim ▪ Gerardo Ledesma-Gil ▪ Lawrence A. Yannuzzi ▪
K. Bailey Freund

History of Present Illness

A case of a 26-year-old female patient with new-onset flashes and floaters in his right eye more than his left eye is reported. He had had similar symptoms a year before presentation that rapidly (over the course of weeks) affected his right eye.

OCULAR EXAMINATION FINDINGS

Visual acuity was 20/25 in the right eye and 20/20 in the left eye. Anterior chambers were quiet bilaterally, and there was no evidence of vitritis. Initial examination revealed an afferent pupillary defect of the right eye. Visual field testing revealed an enlarged blind spot/temporal scotoma of the right eye (Fig. 34.1).

LABORATORY WORKUP

Extensive laboratory workup to exclude systemic diseases, including infectious entities and masquerade syndromes, was performed.

- Antinuclear antibody titer was positive at 1:40, and thyroid-stimulating hormone was low (0.03 mIU/L), indicative of Graves disease.
- Antineutrophil cytoplasmic autoantibody screen, angiotensin-converting enzyme levels, lysozyme, Lyme disease antibody screen, rapid plasma reagin, fluorescent treponemal antibody absorption, interferon gamma release assay for latent tuberculosis, ssDNA autoantibodies, rheumatoid factor (immunoglobulin [Ig]A and IgG), cyclic citrullinated peptide, herpes simplex virus 1 and 2 IgG and IgM antibodies, interleukin-6 serum levels, urinalysis, and hepatitis C antibody were all within normal range.

IMAGING

Brain magnetic resonance imaging at the onset of symptoms was unrevealing. Ophthalmoscopy revealed a zonal, well-demarcated yellowish area centered around the optic nerve, more prominent on confocal color imaging than on standard color fundus photography (Figs. 34.2 and 34.3). Optical coherence tomography (OCT) demonstrated peripapillary outer retinal atrophy with thinning of the outer nuclear layer over disruption of the ellipsoid and interdigitation zones.

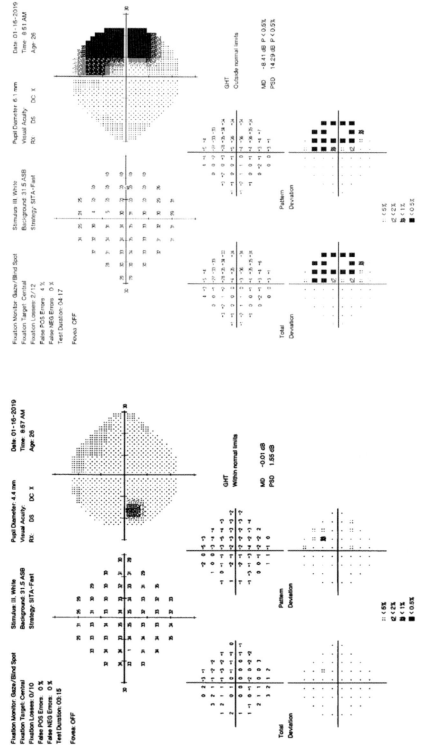

Fig. 34.1 Visual field testing (24–2) of the patient reveals an enlarged blind spot in the right eye.

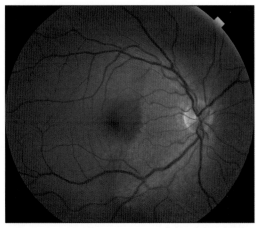

Fig. 34.2 Fundus photograph of affected right eye. Affected retina appears lighter, with a well-demarcated border.

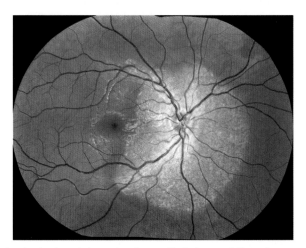

Fig. 34.3 Confocal color fundus photography shows affected area of the retina more clearly than the standard fundus photograph.

The retinal pigment epithelium (RPE) was attenuated (Fig. 34.4). OCT of the left eye appeared normal (Fig. 34.5). Fundus autofluorescence (FAF) showed hypoautofluorescence within the affected region of the right eye with hyperautofluorescence at its margin (Fig. 34.6).

Questions to Ask

- Has the patient had a systemic illness or other autoimmune disease? Systemic or autoimmune diseases have been associated with acute zonal occult outer retinopathy (AZOOR) in some patients.
  - Yes
- Has the patient had a sexually transmitted disease or a history of recent travel, cancer, or exposure to tuberculosis (TB) or Lyme disease? Infections such as syphilis, TB, and Lyme, as well as neoplastic processes, can masquerade as AZOOR.
  - No

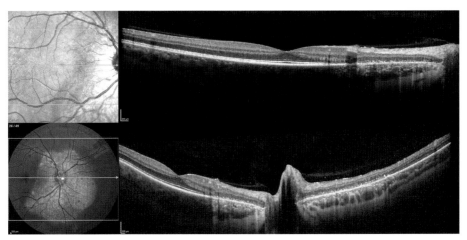

Fig. 34.4 Optical coherence tomography of the affected right eye. Top panel shows outer retinal atrophy with thinning of the outer nuclear layer over disruption of the ellipsoid and interdigitation zones. The retinal pigment epithelium is attenuated. The fovea is spared, which accounts for good visual acuity. Bottom panel shows extent of the outer retinal disruption around the nerve.

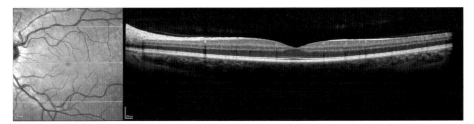

Fig. 34.5 Left eye optical coherence tomography shows normal findings.

- Has the patient had any recurrences? AZOOR is often associated with disease progression.
  - Yes
- Is the patient taking any medications? Toxic retinopathies may mimic AZOOR.
  - No

Assessment

This is a case of a 26-year-old female patient with a history of autoimmune disease presenting with recurrent symptoms of photopsia and floaters in his right eye more than his left and with a well-demarcated region centered around the optic nerve corresponding to outer retinal atrophy and an enlarged blind spot on visual field testing.

Differential Diagnosis

The diagnosis of AZOOR can be missed, particularly at the early stages of the disease. Differential diagnosis includes:
- Other white dot syndromes (e.g., multifocal choroiditis, multifocal evanescent white dot syndrome)

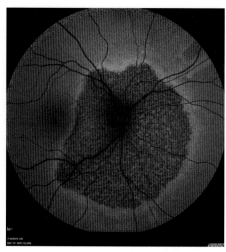

Fig. 34.6 Fundus autofluorescence of the right eye shows hypoautofluorescence within the affected area due to both outer retinal and retinal pigment epithelium involvement. Hyperautofluorescence is seen at the lesion border where the retinal pigment epithelium remains beneath attenuated outer retinal layers.

- Retinitis pigmentosa
- Optic neuropathy
- Masquerade syndromes including syphilitic infection, TB, Lyme disease, and vitreoretinal lymphoma
- Autoimmune retinopathy
- Paraneoplastic disease (e.g., cancer-associated retinopathy, melanoma-associated retinopathy)

Working Diagnosis

Acute zonal occult outer retinopathy (AZOOR)

Multimodal Testing and Results

- Fundus photographs
  - The appearance on ophthalmoscopy will depend on the stage of the disease. In the early stages of AZOOR, the fundus may appear normal. In the active stages of the disease, the affected retina is often demarcated at the leading edge by a yellowish line. In subacute or chronic stages of the disease, the appearance of the affected retina may become trizonal. The zones are concentric and consist of a normal retina (zone 1), followed by a retina with photoreceptor-RPE damage (zone 2), and then a zone of outer retinal and choroidal atrophy (zone 3).[1]
- OCT
  - Like ophthalmoscopy, the extent of damage on OCT will depend on the stage at which the patient presents. Early-stage AZOOR may present only with disruption confined to the photoreceptor layers on OCT.
  - With more advanced disease, retinal architecture in zone 1 should appear as a normal retina. Zone 2 will show photoreceptor-RPE disruption, as well as possible subretinal

deposits that appear drusenoid in nature. Zone 3 is represented by outer retinal and choroidal atrophy.[1]

- FAF
  - FAF is important in demarcating the areas of involvement in AZOOR and looking for evidence of recurrence. The retina is usually hypoautofluorescent within the affected area secondary to RPE and photoreceptor atrophy, with hyperautofluorescence at the leading edge of the zone. Recurrence or activity may be detected with new areas of hyperautofluorescence at the edge of the affected area. This leading edge of hyperauto-fluorescence may become beaded or less hyperautofluorescent during less active phases of the disease.[1]
- Indocyanine green angiography (ICGA)
  - ICGA may show areas of hypofluorescence within areas of affected retina, secondary to atrophy of the choriocapillaris.
- Visual field testing
  - Visual field deficits may show an enlarged blind spot or peripheral defects secondary to the affected areas being commonly centered around the optic nerve.
- Electroretinography (ERG)
  - Full-field ERG may be abnormal if large areas of the retina area are affected.[2]
- Fluorescein angiography (FA)
  - FA may appear normal at the beginning stages of the disease; however, as the disease progresses, window defects may be seen within the areas of RPE atrophy.

Management

No proven therapy exists for AZOOR. Immunosuppressive therapy, though of unproven benefit, has often been trialed in cases of progressive disease. The prognosis of the disease may depend on its extent and whether there is progression into the fovea. Few studies exist that look at the long-term outcomes of patients with AZOOR.

Follow-up Care

- There are no previously established guidelines for follow-up.
- Our patient is followed every 3 months with instructions to return sooner if any further worsening of vision is noted.
- Involvement of the other eye may be delayed by several years.[3]

Algorithm 34.1: Algorithm for Differential Diagnosis for Acute Zonal Occult Outer Retinopathy

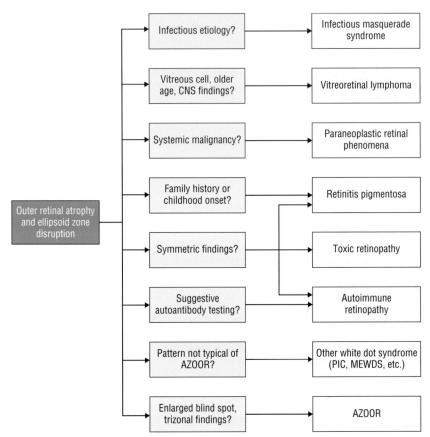

Algorithm 34.1 Algorithm for differential diagnosis for acute zonal occult outer retinopathy. *AZOOR*, acute zonal occult outer retinopathy; *CNS*, central nervous system; *MEWDS*, multiple evanescent white dot syndrome; *PIC*, punctate inner choroidopathy.

Key Points

- The diagnosis of AZOOR can be difficult to make in the early stages of the disease.
- The disease usually affects young to middle-aged individuals, predominantly women, some with a history of autoimmune disease.
- Progression is common with this entity, and the patient needs to be followed to document changes in the symptoms and examination.

References

1. Mrejen S, Khan S, Gallego-Pinazo R, et al. Acute zonal occult outer retinopathy: a classification based on multimodal imaging. *JAMA Ophthalmol*. 2014;132(9):1089-1098.
2. Gass JD, Agarwal A, Scott IU. Acute zonal occult outer retinopathy: a long-term follow-up study. *Am J Ophthalmol*. 2002;134(3):329-339.
3. Agarwal A. *Inflammatory Diseases of the Retina. Gass' Atlas of Macular Diseases*. Vol 1. Elsevier Saunders; 2012.

CHAPTER 35

Acute Vision Loss in a Pregnant Woman Associated With Bilateral Serous Retinal Detachment

David Sarraf ▪ SriniVas Sadda ▪ Meira Fogel-Levin

History of Present Illness

A 32-year-old healthy female patient presented at 22 weeks' gestation with abdominal pain and acute vision loss in the left eye (OS). Past medical history was remarkable for treated hypothyroidism with no personal or family ocular history.

OCULAR EXAMINATION FINDINGS

On examination, visual acuity was 20/20 right eye (OD) and 20/30 OS. Intraocular pressure and anterior chambers of both eyes (OU) were within normal limits. Dilated fundus examination demonstrated normal optic nerve and vessels with a clear vitreous OU; however, a serous retinal detachment was noted OS.

IMAGING

Spectral-domain optical coherence tomography (SD-OCT) demonstrated extrafoveal subretinal fluid OD and central subretinal fluid OS with no evidence of retinal pigment epithelium (RPE) detachment or RPE mottling OU (Fig. 35.1).

Questions to Ask

- What medications does the patient take?
  - Only levothyroxine. Steroid use in any form (e.g., oral, nasal, topical) is an important risk factor for central serous chorioretinopathy (CSC), which must be excluded.
- Does the patient have any neurological symptoms (e.g., meningismus), headaches, hearing abnormalities such as tinnitus, or skin color changes or hair loss?
  - No. Vogt-Koyanagi-Harada (VKH) disease can cause bilateral multifocal serous retinal detachments due to inflammatory choroidal infiltration.
- Does the patient have any current evidence or history of high blood pressure? Hypertensive choroidopathy and preeclampsia can be the cause of subretinal fluid especially in a pregnant patient.
  - No. The patient's blood pressure was normal.

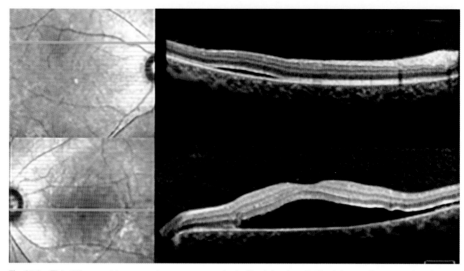

Fig. 35.1 This 32-year-old pregnant woman presented with vision loss in the left eye. Cross-sectional spectral domain optical coherence tomography B scans through the superior macula of the right eye and central fovea of the left eye shows subretinal fluid.

- Does the patient have any remarkable obstetrical history?
  - Yes, this patient endorsed a history of three pregnancy losses (9–13 weeks), and, given her abdominal pain, suspicion for pregnancy complication should be investigated.

Assessment

- This is a case of a 32-year-old pregnant woman with a history of three pregnancy losses who presented with acute abdominal pain and unilateral vision loss. SD-OCT demonstrated bilateral serous retinal detachment.

Differential Diagnosis

- Central serous chorioretinopathy (CSC)
- VKH disease
- Hypertensive choroidopathy
- Macular (i.e., choroidal) neovascularization or macular neovascularization (MNV) (possible causes in this demographic include idiopathic, myopia, multifocal choroiditis)
- Optic disc pit or coloboma
- Posterior scleritis
- Choroidal tumor (e.g., choroidal hemangioma or metastasis)
- Idiopathic uveal effusion syndrome

Working Diagnosis

- Pregnancy-related HELLP syndrome (hemolysis, elevated liver enzymes, and low platelets). These patients may also have evidence of antiphospholipid syndrome (APS).

Multimodal Testing and Results

- SD-OCT
  - As mentioned, SD-OCT showed extrafoveal subretinal fluid superotemporally OD and macular detachment with subretinal fluid centrally OS. Serous retinal detachment can complicate HELLP syndrome in 3.7% of cases.[1]
  - The SD-OCT failed to show any evidence of pigment epithelial detachment typical of CSC or type 1 MNV.
- Wide-field fluorescein angiography (WF-FA)
  - WF-FA illustrated superotemporal choroidal hypoperfusion OD and severe central choroidal ischemia OS with subretinal leakage temporal to the macula OS (Fig. 35.2). Choroidal ischemia, leading to vascular permeability and RPE pump impairment, is the cause of serous retinal detachment and subretinal fluid in patients with HELLP syndrome.[2]
  - FA failed to show the starry-sky pattern of subretinal leakage, typical of VKH, and there was no evidence of inflammatory findings such as disc leakage or papillitis. Gravitational gutters from RPE disturbance, typical of CSC, were also notably absent. CNV and polypoidal choroidal vasculopathy were also excluded.
- Optical coherence tomography angiography (OCTA)
  - MNV was excluded OU
- Laboratory tests
  - This patient had the following confirmatory lab values: low platelets (100,000/μL), high lactate dehydrogenase (LDH; 600 IU/L), and elevated liver function test values with alanine transaminase of 949 U/L and aspartate aminotransferase (AST) of 633 U/L.
    - Up to 90% of patients with HELLP present with abdominal pain, and as many as 20% may report visual disturbance.[3,4] Abdominal pain is due to liver ischemia.
    - The Mississippi severity classification for HELLP syndrome is determined on the basis of the platelet count along with the LDH and AST values.[3,4] Our patient had a Mississippi class score of 2 to 3.
  - Antinuclear antibodies, anti–Sjögren's syndrome antibodies, ribonucleoprotein antibodies, and lupus anticoagulant were positive.
    - These results, with the history of multiple pregnancy losses, indicates an additional possible diagnosis of APS. A study found that 10.5% of patients with APS can develop

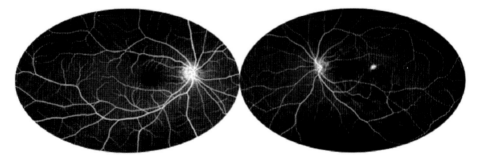

Fig. 35.2   Wide-field fluorescein angiography of both eyes, at baseline presentation, demonstrates choroidal nonperfusion superotemporal to the macula right eye and central left eye (OS) with late leakage in the temporal macula OS.

HELLP syndrome, typically those at an earlier stage of gestation (<24 weeks) and with a more severe clinical course.[5]

- Systemic lupus erythematosus, idiopathic thrombocytopenic purpura, and disseminated intravascular coagulation are additional systemic causes of ischemic choroidopathy and exudative retinal detachment.
- Abdominal imaging (magnetic resonance imaging/computed tomography)
  - Because of the patient's severe abdominal pain, imaging was performed; hepatic, splenic, and renal infarcts were identified.
    - Catastrophic antiphospholipid syndrome (CAPS) is a life-threatening condition associated with simultaneous multiple organ infarcts (spleen, liver, kidney, and placenta in our case).[6]

Management

- Our patient suffered from undiagnosed APS and developed HELLP syndrome, which is more prevalent in early-stage pregnancy in APS patients. Because of multiple systemic organ infarcts, she was later diagnosed with CAPS, which is associated with high maternal mortality risk.
  - Because of the severity of this patient's presentation and the fact that the patient's fetus was below the age of viability, and because delivery was not a short-term option, medical termination of pregnancy was elected. Pathological examination of the placenta showed extensive infarction with fibrin thrombi and areas of decidual necrosis.
  - After the termination of the pregnancy, the patient's systemic and ocular status slowly improved. Because of the continued high mortality risk, she was treated with intravenous steroids, hyperbaric oxygen, urgent plasmapheresis, and anticoagulation (warfarin), and further improvement was noted.

Follow-up Care

- Twenty days after the urgent delivery, the ocular status was notably improved. The subretinal fluid and the choroidal ischemia were resolved OU, although a legacy of RPE disruption was noted OS (Figs. 35.3 and 35.4). Two years from presentation, visual acuity was 20/20 OU, and retinal status was stable and unchanged.
- Rheumatology follow-up is essential:
  - APS can be a component of systemic lupus erythematosus, which requires appropriate rheumatological management and care. This patient was treated with hydroxychloroquine (Plaquenil) 300 mg daily.
  - Anticoagulation therapy should be continued and monitored; sometimes lifelong therapy is necessary.

Key Points

- Subretinal fluid in a pregnant woman should raise suspicion for HELLP syndrome.
- Choroidal ischemia and exudative retinal detachments will improve with urgent delivery of the fetus or termination of the pregnancy if necessary.
- HELLP syndrome may develop in patients with CAPS and is a dangerous complication with simultaneous multiple organ infarcts.

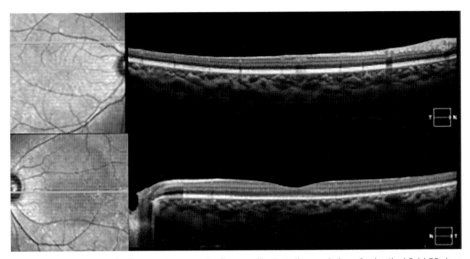

Fig. 35.3 Tracked optical coherence tomography B scans illustrate the resolution of subretinal fluid 20 days after pregnancy termination. Near-infrared reflectance image of the left eye still displays the area affected by the macular detachment.

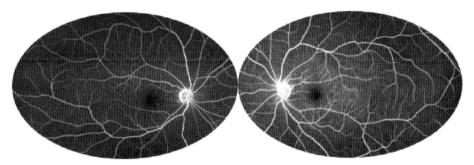

Fig. 35.4 Wide-field fluorescein angiography of both eyes 20 days after termination of the pregnancy illustrates resolution of the choroidal ischemia and leakage. Mild retinal pigment epithelial mottling is noted in the temporal macula in the left eye.

Algorithm 35.1: Algorithm for Bilateral Subretinal Fluid in a Young Patient

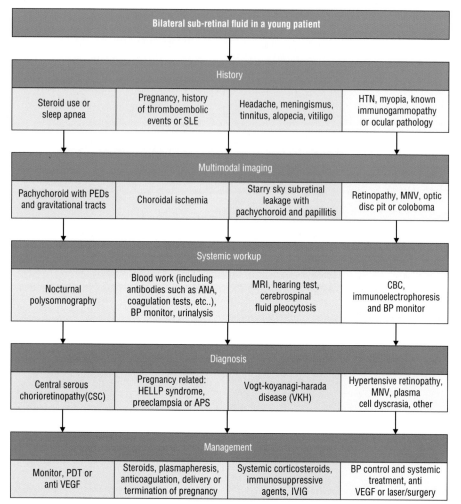

Algorithm 35.1 Algorithm for bilateral subretinal fluid in a young patient. *ANA,* antinuclear antibody; *APS,* antiphospholipid syndrome; *BP,* blood pressure; *CBC,* complete blood count; *HELLP,* hemolysis, elevated liver enzymes, and low platelets; *HTN;* hypertensive retinopathy; *IVIG,* intravenous immunoglobulin; *MNV,* macular neovascularization; *MRI,* magnetic resonance imaging; *PDT,* photodynamic therapy; *PED,* pigment epithelial detachment; *SLE,* systemic lupus erythematosus; *VEGF,* vascular endothelial growth factor.

References

1. Erbagci I, Karaca M, Ugur MG, Okumus S, Bekir N. Ophthalmic manifestations of 107 cases with hemolysis, elevated liver enzymes and low platelet count syndrome. *Saudi Med J.* 2008;29(8):1160-1163.
2. Iida T, Kishi S. Choroidal vascular abnormalities in preeclampsia. *Arch Ophthalmol.* 2002;120(10):1406-1407.
3. Khalid F, Tonismae T. HELLP syndrome. [Updated 2020 Jul 31]. In: *StatPearls.* StatPearls Publishing; Updated June 16, 2022. Available at: https://www.ncbi.nlm.nih.gov/books/NBK560615/#. Accessed May 10, 2023.
4. Dusse LM, Alpoim PN, Silva JT, Rios DR, Brandão AH, Cabral AC. Revisiting HELLP syndrome. *Clin Chim Acta.* 2015;451(Pt B):117-120.
5. Le Thi Thuong D, Tieulié N, Costedoat N, et al. The HELLP syndrome in the antiphospholipid syndrome: retrospective study of 16 cases in 15 women. *Ann Rheum Dis.* 2005;64(2):273-278.
6. Aguiar CL, Erkan D. Catastrophic antiphospholipid syndrome: how to diagnose a rare but highly fatal disease. *Ther Adv Musculoskelet Dis.* 2013;5(6):305-314.

Infectious Macular Diseases

CHAPTER 36

Unilateral Vision Loss in a 45-Year-Old Woman

Emily Cole ■ Pooja Bhat ■ Ann-Marie Lobo ■ Jennifer I. Lim

History of Present Illness

A 45-year-old woman with a past medical history of chronic alcoholism, gastric bypass surgery, and multiple psychiatric conditions noted painless decreased vision in the right eye approximately 1.5 weeks earlier, which had remained stable since initial decrease in vision. She had no previous ocular history, though she noted that she may have had a lazy eye as a child. Review of systems was unremarkable.

OCULAR EXAMINATION FINDINGS

Visual acuity without correction was hand motions in the right eye and 20/20 in the left eye. Both pupils were round and reactive to light, and there was no afferent pupillary defect. Color plates could not be assessed in the right eye because of the degree of vision loss and were full in the left eye. Confrontational visual fields were constricted in the right eye and full in the left. Anterior segment examination was unremarkable except for trace nuclear sclerosis. Dilated fundus examination was notable for a placoid, well-circumscribed yellow-white lesion involving the macula of the right eye.

Questions to Ask

- Does the patient have a history of sexually transmitted infection(s) or multiple sexual partners?
  - She has had multiple sexual partners.
- Is there a history of HIV and/or immunosuppression?
  - None known; HIV test ordered
- Does the patient have an autoimmune disease?
  - No
- Is there a history of systemic malignancy?
  - No
- Has the patient had any recent exposure to an infectious disease?
  - None that she can recall
- Has the patient had any recent flu-like illness?
  - Patient denies any symptoms.

Assessment

This is a case of a 45-year-old woman with a past medical history of chronic alcoholism, gastric bypass surgery, and multiple psychiatric conditions who presents with decreased vision in the right eye, examination and imaging notable for a placoid chorioretinitis in the right eye, and multiple punctate areas of chorioretinitis in the periphery of both eyes.

Differential Diagnosis

- Acute syphilitic posterior placoid chorioretinitis
- Early acute zonal occult outer retinopathy
- Sarcoidosis
- Tuberculous choroidopathy
- Metastases
- Acute posterior multifocal placoid pigment epitheliopathy
- Serpiginous choroidopathy

Working Diagnosis

Acute syphilitic posterior placoid chorioretinitis

Multimodal Testing and Results

- Widefield fundus imaging
  - Our patient's imaging demonstrated a yellow-white placoid lesion in the posterior pole with multiple subtle punctate white lesions in the periphery of both eyes.
  - A wide range of inflammatory changes in the retina can also be present, including phlebitis, retinitis, retinal infiltrates, vitritis, optic neuritis, and/or atrophy.
- Fluorescein angiography
  - Our patient's imaging demonstrates early hypofluorescence and late staining of the plac-oid lesion in the right eye without any areas of hypofluorescence or staining noted in the left eye.
- Fundus autofluorescence
  - Our patient's imaging demonstrated a well-circumscribed area of hyperautofluorescence corresponding to the yellow-white placoid lesion with adjacent irregular mottling in the right eye (Figs. 36.1 and 36.2). The periphery of both eyes demonstrated multiple punc-tate hyperautofluorescent lesions in a 360-degree distribution.
- Optical coherence tomography (OCT)
  - Our patient's OCT showed diffuse ellipsoid loss with nodular irregularity of the outer retina and retinal pigment epithelium (RPE), which is pathognomonic for acute syphi-litic posterior placoid chorioretinitis.[1]
- Optical coherence tomography angiography (OCTA)
  - *En face* swept-source OCTA imaging using a choroidal slab adjacent to the RPE in the region of the choriocapillaris shows decreased flow associated with the placoid lesion.[2,3]

Management

- QuantiFERON-TB Gold
- Angiotensin-converting enzyme
- Lysozyme
- Chest x-ray
- Fluorescent treponemal antibody absorption (FTA-ABS), followed by rapid plasma reagin (RPR)

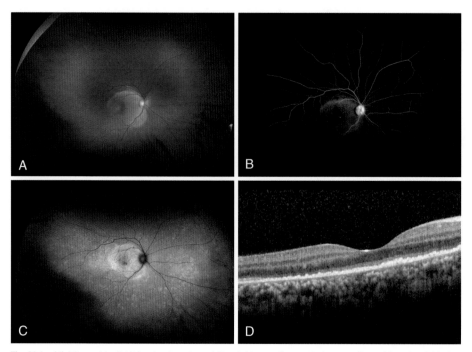

Fig. 36.1 (A) Ultra–wide field fundus imaging of the right eye demonstrates a yellow-white placoid lesion in the macula. (B) Mid-late phase fluorescein angiography at 2 minutes and 11 seconds demonstrates corresponding late staining in the area of the placoid lesion with areas of mottling in the fovea. (C) Fundus autofluorescence shows a placoid area of hyperautofluorescence with multiple punctate areas of hyperauto-fluorescence throughout the entire periphery. (D) Spectral domain optical coherence tomography of the macula reveals diffuse ellipsoid loss with nodular irregularity of the retinal pigment epithelium.

- HIV
- Recommend infectious disease consultation, brain magnetic resonance imaging, and lumbar puncture

Serology testing via the reverse algorithm has become more common for syphilis. Reverse algorithm testing consists of a treponemal test for screening, such as the FTA-ABS or micro-hemagglutination test, followed by a treponemal test, such as the Venereal Disease Research Laboratory (VDRL) or RPR. The use of the traditional versus reverse algorithm depends on disease prevalence, test cost, test volume, and workflow.[4] Use of the traditional or reverse algorithm is ultimately institution dependent based on patient population, test cost, volume, and workflow.

- In patients with suspected neurosyphilis, cerebrospinal fluid VDRL testing should be performed.
- Concurrent HIV testing should be performed in all patients with suspected ocular syphilis, given the high degree of coinfection.[5]

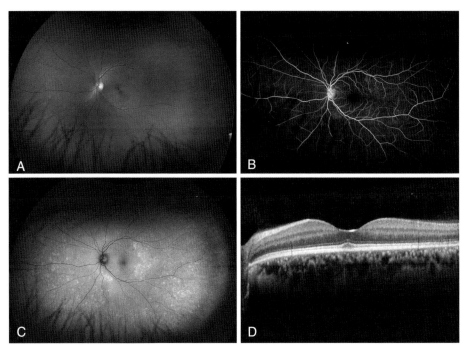

Fig. 36.2 (A) Ultra–wide field fundus imaging of the left eye does not show any obvious retinal lesions. (B) Mid-phase fluorescein angiography at 1 minute shows no evidence of hyper or hypofluorescent lesions. (C) Fundus autofluorescence demonstrates multiple peripheral punctate areas of hyperautofluorescence throughout the entire periphery. (D) Spectral domain optical coherence tomography reveals temporal ellipsoid loss.

- Intravenous penicillin G (3–4 million units every 4 hours) for 10 to 14 days is usually an effective treatment.

Follow-up Care

- Visual prognosis is good if the disease is caught early and promptly treated, with full visual recovery and resolution of symptoms possible.
- If untreated, worsening of ocular inflammation can limit visual potential via development of outer retinal atrophy, vitritis, and optic atrophy.
- Nonspecific treponemal titers (RPR) can be used to measure treatment response, whereas treponemal titers will remain positive throughout the patient's life after a syphilis infection.

Algorithm 36.1: Algorithm for Differential Diagnosis for Placoid Retinal Lesions

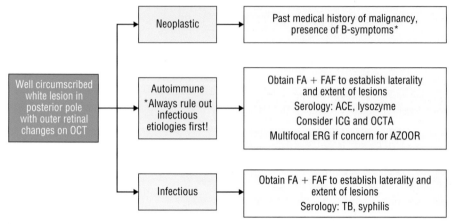

Algorithm 36.1 Algorithm for differential diagnosis for placoid retinal lesions. *FA,* fluorescein angiography; *FAF,* fundus autofluorescence; *OCT,* optical coherence tomography; *ICG,* indocyanine green angiography; *OCTA,* optical coherence tomography angiography; *TB,* tuberculosis; *AZOOR,* acute zonal occult outer retinopathy. B symptoms = systemic symptoms of fever, night sweats, and weight loss.

Key Points

- Presence of a yellow-white placoid lesion in the posterior pole with corresponding ellipsoid loss and outer retina change on the OCT is pathognomonic for acute syphilitic posterior placoid chorioretinitis. Disease can be very asymmetrical between the eyes.[6]
- Prompt recognition and antibiotic therapy of this treatable condition can result in rapid resolution of the patient's vision loss.
- HIV testing should be performed in all patients with suspected ocular syphilis and additional workup for neurosyphilis including cerebrospinal fluid VDRL should also be completed.
- Syphilis can present with virtually any manifestation of anterior or posterior segment inflammation.

References

1. Pichi F, Ciardella AP, Cunningham Jr ET, et al. Spectral domain optical coherence tomography findings in patients with acute syphilitic posterior placoid chorioretinopathy. *Retina.* 2014;34(2):373-384.
2. Barikian A, Davis J, Gregori G, Rosenfeld P. Wide field swept source OCT angiography in acute syphilitic placoid chorioretinitis. *Am J Ophthalmol Case Rep.* 2020;18:100678.
3. Herbort Jr CP, Papasavvas I, Mantovani A. Choriocapillaris involvement in acute syphilis posterior placoid chorioretinitis is responsible for functional impairment and points towards an immunologic mechanism: a comprehensive clinicopathological approach. *J Curr Ophthalmol.* 2020;32(4):381-389.
4. Ortiz DA, Shukla MR, Loeffelholz MJ. The traditional or reverse algorithm for diagnosis of syphilis: pros and cons. *Clin Infect Dis.* 2020;71(suppl 1):S43-S51.
5. Queiroz RP, Smit DP, Peters RPH, Vasconcelos-Santos DV. Double trouble: challenges in the diagnosis and management of ocular syphilis in HIV-infected individuals. *Ocul Immunol Inflamm.* 2020;28(7):1040-1048.
6. Eandi CM, Neri P, Adelman RA, Yannuzzi LA, Cunningham Jr ET, International Syphilis Study Group. Acute syphilitic posterior placoid chorioretinitis: report of a case series and comprehensive review of the literature. *Retina.* 2012;32(9):1915-1941.

CHAPTER 37

Unilateral Painless Vision Loss With Retinal Detachment

Edward L. Randerson ▦ Jihun Song ▦ Debra A. Goldstein

History of Present Illness

An 84-year-old woman from India presented with blurred vision in the left eye (OS). She is asymptomatic in the right eye (OD). She is in overall good health with medically managed hypertension and low back pain. She is known to have a cystic mass in L1 reportedly stable for years. She is pseudophakic in both eyes (OU) after cataract surgery more than 21 years ago. She also has reportedly well-managed glaucoma and is status posttrabeculectomy OS.[1]

Questions to Ask

- When did you first notice the vision change?
  - "Two weeks ago."
- What associated symptoms are present? Any pain or light sensitivity? Any floaters?
  - Patient noted that her vision was very blurry in the left eye and there was no pain, light sensitivity, or floaters.
- Any prior symptoms?
  - None
- Is there any history of surgery or trauma to OS?
  - Yes, trabeculectomy years ago for glaucoma in the left eye. The glaucoma has been well managed since then. No history of trauma.
- Any systemic symptoms? Fever, chills, weight loss, cough, or shortness of breath?
  - Chronic low back pain
- Any family have a history of eye disease? Inflammatory disease?
  - None
- Any recent travel?
  - Yes, patient came to the United States from India 6 months ago to stay with her son.
- Any prior testing for tuberculosis (TB)?
  - Yes, recently had a purified protein derivative (PPD) test, as required for immigration; it was negative.
- Did patient have the bacillus Calmette–Guérin (BCG) vaccine?
  - Yes. Patient noted that everyone where she grew up got this vaccine.

Ocular Exam Findings and Imaging

Best-corrected visual acuity in OD was 20/50 and in OS was hand motion. Intraocular pressure OD was 22 mm Hg and OS was 2 mm Hg. Slit-lamp examination revealed a flat trabeculectomy bleb OS. Examination of the anterior chambers (ACs) revealed bilateral granulomatous keratic precipitates (KPs) with 4+ AC cell and both Koeppe and Busacca nodules of the iris OU. The

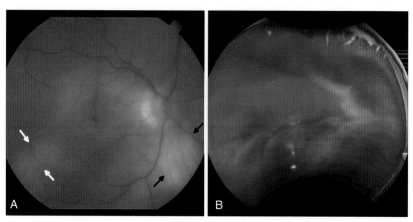

Fig. 37.1 Fundus photography. (A) Orange subretinal lesions in the right eye *(white arrows)* and a yellow-white choroidal nodule *(black arrows)* inferior to the optic disc. (B) Bullous exudative retinal detachment in the left eye on ultra–wide field fundus imaging.

anterior vitreous OD had 2+ cells with 2+ haze and OS had 3+ cells with 4+ haze. Fundus examination OD revealed multiple orange subretinal lesions in the posterior pole and a larger yellow-white choroidal nodule inferior to the optic disc in the midperiphery. OD also had mild optic disc edema and a shallow peripheral retinal detachment (RD) inferiorly. Fundus examination OS revealed a total bullous RD. No retinal breaks were noted on careful examination Fig. 37.1.

Differential Diagnosis

The differential can be broken down into infectious and noninfectious causes of granulomatous panuveitis (see, Algorithm 37.1). At the top of the infectious differential is TB; most other infections (except syphilis) are ruled out by the subacute (rather than hyperacute) presentation in an otherwise healthy patient. Ocular TB can affect all orbital and ocular tissues. When intraocular, TB typically manifests as a granulomatous panuveitis. Choroidal lesions may be small, known as tubercles, or large, referred to as tuberculomas. There may also be iris nodules, anterior and intermediate uveitis, and retinal vasculitis.

The most likely noninfectious etiology in this case is Vogt-Koyanagi-Harada disease, a granulomatous autoimmune panuveitis that often presents after a prodrome of tinnitus and meningitis. Ocular findings at onset include granulomatous KPs, ACs, and vitreous cells; an inflamed optic nerve ("cherry red" disc); and exudative retinal detachments (ERDs). Later, small or large choroidal nodules may be seen. Another granulomatous uveitis would be sarcoidosis, although this presentation was much more dramatic than is typically seen.

Certainly, malignancy can present with choroidal nodules, but one would not expect the bilateral granulomatous panuveitis presentation.

Working Diagnosis

Bilateral painless granulomatous panuveitis with choroidal lesions OD, subretinal fluid (SRF) peripherally OD, and ERD OS in a patient from an endemic area, most likely tuberculous despite the negative PPD.

Algorithm 37.1: General Posterior Uveitis Differential Diagnosis

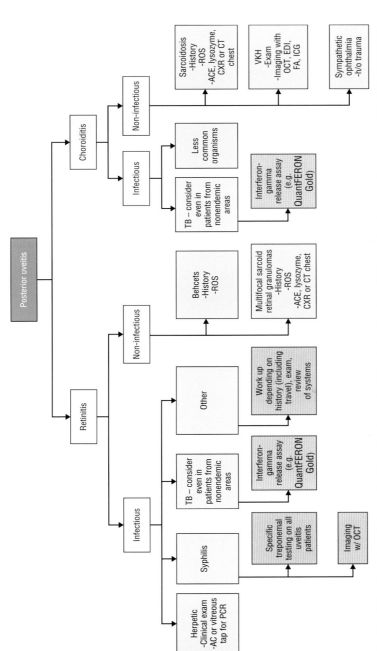

Algorithm 37.1 General posterior uveitis differential diagnosis. *AC*, anterior chamber; *ACE*, angiotensin-converting enzyme; *CT*, computed tomography; *CXR*, chest x-ray; *EDI*, enhanced-depth imaging; *FA*, fluorescein angiography; *ICG*, indocyanine green angiography; *OCT*, optical coherence tomography; *PCR*, polymerase chain reaction; *ROS*, reactive oxygen species; *TB*, tuberculosis; *VKH*, Vogt-Koyanagi-Harada disease.

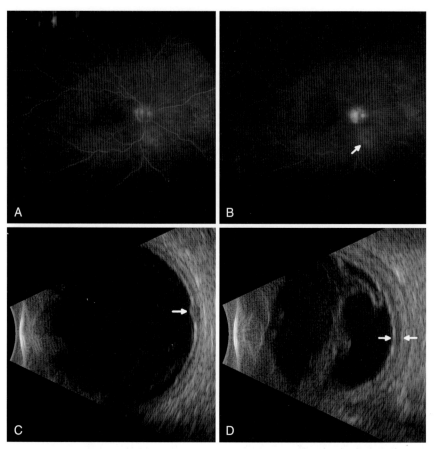

Fig. 37.2 Fluorescein angiography (FA) and ultrasonography. (A) Early-phase FA in the right eye showed mottled hyperfluorescence in the posterior pole. (B) Late-phase FA showed mild leakage from the choroidal nodule *(arrow)* and optic disc. (C) B-scan ultrasound in the right eye demonstrated a nodular elevation *(arrow)* of the choroid with medium to low internal echogenicity. (D) B-scan ultrasound image OS showed diffuse choroidal thickening *(between arrows)* and bullous retinal detachment visible in the vitreous cavity.

Multimodal Testing and Results

Multimodal imaging with fundus photography, fluorescein angiography, and ultrasound confirmed the examination findings and assisted in creating a focused differential (Figs. 37.1, 37.2, and algorithm 37.1).

Management

This complex case requires a high suspicion for ocular TB, as well as a detailed understanding of current lab testing. PPD was negative. A positive test is based on type IV hypersensitivity reaction to the injected tuberculin antigen. However, in this case our 84-year-old patient was likely anergic; we suspected this during our initial questioning because it is highly unlikely that an 84-year-old from India had never been exposed to TB.

Detection of TB in this case is best tested by an interferon-gamma release assay (IGRA) test such as T-SPOT.TB test (Oxford Immunotec Ltd, Oxford, UK) or QuantiFERON-TB GOLD (QFT-G:Cellestis Ltd, Carnegie, Australia). Ocular TB is a paucibacillary infection, and vitreous sampling with polymerase chain reaction (PCR) and culture are notoriously negative and have a very low sensitivity.[2] Additional workup includes testing for pulmonary involvement with chest imaging (x-ray or computed tomography [CT] scan). Syphilis is much less likely but should be tested for simultaneous to the IGRA blood draw.

In this case the QuantFERON Gold test returned positive, and syphilis testing was negative. Imaging with chest x-ray and CT chest were without pulmonary infection but did reveal a cystic spinal mass lesion in L1. The patient was started on four-drug anti-TB treatment (ATT) with rifampicin, isoniazid, pyrimethamine, and ethambutol. Simultaneous oral and topical steroids were given to reduce ocular inflammation and prevent further a Jarisch-Herxheimer–like reaction upon initiation of ATT.

Follow-up Care

Over the course of the next year with long-term ATT and titration of steroids, the patient's vision improved OD to 20/30 and OS to 20/25 (Fig. 37.3).

The cystic L1 spinal lesion was also noted to resolve with ATT. This likely represented an extrapulmonary manifestation of TB known as Pott disease and was another site of active infection.

Algorithms

For all types of uveitis:
- Determine the type
  - Granulomatous
  - Nongranulomatous
- Determine the location of inflammation
  - Anterior

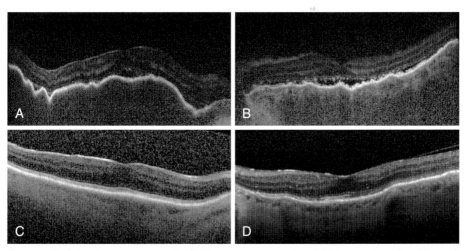

Fig. 37.3 Optical coherence tomography (OCT) imaging progression. OCT images through a 12-month follow-up period. (A) Right eye (OD) at presentation with multiple nodular choroidal elevations (tuberculoma) and a small amount of subretinal fluid (SRF). The left eye (OS) was not imaged on presentation because of the total retinal detachment (RD). (B) OS 3 weeks on anti-TB treatment (ATT), first obtainable OCT image OS demonstrating resolution of the RD, now with small central SRF and nodular-thickened choroid. (C–D) 12 months on ATT with normalization of choroid and complete resolution of SRF OU; mild postinflammatory damage is noted by the mild ellipsoid zone (EZ)/interdigitation zone (IZ) irregularity OS > OD.

- Intermediate
- Posterior
- Pan (all of the above)
- Create a broad differential diagnosis
  - Infectious
  - Autoimmune
  - Malignant
    - Use history, clinical examination, and multimodal imaging to create a differential diagnosis.
    - Send the patient for laboratory work-up; consider admission in cases with precipitous visual decline and/or significant concern for extent of systemic involvement.
  - Start treatment based on testing results; use extreme caution if starting high-dose systemic steroids while infectious labs are pending

Key Points

- A high suspicion for ocular TB is needed to recognize and appropriately treat the disease.
- PPD testing is sensitive and useful in countries where TB is not endemic, but it cannot be used reliably in patients who have had the BCG vaccine or who are anergic.
- Ocular TB is a paucibacillary infection; culture and PCR are frequently falsely negative and have a low sensitivity.
- Long-term ATT is best completed and monitored by an infectious disease specialist.
- A Jarisch-Herxheimer–like reaction can develop during ATT; simultaneous steroids can help prevent vision loss from inflammation.

References

1. Song JH, Koreishi AF, Goldstein DA. Tuberculous uveitis presenting with a bullous exudative retinal detachment: a case report and systematic literature review. *Ocul Immunol Inflamm*. 2019;27(6):998-1009.
2. Agarwal A, Agrawal R, Gunasekaran DV, et al. The Collaborative Ocular Tuberculosis Study (COTS)-1 report 3: polymerase chain reaction in the diagnosis and management of tubercular uveitis: global trends. *Ocul Immunol Inflamm*. 2019;27(3):465-473.

CHAPTER 38

Unilateral Vitreous Cell and Chorioretinal Lesions in an Asymptomatic Woman

Karl N. Becker ▪ Norbert M. Becker

History of Present Illness

A 49-year-old woman with type 2 diabetes mellitus (DM), hypertension, earlier fever of unknown origin, and hand numbness presented for her yearly diabetic eye examination. Her last dilated eye examination was 2 years earlier and had been unremarkable at that time. She reports stable vision with no ocular symptoms, including no flashes, floaters, pain, redness, or photophobia. She denies any family history of blindness or glaucoma.

OCULAR EXAMINATION FINDINGS

Visual acuity uncorrected was 20/25 in the right eye and 20/20 in the left eye. Intraocular pressures were 20 mm Hg in both eyes. External and anterior segment examinations were unremarkable except for bilateral trace nuclear sclerotic cataracts. Anterior chambers were quiet in both eyes, but dilated examination revealed 1+ anterior vitreous cell in the right eye with no vitreous haze. Both eyes had healthy optic discs, unremarkable macular areas, and a few dot-blot hemorrhages in two quadrants. The right eye had multiple flat, punched-out white lesions that were most prominent nasally and superiorly (Fig. 38.1).

IMAGING

Optical coherence tomography (OCT) (Fig. 38.2) was obtained, which demonstrated a normal foveal contour without macular edema or disruption of the retinal layers in both eyes.

Questions to Ask

- Does the patient have a history of systemic inflammatory disease, including sarcoidosis, systemic lupus erythematosus, rheumatoid arthritis, or other autoimmune disease that may be related to intraocular inflammatory disease? Does the patient have a history of symptoms consistent with the above diseases, including shortness of breath, cough, rashes, or joint pain and swelling?
  - No
- Does the patient have a family history of systemic inflammatory disease?
  - No

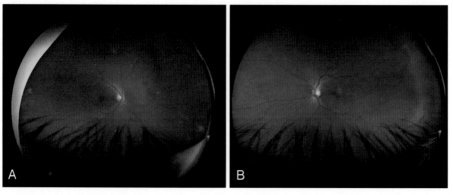

Fig. 38.1 Optos wide field images of both eyes. (A) shows the punched-out white lesions in the nasal midperiphery of the right eye. (B) shows few dot-blot hemorrhages but no punched-out lesions.

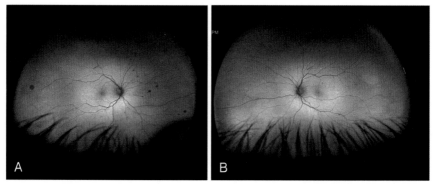

Fig. 38.2 Optos fundus autofluorescence of both eyes. (A) demonstrates the hypoautofluorescent lesions in the nasal midperiphery of the right eye. (B) shows now abnormal findings on autofluoresence.

- Does the patient have a history of systemic infection, including tuberculosis (TB), syphilis, histoplasmosis, or toxoplasmosis? Does the patient have risks for exposure to these infections, including being from an endemic area (another country for TB, the Ohio and Mississippi River valleys for histoplasmosis), high-risk sexual behavior, or pet ownership? Does the patient have a history of symptoms consistent with these infections?
  - No
- Does the patient have a history of viral infection, including herpes simplex virus 1 or 2, varicella zoster, or West Nile virus?
  - Yes, the patient was hospitalized a year earlier with complications from West Nile virus, with positive serology testing at that time.

Assessment

- This is a case of a 49-year-old woman with type 2 DM and history of hospitalization for West Nile fever presenting without ocular symptoms but with multiple chorioretinal lesions and vitreous cell in the right eye.

Differential Diagnosis

- Multifocal choroiditis with panuveitis
- Ocular histoplasmosis syndrome
- Syphilitic uveitis
- Sarcoid uveitis
- TB uveitis
- Hypertensive retinopathy
- Diabetic retinopathy
- Ocular toxoplasmosis
- West Nile virus chorioretinitis

Working Diagnosis

- Inactive West Nile virus chorioretinitis

Multimodal Testing and Results

- Fundus photographs
  - Active disease has creamy white-yellow targetoid lesions 200 to 1000 μm in diameter in the midperiphery. Inactive disease has pigmented and atrophic punched-out chorioretinal scars. Lesions are typically clustered with curvilinear distribution along the course of nerve fibers[1] (Fig. 38.1). Mild vitritis is typical. Retinal hemorrhages and cotton wool spots are possible. Optic nerve involvement with optic neuritis or neuroretinitis are possible, as are retinal vasculitis and serous retinal detachment.
- OCT
  - Our patient showed an unremarkable OCT. Lesions are typically outside the macula. OCT through lesions can show outer retinal disruption, including of the ellipsoid zone with possible hyperreflective outer retinal deposits.[1]
- Fundus autofluorescence
  - Hyperautofluorescent lesions in active disease and hypoautofluorescent lesions in inactive disease in the typical distribution[1] (Fig. 38.2).
- Fluorescein angiography (FA)
  - FA showed typical distribution of inactive lesions with central hypofluorescence and a surrounding ring of staining, as well as areas of diabetes-related peripheral capillary nonperfusion in the right eye (Fig. 38.3). The left showed microaneurysms consistent with nonproliferative diabetic retinopathy. Active lesions show early hypofluorescence and late staining.[1] Choroidal neovascular membrane (CNVM) is possible at the site of lesions.[2] Retinal vascular leakage is possible.[2] Macular ischemia is a rare complication.[2]
- Indocyanine green angiography (ICGA)
  - ICGA was not performed in our patient; however, lesions are in the typical distribution with hypocyanescent choroidal lesions.[1]

Management

- The patient had inactive chorioretinal lesions. The vitreous cell was likely a result of the earlier active inflammation at the time of infection. No treatment was indicated in this case, as in the majority of cases.

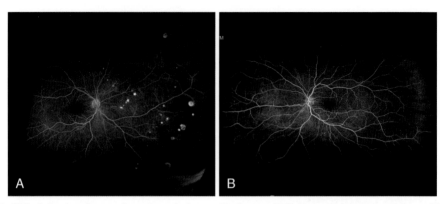

Fig. 38.3 Late-stage fluorescein angiography image of both eyes. (A) Right eye demonstrating staining of the midperipheral lesions and findings of non-proliferative diabetic retinopathy including capilllary non-perfusion. (B) Left eye demonstrating microaneurysms consistent with non-proliferative diabetic retinopathy.

- If CNVM develops, anti–vascular endothelial growth factor therapy may be used to manage vision-threatening lesions. If severe, vitreous hemorrhage or retinal detachment may occur.[2]
- Ischemic maculopathy, a rare complication, does not have effective intervention.
- Chorioretinitis is more common in older patients and in those with concurrent diabetic retinopathy.[2]
- If lesions appear inactive and are in the typical distribution for West Nile chorioretinitis, no testing may be indicated. Confirmation of earlier infection can be obtained with serum immunoglobulin (Ig)G testing. IgM testing can be performed during the acute phase of the disease but may be negative early in the disease.[3]
- If lesions are in a different distribution, evaluation should be done for the above diagnoses that remain on the differential, with guidance of clinical history and other examination findings.

Follow-up Care

- There are no previously established guidelines for follow-up.
- Our patient is followed on a biannual basis for her diabetic retinopathy.

Key Points

- West Nile virus can present with numerous ophthalmic manifestations, the most common being chorioretinal lesions in curvilinear clusters along the nerve fibers in the midperiphery.
- Complications are rare but include CNVM and ischemic maculopathy.

Algorithm 38.1 Algorithm for Differential Diagnosis of Chorioretinal Lesions

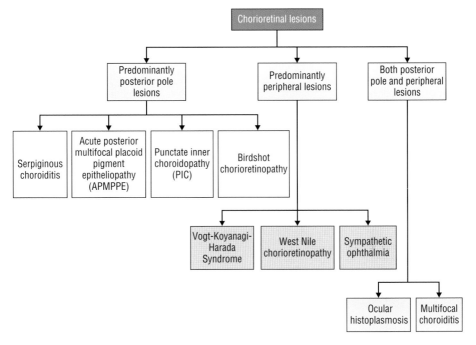

Algorithm 38.1   Algorithm for differential diagnosis of chorioretinal lesions.

References

1. Learned D, Nudleman E, Robinson J, et al. Multimodal imaging of West Nile virus chorioretinitis. *Retina.* 2014;34(11):2269-2274.
2. Lee JH, Agarwal A, Mahendradas P, et al. Viral posterior uveitis. *Surv Ophthalmol.* 2016;62(4):404-445.
3. Centers for Disease Control and Prevention. *West Nile Virus.* Updated March 29, 2023. Available at: https://cdc.gov/westnile. Accessed May 10, 2023.

CHAPTER 39

Bilateral Chorioretinal Scars and Pigment Mottling in a Newborn

Camila V. Ventura ■ Thayze Martins

History of Present Illness

We present a case of a 2.5-month-old female newborn (gestational age at birth of 39 weeks, weight at birth of 2.580 g, and cephalic perimeter of 27 cm). Microcephaly was detected at birth and classified as severe. Mother did not recall any symptoms such as rash, malaise, fever, and arthralgia during the pregnancy.

OCULAR EXAMINATION FINDINGS

Initial ophthalmological examination included biomicroscopy and fundus examination. The anterior segment was unremarkable. Dilated fundus examination showed small and pale optic disc, increased disc cupping (0.6), temporal peripapillary atrophy, and absence of a double-ring sign in both eyes. Well-defined foveal chorioretinal atrophy with pigmented margins and associated macular pigment mottling were detected bilaterally. Bilateral vascular attenuation was also noted.

The follow-up examination at 3 months did not reveal nystagmus or strabismus. No refractive errors were detected except for the presence of hypoaccommodation. Monocular visual acuity using Teller acuity cards performed at 38 cm was 0.86 cy/cm in both eyes, which revealed near-blindness visual impairment. The patient was prescribed +3.00 D spectacles for hypoaccommo-dation and referred for early low vision intervention.

IMAGING

Retinal imaging using a wide-angle digital fundus camera with a 130-degree lens (RetCam digital imaging system, Natus Medical, Pleasanton, CA) was performed for documentation and follow-up.

The comparison of the chorioretinal atrophy at 3 and 21 months of age revealed an increase of the chorioretinal atrophy area from 7.197 mm^2 to 7.851 mm^2 in the right eye and from 4.052 mm^2 to 4.727 mm^2 in the left eye. An increase of the pigmentation around the margin of the chorioretinal atrophy was also noted in both eyes (Fig. 39.1).

Questions to Ask

- What is the pregnancy history of the newborn? Did the mother have any symptoms of arboviruses?
  - No. The mother did not report complications or symptoms during pregnancy.

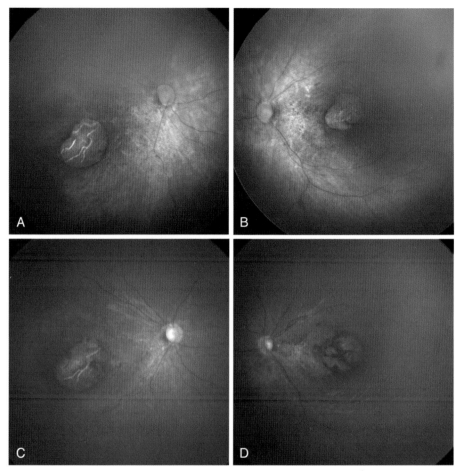

Fig. 39.1 (A–B) Initial assessment. Small and pale optic disc, increased disc cupping (0.6), temporal peripap-illary atrophy, and well-defined chorioretinal atrophy with pigmented margins affecting the fovea associated with pigment mottling in the macular region. (C–D) Follow-up images showing an increase in size of the chorioretinal atrophy and of the pigmentation on its margin.

- Was any systemic infection detected during pregnancy? Congenital toxoplasmosis, rubella, cytomegalovirus, varicella-zoster virus, herpes simplex, syphilis, and human immunodeficiency virus (HIV) could cause funduscopic findings associated with microcephaly.
  - No. Congenital infectious diseases (TORCHs) were ruled out. When the child was born, cerebrospinal fluid sample testing revealed Zika virus infection. Notably, this infant was born during the Zika virus outbreak in Brazil, and at the time there were no reports on congenital Zika syndrome (CZS).
- Did the mother use alcohol or any illicit drug during pregnancy that is associated with microcephaly? Is there any family history of consanguinity, microcephaly, or genetic diseases?
  - No.

Assessment

- This is a case of a female newborn with severe microcephaly and who was found on ophthalmological examination to have bilateral optic disc pallor and chorioretinal atrophy associated with pigment mottling in the macula.

Differential Diagnosis

- Congenital infectious diseases (toxoplasmosis, rubella, cytomegalovirus, varicella-zoster virus, herpes simplex, syphilis, and HIV)
- Genetic etiologies (Aicardi-Goutières syndrome, pseudo-TORCH syndrome, and mutations in the *JAM3*, *NDE1*, and *ANKLE2* genes)
- Torpedo-like maculopathy
- Illicit drugs or alcohol abuse during pregnancy. Illicit drugs such as cocaine, when taken during pregnancy, may cause optic nerve abnormalities, including optic disc hypoplasia and optic disc atrophy, as well as delayed visual maturation.[1] Alcohol abuse during pregnancy may lead to fetal alcohol syndrome, which is associated with optic nerve hypoplasia and decreased vision.[2]

Working Diagnosis

- Congenital Zika syndrome (CZS)

Multimodal Testing and Results

- Fundus photographs
  - A well-defined chorioretinal atrophy and gross macular pigment mottling is visualized but may not be present in all affected newborns.[3]
- Optical coherence tomography (OCT)
  - OCT imaging of the macula can be performed in the affected eyes and shows significant retinal thinning where the scar is located, discontinuation of the ellipsoid zone, hyperreflectivity underlying the retinal pigment epithelium, and choroidal thinning (Fig. 39.2).[4]
- Fluorescein angiography (FA)
  - FA shows a window defect corresponding to the chorioretinal atrophy, as well as hypofluorescent dots at the site of pigment dispersion in the macula (Fig. 39.3).[5]

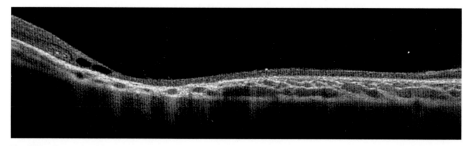

Fig. 39.2 Example of the ocular coherence tomography imaging of a chorioretinal scar in the macula caused by congenital Zika infection.

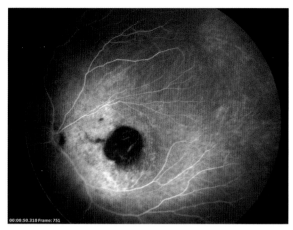

Fig. 39.3   Fluorescein angiography imaging of the child's left eye showing window defect and hypofluorescent dots in the macula corresponding to the chorioretinal atrophy and pigment mottling, as well as an avascularity of the peripheral retina.

- Neuroimaging
  - Neuroimaging (computed tomography and magnetic resonance imaging) will typically show cortical and subcortical calcifications, increased ventricles, marked cortical thinning, and hypoplasia or absence of the corpus callosum. In addition, cranial deformities such as severe microcephaly, overlapping cranial sutures, and craniofacial disproportion can also be noted.[6]
- Laboratory and genetic testing
  - The gold-standard examination to confirm Zika virus infection is real-time polymerase chain reaction and should be performed in both mother and child when CZS is suspected. The laboratory investigation of other congenital infectious diseases should be performed, and genetic testing is also recommended.[6]

Management

- General management for CZS includes managing the complications related to the neurological, ocular, and skeletal findings. Initially, these infants need to have their seizures controlled and dysphagia assessed by pediatric neurologists and pediatric gastroenterologists, respectively. These infants also require special attention regarding their limbs because congenital contractures and hypertonia are commonly observed.[7]
- Given that the fundus findings did not show any signs of uveitis or inflammatory activity, no treatment was required for retinal findings.
- Given that the newborn presented with hypoaccommodation, magnification spectacles were prescribed.[8]
- Given that the newborn presented with severe visual impairment, early intervention low vision therapy was initiated.[9]

Follow-up Care

- Given the novelty of this entity, there are no previously established guidelines for follow-up.

- Given the lack of knowledge on progression of lesions and findings, the newborn was closely followed during her first year of life and then yearly after that.
- Ophthalmological examinations should include structural examination and functional assessments.[10]
- Early intervention program including visual, motor, hearing, and intellectual therapies is of great value when managing these children.[9]

Algorithm 39.1: Differential Diagnosis for Congenital Chorioretinal Scar

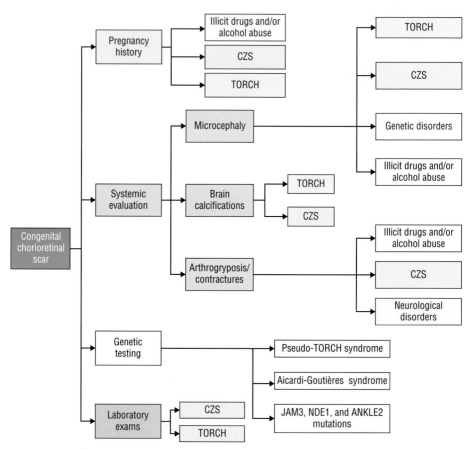

Algorithm 39.1 Differential diagnosis for congenital chorioretinal scar. *CZS,* congenital Zika syndrome; *TORCHS,* toxoplasmosis, other agents, rubella, cytomegalovirus, herpes simplex.

Key Points

- Consider CZS when there are arbovirus symptoms during any trimester of pregnancy or there is a history of Zika virus infection, as well as in all children born in regions with endemic microcephaly or any other cranial or neurological findings.
- One-third of children with CZS present structural ocular findings, of which funduscopic findings are the most observed.

- Visual impairment is commonly observed in children with CZS.
- A multidisciplinary team and early intervention therapies are essential when managing these children to promote better visual and neurodevelopment.

References

1. Good WV, Ferriero DM, Golabi M, et al. Abnormalities of the visual system in infants exposed to cocaine. *Ophthalmology*. 1992;99:341-346.
2. Strömland K. Ocular abnormalities in the fetal alcohol syndrome. *Acta Ophthalmol Suppl (1985)*. 1985;171:1-50.
3. Ventura CV, Zin A, Paula Freitas B, et al. Ophthalmological manifestations in congenital Zika syndrome in 469 Brazilian children. *J AAPOS*. 2021;25(3):158.e1-158.e8.
4. Ventura CV, Ventura LO, Bravo-Filho V, et al. Optical coherence tomography of retinal lesions in infants with congenital Zika syndrome. *JAMA Ophthalmol*. 2016;134(12):1420-1427.
5. Ventura CV, Gois AL, Freire BO, et al. Fluorescein angiography findings in children with congenital Zika syndrome. *Ophthalmic Surg Lasers Imaging Retina*. 2019;50:702-708.
6. Moore CA, Staples JE, Dobyns WB, et al. Characterizing the pattern of anomalies in congenital Zika syndrome for pediatric clinicians. *JAMA Pediatr*. 2017;171:288-295.
7. Bailey Jr DB, Ventura LO. The likely impact of congenital Zika syndrome on families: considerations for family supports and services. *Pediatrics*. 2018;141(suppl 2):S180-S187.
8. Ventura LO, Lawrence L, Ventura CV, et al. Response to correction of refractive errors and hypoaccommodation in children with congenital Zika syndrome. *J AAPOS*. 2017;21(6):480-484.e1.
9. Ventura CV, Ventura LO. Ophthalmologic manifestations associated with Zika virus infection. *Pediatrics*. 2018;141(suppl 2):S161-S166.
10. de Oliveira Dias JR, Ventura CV, de Paula Freitas B, et al. Zika and the eye: pieces of a puzzle. *Prog Retin Eye Res*. 2018;66:85-106.

CHAPTER 40

Unilateral Floaters and Vitreous Cells

Ali R. Salman ■ Wendy M. Smith ■ Diva R. Salomao ■
Lauren A. Dalvin ■ Timothy W. Olsen

History of Present Illness

We present a case of a 58-year-old woman referred for treatment-refractory anterior uveitis and vitritis of her left eye after cataract surgery 2 years earlier. She also reported inflammatory arthritis (seronegative) and abdominal pain with nausea and vomiting for over 10 years. She was HLA-B27 positive. Subjectively, she reported persistent, symptomatic floaters in the left eye with blurry vision. Previously, she was managed with topical and intravitreal corticosteroids and systemic immune suppression.

OCULAR EXAMINATION FINDINGS

Visual acuity with pinhole correction was 20/20 in the right eye and 20/30 in the left eye. Intraocular pressures were normal. External and anterior segment examinations were normal in the right eye. There were 1+ anterior chamber cells of the pseudophakic left eye along with diffuse vitreous cells, but no chorioretinal lesions or vitreous opacities were present.

IMAGING

Optical coherence tomography (OCT) of the left eye showed irregular macular thickening, an epiretinal membrane with flattening of the foveal depression and inner retinal striae, and no subretinal deposits or intraretinal fluid. The choroid had normal thickness.

Questions to Ask

- Was the cataract surgery complicated? Certain complications increase the risk of postoperative indolent endophthalmitis.
  - No
- Has the patient experienced neurological symptoms, fevers, chills, or night sweats? Vitreoretinal lymphoma should be considered in the differential diagnosis for treatment-refractory uveitis and frequently has concurrent central nervous system lesions.
  - No
- Has the patient had a high-risk infectious exposure? Multiple infectious etiologies may present with chronic uveitis, including tuberculosis and Lyme disease.
  - No
- Has the patient experienced weight loss from her gastrointestinal symptoms? Whipple disease affects gastrointestinal absorption, leading to diarrhea and potential weight loss.
  - Yes

Assessment

- A 58-year-old woman with a history of seronegative inflammatory arthritis and GI symptoms is referred for treatment of a refractory anterior uveitis and vitritis in her left eye after cataract surgery 2 years earlier. Examination revealed left eye anterior chamber cells, vitreous cells, and an epiretinal membrane with inner retinal striae.

Differential Diagnosis

- Chronic endophthalmitis
- Vitreoretinal lymphoma
- Sarcoidosis
- *Mycobacterium avium-intracellulare* complex
- Tuberculosis
- Presumed ocular histoplasmosis
- Multifocal choroiditis and panuveitis—no chorioretinal lesions were present in this patient
- Amyloidosis—vitreous does not show glass wool opacities, and no material is seen emanating from the retinal vessels
- Lyme disease

Working Diagnosis

- Ocular Whipple disease
  - Whipple disease can present with seronegative inflammatory arthritis, diarrhea, weight loss, chronic anterior uveitis, vitritis, and typically follows an indolent course.[1]

Examination/Multimodal Testing and Results

- Slit lamp examination
  - The left eye had 1+ anterior chamber cells, diffuse vitreous cells, and 1+ vitreous haze. Other possible findings may include corneal keratic precipitates, crystalline keratopathy, and iris or lens deposits.[1]
- Fundus photographs
  - There was an epiretinal membrane with traction on the retina. Patients may also exhibit vitreous infiltrates, chorioretinal lesions, periphlebitis, macular edema, optic disc edema, and optic atrophy.[1]
- Neuroophthalmic examination
  - Neuroophthalmic findings were not noted. Oculomasticatory myorhythmia, which involves a smooth pendular convergent-divergent nystagmus with concurrent contractions of the masticatory muscles, is considered a pathognomonic sign of Whipple disease.[2]
- OCT
  - An OCT of the left eye showed macular thickening, an epiretinal membrane, flattening of the foveal depression, and inner retinal striae without cystoid macular edema.
- Vitreous biopsy
  - The patient had a therapeutic and diagnostic pars plana vitrectomy. The specimen demonstrated the classic finding of foamy histiocytes with intracytoplasmic, PAS+ gram-positive rods consistent with *Tropheryma whipplei*[3] (Fig. 40.1). *T. whipplei* was then confirmed in the specimen by polymerase chain reaction (PCR).
  - Aqueous humor may be sampled when uveitis is primarily localized to the anterior chamber.

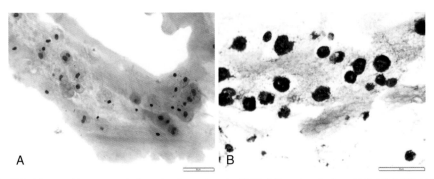

Fig. 40.1 Vitreous biopsy sample hematoxylin and eosin (H&E) *(left)* and periodic acid–Schiff (PAS) *(right)* stains. The *left* image highlights the classic finding of "foamy" histiocytes, so named for the abundant clear bubbly cytoplasm on H&E staining. The *right* image depicts the presence of PAS+ intracellular *T. whipplei* organisms.

- Extraocular biopsy
  - Over 70% of patients with ocular Whipple's disease also experience systemic findings.[1]
  - Initially known as "intestinal lipodystrophy," Whipple's disease is most commonly diagnosed from small bowel biopsy samples using PAS staining and PCR assays.[4]
  - Other sites may be biopsied depending on suspected areas of involvement (e.g., synovial fluid may be sampled in patients with arthritis) (Fig. 40.2).

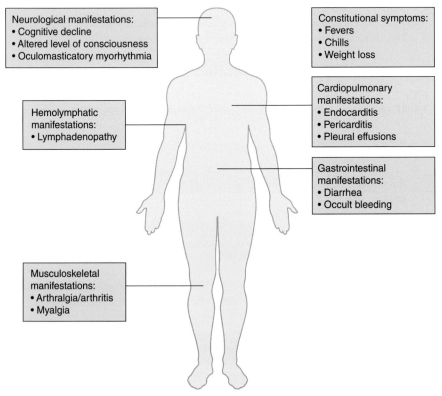

Neurological manifestations:
• Cognitive decline
• Altered level of consciousness
• Oculomasticatory myorhythmia

Constitutional symptoms:
• Fevers
• Chills
• Weight loss

Cardiopulmonary manifestations:
• Endocarditis
• Pericarditis
• Pleural effusions

Hemolymphatic manifestations:
• Lymphadenopathy

Gastrointestinal manifestations:
• Diarrhea
• Occult bleeding

Musculoskeletal manifestations:
• Arthralgia/arthritis
• Myalgia

Fig. 40.2 Systemic manifestations of Whipple disease.

Management

- Without treatment, Whipple's disease is fatal.[5]
- Immediately after diagnosis, patients should be started on at least a 2-week course of intravenous (IV) ceftriaxone or a combination of IV streptomycin and penicillin G.
- After the acute phase of treatment, patients require a long course of oral antibiotics, typically oral trimethoprim/sulfamethoxazole. Secondary options include a tetracycline, such as doxycycline, or rifampin.[4]
- Oral antibiotics must be continued for at least 1 to 2 years.[6]
- After PCR confirmation of the diagnosis, the patient was started on 4 weeks of IV ceftriaxone followed by 1 year of oral trimethoprim/sulfamethoxazole.

Follow-up Care

- There are no previously established guidelines for follow-up.
- Our patient has been followed on a biannual basis and has continued to improve from her systemic and ocular symptoms.
- Follow-up intervals vary according to the presence and nature of complications, such as uveitis and glaucoma.

Algorithm 40.1: Algorithm for Chronic Uveitis

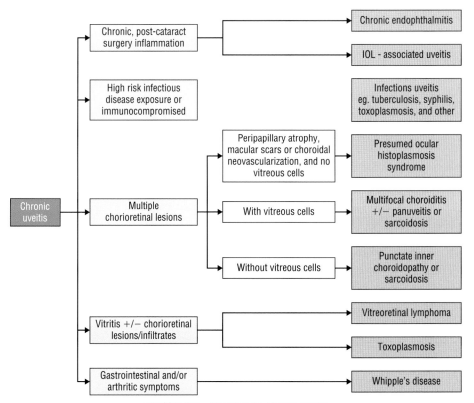

Algorithm 40.1   Algorithm for chronic uveitis.

Key Points

- Consider Whipple disease in patients with chronic recalcitrant uveitis, especially in the setting of systemic symptoms such as diarrhea, weight loss, and arthralgias.
- Left untreated, Whipple disease can be fatal.
- Given the chronic nature of the infection, a prolonged course of systemic, oral antibiotics are required after an initial phase of IV treatment.

References

1. Chan R, Yannuzzi L, Foster C. Ocular Whipple's disease. *Ophthalmology*. 2001;108;2225-2231.
2. Schwartz MA, Selhorst JB, Ochs AL, et al. Oculomasticatory myorhythmia: a unique movement disorder occurring in Whipple's disease. *Ann Neurol*. 1986;20(6):677-683.
3. Raoult D, Birg M, La Scola B, et al. Cultivation of the bacillus of Whipple's disease. *N Engl J Med*. 2000;342:620-625.
4. Fenollar F, Puéchal X, Raoult D. Whipple's disease. *N Engl J Med*. 2007;356:55-66.
5. Dutly F, Altwegg M. Whipple's disease and *"Tropheryma whippelii"*. *Clin Microbiol Rev*. 2001;14:561-583.
6. Touitou V, Fenollar F, Cassoux N, et al. Ocular Whipple's disease: therapeutic strategy and long-term follow-up. *Ophthalmology*. 2012;119:1465-1469.

Retinovascular

CHAPTER 41

Bilateral Retinal Hemorrhages in a Young Man

David Sarraf ■ Meira Fogel-Levin ■ SriniVas Sadda ■ Sushant Wagley

History of Present Illness

A 19-year-old male patient woke up with bilateral blurred vision. Past medical history was positive for ventriculoperitoneal (VP) shunt inserted 11 years earlier due to secondary hydrocephalus caused by traumatic head injury.

OCULAR EXAMINATION FINDINGS

On examination, visual acuity was 20/150 in the right eye (OD) and 20/60 in the left eye (OS). Extraocular muscle examination revealed a bilateral abduction deficit. Intraocular pressures and anterior segment examination were unremarkable. Dilated fundus examination demonstrated retinal venous engorgement and tortuosity associated with multilayered retinal hemorrhages, retinal exudates, and optic disc edema in each eye (Fig. 41.1).

IMAGING

Spectral-domain optical coherence tomography (OCT) of the nerve demonstrated bilateral optic disc elevation (Fig. 41.2A, B). OCT B scan through the macula showed multiple retinal hemorrhages OU, including subretinal, intraretinal, and sub–internal limiting membrane (ILM) hemorrhages (Fig. 41.2C, D).

Questions to Ask

- Did the patient report any neurological signs (e.g., headache, nausea, weakness)?
  - Yes. The patient reported occasional headaches, vomiting with abdominal distention, and lower extremity weakness. Elevated intracranial pressure (ICP) can be an important cause of bilateral optic disc edema and bilateral sixth nerve palsy.[1,2] Retinal hemorrhages can be noted adjacent to the nerve in cases of elevated ICP.[3]
- Did the patient report any history of recent head trauma? Head trauma is one of the most common etiologies of bilateral sixth nerve palsy.[1,2]
  - The patient denied any history of recent head trauma.
- Did the patient endorse any history of high blood pressure? Severe (grade 4) malignant hypertension can cause optic nerve edema and multilayered retinal hemorrhages.[4]
  - The patient's blood pressure was normal by history and examination.

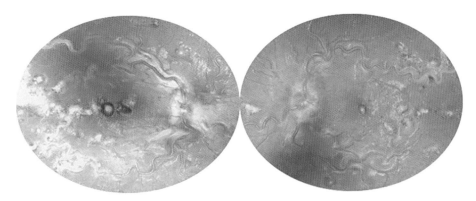

Fig. 41.1 Ultrawide-field color fundus images of both eyes illustrate bilateral tortuous and engorged retinal veins, retinal hemorrhages, and exudates associated with optic disc edema. Note the white centered hemorrhages in both eyes.

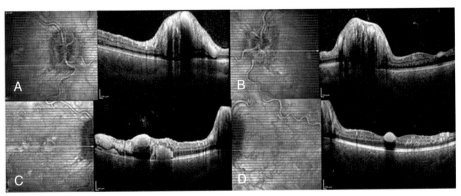

Fig. 41.2 Cross-sectional spectral-domain optical coherence tomography (OCT) B scans of both eyes (OU) through the optic disc (in A and B) and central fovea (in C and D). (A, B) OCT shows elevated optic discs OU. (C, D) OCT of the right eye shows hyperreflective multilayered retinal hemorrhages, including intraretinal and subretinal hemorrhages, and OCT of the left eye shows central hyperreflective sub–ILM hemorrhage.

- Did the patient have any history of blood clotting or hematological disorders? Central retinal vein occlusion (CRVO) can cause venous engorgement and tortuosity with retinal hemorrhages. Simultaneous bilateral CRVO in a young adult should raise the possibility of systemic conditions leading to a hyperviscosity syndrome such as immunogammopathy or leukemia.[5-8]
  - No. The patient denied any personal or familial history of hypercoagulation disorders or hematological diseases.

Assessment

This is a case of a 19-year-old male patient with history of VP shunt who presented with bilateral vision loss, vomiting, abdominal distention, headaches, and leg weakness. Examination revealed bilateral sixth nerve palsy, optic disc edema, and engorged retinal veins with retinal exudation and multilayered retinal hemorrhages.

Differential Diagnosis

- Elevated ICP (possible causes in this case include VP shunt obstruction or infection)
- Hypertensive retinopathy
- Diabetic retinopathy
- Retinitis (infectious, infiltrative)
- Optic neuritis (infectious, infiltrative)
- CRVO
- Hyperviscosity syndrome

Working Diagnosis

Hyperviscosity syndrome OU

Systemic Investigation

- VP shunt imaging (with computed tomography [CT]/magnetic resonance imaging)
  - Imaging was unremarkable and there were no signs of VP shunt catheter malfunction or obstruction
- Basic laboratory tests
  - White blood count (WBC): 697,000/μL
  - Hemoglobin: 8.4 g/L
  - Platelets: 387,000/μL
    - Up to half of the patients with leukemia may demonstrate ocular involvement.[9] CRVO is reported in conjunction with an extremely high WBC blood count causing a hyperviscosity syndrome.[10]
- Abdomen CT
  - CT showed an enlarged spleen. Leukemic cells can accumulate in the spleen leading to splenic enlargement and abdominal distention.

New Working Diagnosis

After ruling out VP shunt obstruction and given the abnormal blood count, a diagnosis of hyperviscosity syndrome secondary to blood dyscrasia was rendered.

Multimodal Retinal Imaging

- OCT
  - OCT showed multiple levels of retinal hemorrhage, including sub-ILM, intraretinal, and subretinal hemorrhages (Fig. 41.2).
- Fundus autofluorescence (FAF)
  - FAF displayed hypoautofluorescent blockage corresponding to the retinal hemorrhages (Fig. 41.3).
- Wide-field fluorescein angiography (WF-FA)
  - WF-FA confirmed the presence of retinal venous tortuosity OU. Blockage corresponding to the retinal hemorrhages was noted OU (Fig. 41.4).
  - Nonperfusion was identified in the temporal peripheral retina OU (Fig. 41.4). Bilateral peripheral retinal nonperfusion with secondary collaterals and retinal neovascularization has been described in cases of chronic myelogenous leukemia (CML) and attributed to complications of hyperviscosity.[11,12]

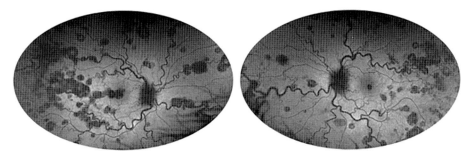

Fig. 41.3   Ultrawide-field autofluorescence of both eyes (OU) shows round hypoautofluorescent lesions corresponding to the retinal hemorrhages OU. Retinal veinous tortuosity is well illustrated OU.

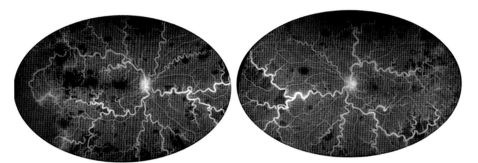

Fig. 41.4   Late ultrawide-field fluorescein angiography illustrates optic disc leakage, retinal venous tortuosity and associated microvascular abnormalities, and peripheral retinal nonperfusion with adjacent leakage in both eyes.

Management

The patient experienced an acute deterioration in his neurological status during the hospitalization course with decreased level of consciousness and fixed pupils. Lumbar puncture showed a high opening pressure (56 cm H_2O) and positive cytology for leukemic cells.

- An emergency shunt surgery was performed, which revealed ventricular catheter obstruction due to the leukemic cells. This was possibly an acute event as previous scans of the shunt were normal.
- Acute treatment was initiated. Intravenous fluids, mannitol, steroids, and hydroxyurea were administered, and leukapheresis was performed.
- Bone marrow biopsy was completed and confirmed a myeloid profile consistent with the diagnosis of CML.
- The patient was treated with dasatinib, a tyrosine kinase inhibitor for CML.

Follow-up Care

- Vision improved to 20/40 OD and 20/20 OS just 2 weeks after the baseline presentation. Ophthalmic examination showed significant improvement of the bilateral abduction deficit and resolution of the optic disc edema.
- No ocular intervention was necessary during the acute phase.

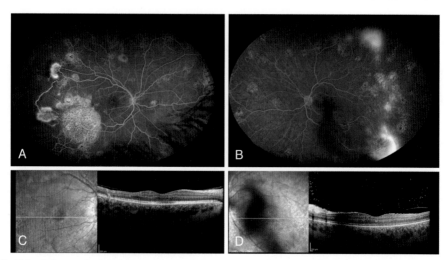

Fig. 41.5 Follow-up 8 months later. Ultrawide-field fluorescein angiography (FA) of the right (A) and left (B) eyes and follow-up cross-sectional spectral-domain optical coherence tomography (OCT) B scans through the central macula of the right (C) and left (D) eyes. (A, B) FA demonstrates multiple fronds of retinal neovascularization with late leakage at the margins of retinal nonperfusion in both eyes (OU). Note the collateral formation temporal in the right eye (OD). Large patches of retinal pigment epithelium mottling are present OU. There is marked improvement of the retinal venous tortuosity and resolved optic disc edema OU. (C, D) OCT shows resolution of the retinal hemorrhages OU, with no evidence of subretinal or intraretinal fluid. Focal disruption of the ellipsoid zone is noted temporal to the fovea OD. Thinning of the inner nuclear layer can also be appreciated temporal OD corresponding to an earlier paracentral acute middle maculopathy lesion.

- Close follow-up to assess for the development of macular edema, retinal ischemia, and secondary retinal neovascularization is essential. Treatments with intravitreal anti–vascular endothelial growth factor injection, panretinal laser photocoagulation (PRP), and even vitrectomy, for severe cases, can be indicated.[13,14]
- The patient was lost to follow-up but returned 8 months later. Examination and ultrawide-field fluorescein angiography (FA) showed the development of bilateral retinal neovascularization at the margins of peripheral retinal nonperfusion. OCT demonstrated complete resolution of the multilayered hemorrhages with no evidence of edema in either eye. Urgent PRP was performed in each eye, and the patient was followed to ensure regression of the neovascularization (Fig. 41.5).

Key Points

- The combination of bilateral retinal venous tortuosity associated with multilayered retinal hemorrhages and exudates and optic disc edema should raise the possibility of a hyperviscosity syndrome due to an immunogammopathy, such as Waldenström macroglobulinemia, or a blood dyscrasia, such as leukemia.
- OCT is an essential tool to detect macular edema, and FA is an important modality to detect peripheral nonperfusion and retinal neovascularization. Early detection and close follow-up are recommended.

Algorithm 41.1: Algorithm for Bilateral Retinal Hemorrhages in a Young Patient

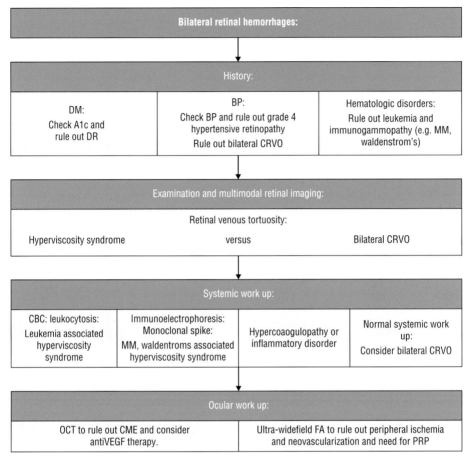

Algorithm 41.1   Algorithm for bilateral retinal hemorrhages in a young patient. *antiVEGF*, Anti–vascular endo-thelial growth factor; *BP*, blood pressure; *CBC*, complete blood count; *CME*, cystoid macular edema; *CRVO*, central retinal vein occlusion; *DM*, diabetes mellitus; *DR*, diabetic retinopathy; *FA*, fluorescein angiography; *MM*, multiple myeloma; *OCT*, optical coherence tomography; *PRP*, panretinal photocoagulation.

References

1. Rigi M, Almarzouqi SJ, Morgan ML, Lee AG. Papilledema: epidemiology, etiology, and clinical management. *Eye Brain*. 2015;7:47-57.
2. Durkin SR, Tennekoon S, Kleinschmidt A, Casson RJ, Selva D, Crompton JL. Bilateral sixth nerve palsy. *Ophthalmology*. 2006;113(11):2108-2109.
3. Binenbaum G, Rogers DL, Forbes BJ, et al. Patterns of retinal hemorrhage associated with increased intracranial pressure in children. *Pediatrics*. 2013;132(2):e430-e434.
4. Chatterjee S, Chattopadhyay S, Hope-Ross M, Lip PL. Hypertension and the eye: changing perspectives. *J Hum Hypertens*. 2002;16(10):667-675. [Erratum in: J Hum Hypertens. 2002;16(12):901].
5. Golesic EA, Sheidow TG. An otherwise healthy young man presents with bilateral CRVO as the first sign of hyperviscosity syndrome in the setting of new multiple myeloma. *Retin Cases Brief Rep*. 2015; 9(1):38-40.
6. Tomasini DN, Segu B. Systemic considerations in bilateral central retinal vein occlusion. *Optometry*. 2007;78(8):402-408.

7. Gelman R, DiMango EA, Schiff WM. Sequential bilateral central retinal vein occlusions in a cystic fibrosis patient with hyperhomocysteinemia and hypergamma-globulinemia. *Retin Cases Brief Rep.* 2013; 7(4):362-367.

8. Rajagopal R, Apte RS. Seeing through thick and through thin: retinal manifestations of thrombophilic and hyperviscosity syndromes. *Surv Ophthalmol.* 2016;61(2):236-247.

9. Schachat AP, Markowitz JA, Guyer DR, Burke PJ, Karp JE, Graham ML. Ophthalmic manifestations of leukemia. *Arch Ophthalmol.* 1989;107(5):697-700.

10. Narang S, Gupta P, Sharma A, Sood S, Palta A, Goyal S. Bilateral central retinal vein occlusion as presenting feature of chronic myeloid leukemia. *Middle East Afr J Ophthalmol.* 2016;23(3):253-255.

11. Reddy SC, Jackson N, Menon BS. Ocular involvement in leukemia: a study of 288 cases. *Ophthalmologica.* 2003;217(6):441-445.

12. Nobacht S, Vandoninck KF, Deutman AF, Klevering BJ. Peripheral retinal nonperfusion associated with chronic myeloid leukemia. *Am J Ophthalmol.* 2003;135(3):404-406.

13. Huynh TH, Johnson MW, Hackel RE. Bilateral proliferative retinopathy in chronic myelogenous leukemia. *Retina.* 2007;27(1):124-125.

14. Almeida DR, Chin EK, Grant LW. Chronic myelogenous leukemia presenting with bilateral optic disc neovascularization. *Can J Ophthalmol.* 2014;49(3):e68-e70.

CHAPTER 42

Multiple Branch Retinal Artery Occlusions in a Woman

Anita Agarwal ■ Livia Della Mora

History of Present Illness

A 29-year-old otherwise healthy woman woke up with field loss in her right eye. She denies photopsias, headache, hearing loss, or acute neurological symptoms. She takes a seizure medication but is otherwise healthy.

OCULAR EXAMINATION FINDINGS

Her visual acuities were 20/80 in the right eye and 20/20 in the left eye. She had a relative afferent pupillary defect on the right side, and the anterior segment and vitreous were quiet in each eye. The right fundus examination showed three areas of retinal whitening secondary to multiple branch retinal artery occlusions. The left fundus examination was unremarkable.

IMAGING

Fundus photographs of the right eye eyeshowed retinal opacification in the superior half of the macula, superior and nasal to the disc; these areas correspond to the distribution of the affected branch retinal arterioles (Figs. 42.1 and 42.2). There is evidence of earlier occlusion of two inferonasal branches with sclerosed segments of the arterioles (Fig. 42.2, *arrows*). The left eye (Fig. 42.3) was not involved at this time. Fluorescein angiogram (FA) of the right eye (Fig. 42.4) shows multiple occluded arterioles (Fig. 42.5) and the characteristic finding of arteriolar wall staining of the affected and many of the unoccluded arterioles (Fig. 42.6) in contrast to the left eye (Fig. 42.7). Optical coherence tomography shows inner retinal thickening and opacification of the infarcted retina with shadowing of the underlying outer retina (Figs. 42.8 and 42.9).

Questions to Ask

- Did the patient have a similar episode or symptoms previously? Clotting disorders, related to factor V Leiden deficiency and protein S or protein C abnormalities, may be associated with recurrent thrombosis. The branch retinal artery occlusions recur in Susac syndrome; hence a history is useful.
  - No
- Does the patient have a history of carotid or cardiovascular disease? Branch retinal artery occlusions can result from carotid atherosclerotic disease, cardiac valvular disease, left atrial myxoma, and patent foramen ovale.
  - No

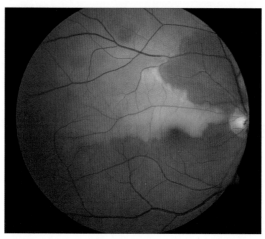

Fig. 42.1 Opacification of the superior macula from occlusion of a branch arteriole close to the optic disc.

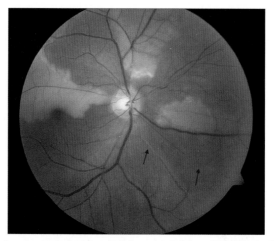

Fig. 42.2 Simultaneous occlusion of multiple branch arterioles with resultant retinal whitening.

- Has the patient had any recent cosmetic procedure? Emboli can result from retrograde embolism from triamcinolone injection to a hemangioma on the face or intranasal injections into a turbinate or from retrograde embolism after injection of fillers in cosmetic surgery.
  - No
- Is there hearing loss? The condition, Susac syndrome, affects arterioles in the retina, brain, and inner ear.
  - Yes
- Any previous focal neurological deficits or behavior alterations?
  - No

Branch retinal arterial occlusions, hearing loss, and focal neurological deficits constitute the triad of Susac syndrome. The involvement of the three different structures could be delayed, and a history related to hearing loss or neurological symptoms is useful. The peri–corpus callosal areas and limbic system are involved; hence patients may have "brain fogginess" or bizarre or unexpected behavior changes.

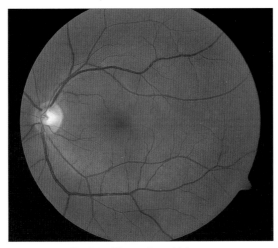

Fig. 42.3   The unaffected left eye.

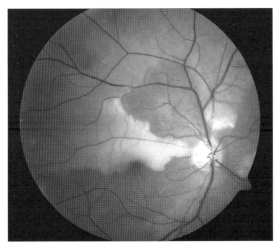

Fig. 42.4   Red-free image of the right eye showing areas of retinal opacification from multiple arteriolar occlusions.

Assessment

This is a case of a 29-year-old woman with recurrent and multiple simultaneous branch retinal artery occlusions with typical fluorescein staining of the affected and some unaffected arterioles. Though she did not have hearing loss or neurological symptoms at the time of presentation, she had peri–corpus callosal infarcts on magnetic resonance imaging (MRI), confirming the clinical diagnosis of Susac syndrome.

Differential Diagnosis

Branch retinal artery occlusions from other causes should be considered.

- *Bartonella henselae* retinitis (cat scratch disease) at the site of a retinal arteriole: neuroretinitis and/or patches of focal white retinitis are typically seen; these are not present in our patient; also no history of owning cats in this patient

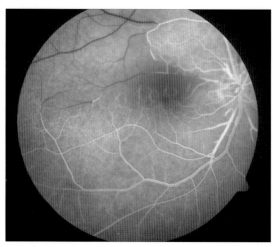

Fig. 42.5 Early phase fluorescein angiogram showing not only the occluded macular arteriole but also early staining of the walls of other arterioles in the vicinity of the optic disc.

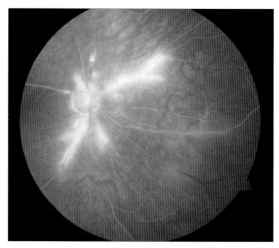

Fig. 42.6 Late-phase angiogram showing fusiform staining of affected arterioles and subsequent leakage of dye into the surrounding retina from many still unoccluded but affected arteriolar walls. Those with total occlusion show boxcarring.

- Toxoplasma retinitis in the vicinity of a retinal arteriole causing occlusion: no areas of retinitis or vitritis in this patient
- Protein S or protein C deficiency: protein C and protein S levels not checked as the patient had the typical fluorescein pattern of fusiform arteriolar wall staining that is unique to Susac syndrome and does not warrant testing for other conditions
- Fat embolism in a patient with persistent foramen ovale: typically posttraumatic or postpartum
- Talc embolism from intravenous drug use in patient with patent foramen ovale: usually multiple crystalline deposits seen in the retina and arteriolar lumen
- Embolism from a carotid plaque: refractile embolus if cholesterol embolus
- Embolism from a left atrial appendage or valvular vegetations: no work-up done to rule out calcific plaques or platelet fibrin emboli as the FA was diagnostic of Susac syndrome

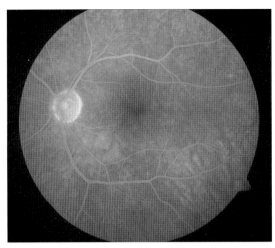

Fig. 42.7 Left eye is not involved. Note the normal retinal vasculature on fluorescein angiogram.

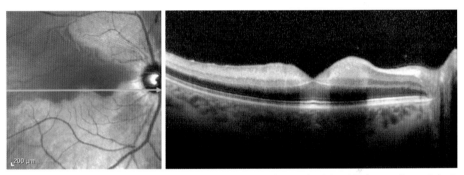

Fig. 42.8 Optical coherence tomography B-scan demonstrating hyperreflectivity of the inner retina and shadowing beneath it corresponding to areas of retinal infarction.

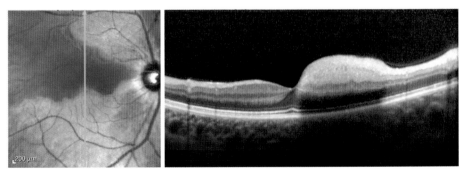

Fig. 42.9 Vertical section through the macula displaying hyperreflectivity of the affected areas.

- Retrograde embolism from triamcinolone injection to a hemangioma on the face or intranasal injections into a turbinate
- Retrograde embolism from injection of fillers in cosmetic surgery
- Branch retinal artery occlusion in a prepapillary loop
- Sickle cell retinopathy with arteriolar occlusion
- Systemic lupus erythematosus (SLE) and, rarely, dermatomyositis

Diagnosis

Susac syndrome (recurrent idiopathic branch retinal artery occlusions)

Multimodal Imaging

- Fundus photographs
  - Multiple areas of retinal whitening in the right eye result from branch retinal artery occlusions. There are almost never any retinal hemorrhages in Susac syndrome, unlike SLE and dermatomyositis.
- FA
  - The appearance on FA of fusiform staining of the affected arterioles and often many of the non-occluded arterioles is a pathognomonic sign in Susac syndrome. Eyes with *Bartonella* or toxoplasma retinitis will show staining of the patch of retinitis in the vicinity of the occluded vessel. An embolus causes occlusion at a bifurcation; however, the occlusion in Susac syndrome is not at a bifurcation, but along a segment of the arteriole. A careful examination of the fundus will reveal emboli, retinitis, periarteriolar plaques, or features of sickle cell retinopathy. Lupus retinopathy and dermatomyositis result in several retinal hemorrhages and the fluorescein leakage is widespread, unlike the isolated fusiform staining of the arteriolar wall in Susac syndrome.
- MRI
  - MRI of the brain, especially sagittal sections to look for peri–corpus callosal white matter changes, helps corroborate the diagnosis.
- Audiogram
  - An audiogram to look for sensory neural hearing loss may be done.
- Lab tests
  - They are not necessary to rule out other causes such as protein C and protein S deficiencies if the typical FA pattern is seen. However, if the affected arteriole is completely occluded preventing the fluorescein from passing beyond the occlusion, and no other arteriole is partly involved, the typical fusiform staining of the arteriole is not seen. Lab tests to rule out protein C and protein S deficiency will be necessary in that situation.

Management

- High-dose systemic steroids tapered over 6 to 8 weeks
- Intravenous immunoglobulin (IVIG)
- Immunomodulatory drugs such as mycophenolate mofetil
- Rituximab

Follow-up Care

- Regular follow-up to see if the lesions recur and wide-field FA imaging to monitor for resolution and disappearance of the arteriolar wall staining and leakage.
- Annual Goldmann visual field to look for asymptomatic field loss.
- Maintenance immunosuppression with mycophenolate mofetil or other immunosuppressives.

Key Points

- Consider Susac syndrome in patients with recurrent and multiple branch retinal artery occlusions with hearing loss and/or neurological changes.
- Sometimes the triad of vision loss, hearing loss, and neurological features can manifest over several years.
- Susac syndrome patients need urgent neurologic evaluation with MRI imaging to look for peri–corpus callosal changes on T2 fluid-attenuated inversion recovery sequences.
- IVIG, high-dose systemic steroids, and immunosuppressive medications are urgently needed.
- Neurology, otolaryngology, and retinal follow-up is needed on a regular basis.
- There is no definitive blood test available to confirm circulating antibodies or other biomarkers.

Algorithm 42.1: Algorithm for Differential Diagnosis for Susac Syndrome

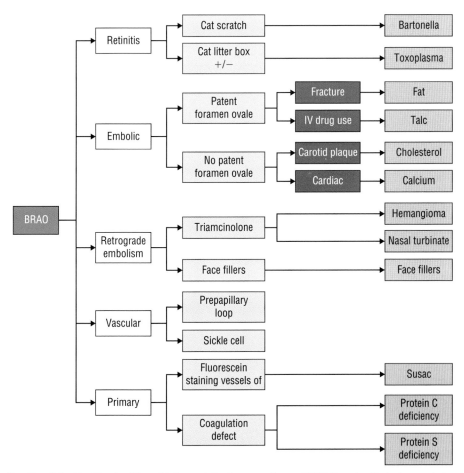

Algorithm 42.1 Algorithm for differential diagnosis for Susac syndrome. *BRAO,* Branch retinal artery occlusion; *IV,* intravenous.

References

1. Agarwal A. Idiopathic recurrent branch retinal arterial occlusion (Susac syndrome). In: *Gass' Atlas of Macular Diseases*. Vol 1. United Kingdom: Elsevier Saunders; 2012:474.
2. Ayache D, Plouin-Gaudon I, Bakouche P, Elbaz P, Gout O. Microangiopathy of the inner ear, retina, and brain (Susac syndrome): report of a case. *Arch Otolaryngol Head Neck Surg*. 2000;126(1):82-84.
3. Eluvathingal Muttikkal TJ, Vattoth S, Keluth Chavan VN. Susac syndrome in a young child. *Pediatr Radiol*. 2007;37(7):710-713.
4. Gass JD, Tiedeman J, Thomas MA. Idiopathic recurrent branch retinal arterial occlusion. *Ophthalmology*. 1986;93(9):1148-1157.
5. Haider AS, Viswanathan D, Williams D, Davies P. Paracentral acute middle maculopathy in Susac syndrome. *Retin Cases Brief Rep*. 2020;14(2):150-156.
6. Johnson MW, Flynn Jr HW, Gass JD. Idiopathic recurrent branch retinal arterial occlusion. *Arch Ophthalmol*. 1989;107(5):757.
7. Pawate S, Agarwal A, Moses H, Sriram S. The spectrum of Susac's syndrome. *Neurol Sci*. 2009;30(1):59-64.
8. Rennebohm RM, Asdaghi N, Srivastava S, Gertner E. Guidelines for treatment of Susac syndrome: an update. *Int J Stroke*. 2020;15(5):484-494.
9. Snyers B, Boschi A, De Potter P, Duprez T, Sindic C. Susac syndrome in four male patients. *Retina*. 2006;26(9):1049-1055.
10. Susac JO, Hardman JM, Selhorst JB. Microangiopathy of the brain and retina. *Neurology*. 1979;29(3):313-316.
11. Susac JO. Susac's syndrome: the triad of microangiopathy of the brain and retina with hearing loss in young women. *Neurology*. 1994;44(4):591-593.
12. Susac JO, Egan RA, Rennebohm RM, Lubow M. Susac's syndrome: 1975–2005 microangiopathy/autoimmune endotheliopathy. *J Neurol Sci*. 2007;257(1-2):270-272.
13. Turczynska MJ, Krajewski P, Brydak-Godowska JE. Widefield fluorescein angiography in the diagnosis of Susac syndrome. *Retina*. 2021;41(7):1553-1561.
14. Vodopivec I, Prasad S. Treatment of Susac syndrome. *Curr Treat Options Neurol*. 2016;18(1):3.

CHAPTER 43

Unilateral Disc Edema in an Elderly Woman

Michael T. Andreoli   ▧   William F. Mieler

History of Present Illness

An 82-year-old female patient with a history of hyperlipidemia and hypertension presented urgently for central and peripheral vision loss in the right eye. She denied pain or visual symptoms in the left eye.

OCULAR EXAMINATION FINDINGS

Visual acuity was 3/200 in the right eye and 20/40 in the left eye with an afferent pupillary defect. Intraocular pressure was normal. External and anterior segment examination showed pseudophakia in each eye. Dilated fundus examination showed disc edema in the right eye. Humphrey visual field testing showed significant field constriction in the right eye.

IMAGING

Optical coherence tomography (OCT) showed nerve edema. Fluorescein angiogram (FA) showed impaired choroidal filling temporally and nasally, extending into the arteriovenous phase in the right eye.

Questions to Ask

- Has the patient had any strokes?
  - No
- Has the patient had recent fevers, chills, night sweats, weight loss, headaches, scalp tenderness, or jaw claudication?
  - No
- Does the patient have a history of rheumatological conditions?
  - No

Assessment

- This is a case of an 82-year-old female patient with hypertension and hyperlipidemia presenting with new-onset pallid disc edema and impaired choroidal filling on FA in the right eye.

Differential Diagnosis[1,2]

- Giant cell arteritis (GCA)

- Lupus retinopathy
- Granulomatosis with polyangiitis
- Nonarteritic anterior ischemic optic neuropathy

Working Diagnosis

- GCA. The patient was found to have elevated erythrocyte sedimentation rate (ESR) and C-reactive protein (CRP). Temporal artery biopsy confirmed the diagnosis of GCA.

Multimodal Testing and Results

- Fundus photographs
  - On fundus examination, disc edema (which may be accompanied by pallor) is often present (Fig. 43.1).[3]
- OCT
  - OCT of the optic nerve may show elevation or retinal nerve fiber layer thickening Figs. 43.2).
- Visual field
  - Severe deficits in the visual field are seen (Fig. 43.3).

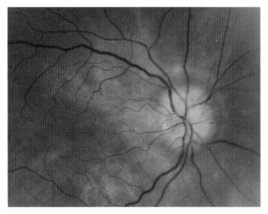

Fig. 43.1 Fundus photograph of the posterior pole shows waxy pallor of the optic nerve.

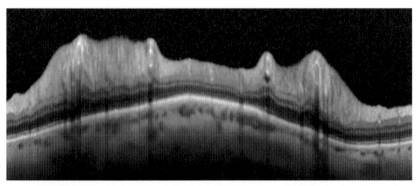

Fig. 43.2 Optical coherence tomography of the optic nerve shows nerve edema with thickening of the retinal nerve fiber layer.

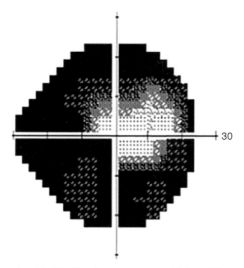

Fig. 43.3 Humphrey visual field testing shows severe constriction of the peripheral visual field.

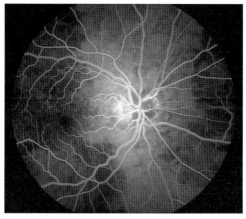

Fig. 43.4 Fluorescein angiography of the arteriovenous phase shows anomalous optic nerve vessels and sectoral choroidal ischemia in a triangular distribution.

- FA
  - Restricted choroidal filling, especially in a triangular distribution called triangular sign of Amalric, is concerning for GCA or other systemic inflammatory conditions (Fig. 43.4).[4]

Management

- An urgent diagnostic workup, including ESR, CRP, and complete blood count, are recommended. When there is concern for GCA, a temporal artery biopsy should be performed, even without abnormalities on blood testing.
- When visual function has been affected, many experts recommend urgent intravenous steroid treatment,[1] which is typically followed by oral steroid taper and possible immunomodulatory therapy.

Follow-up Care

- Systemic care is often provided by a rheumatologist.
- Ocular management is typically performed by an ophthalmologist, often with neurooph-thalmology or retina training.

Algorithm 43.1: Giant Cell Arteritis

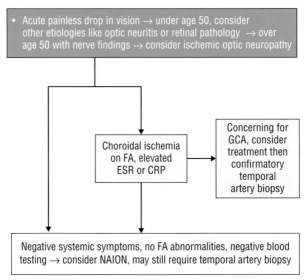

Algorithm 43.1 Giant cell arteritis. *CRP,* C-reactive protein; *ESR,* erythrocyte sedimentation rate; *FA,* fluorescein angiography; *GCA,* giant cell arteritis; *NAION,* nonarteritic anterior ischemic optic neuropathy.

Key Points

- GCA can have a spectrum of ophthalmic findings, but typical findings include optic nerve edema and choroidal ischemia on FA.
- Consider GCA in the setting of acute vision loss in a patient over the age of 50 without other valid explanation.
- Systemic symptoms and blood work can be helpful to risk stratify these patients; however, temporal artery biopsy is crucial to the definitive diagnosis.
- Patients with GCA often require long-term immunosuppression therapy.

References

1. Fein AS, Ko MW. Neuro-ophthalmologic complications of giant cell arteritis: diagnosis and treatment. *Semin Neurol.* 2019;39(6):673-681.
2. Margolin E. The swollen optic nerve: an approach to diagnosis and management. *Pract Neurol.* 2019; 19(4):302-309.
3. McFadzean RM. Ischemic optic neuropathy and giant cell arteritis. *Curr Opin Ophthalmol.* 1998;9(6): 10-17.
4. Valmaggia C, Speiser P, Bischoff P, Niederberger H. Indocyanine green versus fluorescein angiography in the differential diagnosis of arteritic and nonarteritic anterior ischemic optic neuropathy. *Retina.* 1999;19(2):131-134.

CHAPTER 44

Peripheral Transient Fluctuating Retinal Lesion

Talisa E. de Carlo Forest ▪ William F. Mieler

History of Present Illness

A 58-year-old female patient was referred for evaluation of a choroidal mass in the right eye.

OCULAR EXAMINATION AND IMAGING

- Best corrected visual acuity was 20/20 in both eyes.
- Pupils, intraocular pressure, and extraocular motility were all within normal limits.
- External and slit-lamp examination were unremarkable aside from minimal nuclear sclerotic cataracts bilaterally.
- Dilated fundus examination demonstrated mildly pigmented elevations overlying the inferotemporal vortex vein in the right eye (Fig. 44.1). There was no evidence of hemorrhage, subretinal fluid, orange pigment, or other associated pathology. The left eye was unremarkable.
- B-scan ultrasonography demonstrated enlargement of the lesion with Valsalva and downgaze and flattening of the lesion with ocular digital pressure and primary gaze (Fig. 44.2).

Questions to Ask

- Any growth of the lesions over time? Malignant neoplasms will grow over time, but benign lesions such as varix of the vortex vein ampulla, choroidal nevi, and congenital hypertrophy of the retinal pigment epithelium are expected to be stable.
  - No
- Any history of metastatic cancer? Cancer can metastasize to the choroid causing multifocal tumors.
  - No
- Any photopsias or change in subjective vision? Some choroidal melanomas may be symptomatic.
  - No
- Any history of retinal bleeds and peripheral drusen? Subretinal hemorrhage from choroidal neovascularization in eyes with peripheral exudative hemorrhagic chorioretinopathy (PEHCR) can be mistaken for a choroidal mass. This would be expected to change color from red to yellow as the hemorrhage dehemoglobinizes over a few of months.
  - No

Assessment

- This is a 58-year-old female patient with one incidentally noted, stable-appearing, mildly pigmented mass overlying the vortex vein in the right eye.

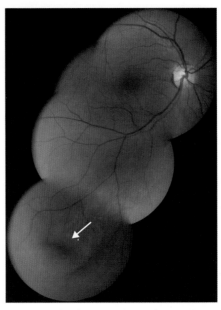

Fig. 44.1 Montage of color fundus photographs demonstrating a pigmented mass *(arrow)* overlying the inferotemporal vortex vein but an otherwise normal retina.

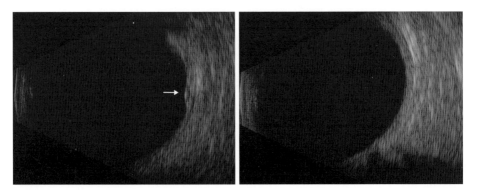

Fig. 44.2 Dynamic B-scan ultrasonography showing that the lesion *(arrow)* is elevated on downgaze *(left)* and flattened in primary gaze *(right)*.

Differential Diagnosis

- Varix of the vortex vein ampulla
- Choroidal nevus
- Choroidal metastasis
- Choroidal melanoma
- Peripheral exudative hemorrhagic chorioretinopathy (PEHCR)

Working Diagnosis

- Varix of the vortex vein ampulla

Multimodal Testing and Results

Additional testing is optional and supportive of the clinical diagnosis.
- Dynamic B-scan ultrasonography
    - The mass will enlarge with Valsalva or altered change in gaze and diminish with ocular digital pressure.[1]
- Color fundus photographs
    - Fundus photography shows the mass(es) overlying the vortex vein with a contiguous mildly pigmented reddish coloration. The mass may have a bilobed appearance. There may be multiple varices.
- Fluorescein angiography and indocyanine green angiography
    - Angiography demonstrates the lesion to fill in the early choroidal phase and outlines the lesion as dilations of the vortex vein ampullae that collapse with digital pressure.[2,3]
- Peripheral optical coherence tomography (OCT)
    - Peripheral OCT demonstrates a hyporeflective choroidal elevation and dilated choroidal vessels.[4,5] No delineated choroidal mass, overlying outer retinal or retinal pigment epithelial changes, or subretinal fluid would be expected. The lesion should diminish with ocular digital pressure.[6]
- Fundus autofluorescence
    - The lesions demonstrate a hypoautofluorescent rings surrounding a mildly hyperautofluorescent center.[7]

Management and Follow-up Care

- No follow-up (except for routine ocular examinations based on age) or treatment is necessary. Correct diagnosis can save a patient from unnecessary testing and frequent follow-up.[8,9]

Algorithm 44.1: Algorithm for Differential Diagnosis

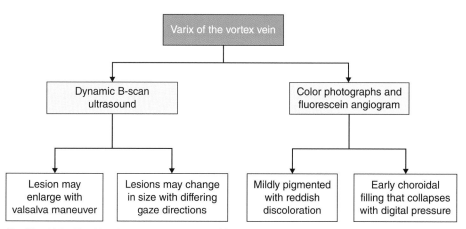

Algorithm 44.1 Algorithm for differential diagnosis.[1,4] Key features include the location overlying the vortex ampulla, changes in size of the lesion with Valsalva maneuver, and possible collapse with digital massage. The other entities in the differential diagnosis do not have similar characteristics.

Key Points

- The patient's condition may mimic a choroidal tumor.
- A varix of the vortex ampulla is generally a harmless finding that can be safely observed and monitored.

References

1. de Carlo TE, Mieler W. Dynamic echography of varix of the vortex vein ampulla. *Retin Cases Brief Rep.* 2021;15(5):548-551.
2. Kang HK, Beaumont PE, Chang AA. Indocyanine green angiographic features of varix of the vortex vein ampulla. *Clin Exp Ophthalmol.* 2000;28(4):321-323.
3. Kang TD, Douglass AM, Ferenczy SR, Say EA, Shields CL. In vivo hemodynamic changes of vortex vein varix on real-time video angiography. *Retina.* 2017;37(2):e8-e9.
4. Ismail RA, Sallam A, Zambarakji HJ. Optical coherence tomographical findings in a case of varix of the vortex vein ampulla. *Br J Ophthalmol.* 2011;95(8):1169-1182.
5. Murtagh P, O'Dwyer G, Horgan N. Vortex vein ampulla. *Ophthalmology.* 2021;128(12):1707.
6. Spiess K, Elgohary MA. Diagnosis of vortex varix using optical coherence tomography and scleral indentation. *Retin Cases Brief Rep.* 2022;16(3):362-364.
7. Veronese C, Staurenghi G, Pellegrini M, et al. Multimodal imaging in vortex vein varices. *Retin Cases Brief Rep.* 2019;13(3):260-265.
8. Al-Dahmash SA, AlBloushi AF, Alsarhani WK. Multiple giant vortex vein varices masquerading as choroidal metastases. *J Fr Opthalmol.* 2021;44(1):e31-e33.
9. Gündüz K, Shields CL, Shields JA. Varix of the vortex vein ampulla simulating choroidal melanoma: report of four cases. *Retina.* 1998;18(4):343-347.

CHAPTER 45

Acute Vision Loss With Peripapillary Cotton Wool Spots

Melissa Yao ▪ Ahmad Santina ▪ SriniVas Sadda ▪ David Sarraf

History of Present Illness

A 26-year-old healthy male patient presented with a 1-week history of acute vision loss. Ocular history was noncontributory.

OCULAR EXAMINATION FINDINGS

Snellen visual acuity was 20/30 in the right eye (OD) and 20/70 in the left eye (OS). Intraocular pressures were normal, and external and anterior segment examination were unremarkable in both eyes (OU). Dilated retinal examination showed multiple cotton wool spots (CWS) in a peripapillary distribution OU and spot retinal hemorrhages in the inferior macula OS (Fig. 45.1).

IMAGING

Optical coherence tomography (OCT) displayed central subretinal fluid (SRF) OU and band-like, hyperreflective infarcts of the inner (CWS) and middle (paracentral acute middle maculopathy [PAMM]) retina OU (Figs. 45.2 and 45.3).

Questions to Ask

- Did the patient endorse a history of diabetes? Diabetic retinopathy can present with CWS and retinal hemorrhage.
  - No. The patient's hemoglobin A_{1C} was 5.1 at the time of the encounter.
- What medications did the patient report taking? Medications such as interferon can cause CWS.
  - None
- Did the patient report a history of trauma? Trauma has been associated with Purtscher retinopathy.
  - No
- Did the patient admit to a history of autoimmune disorders? Systemic lupus erythematosus (SLE), scleroderma, and dermatomyositis can be complicated by a Purtscher-like retinopathy.
  - No. The patient denied any significant medical history.
- Did the patient have any evidence of pancreatitis?
  - Yes. The patient presented to the emergency room 1 week earlier with severe vomiting and cramping and was found to have acute pancreatitis with a serum lipase level of 1721 (10–40 normal).

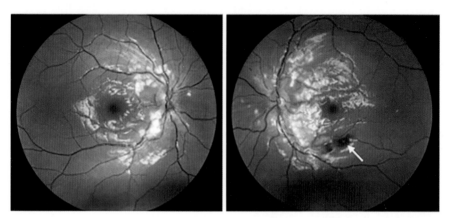

Fig. 45.1 Color fundus photography shows multiple cotton wool spots in a peripapillary distribution. Note the associated large flame hemorrhage inferior to the fovea in the left eye *(right image, white arrow)*.

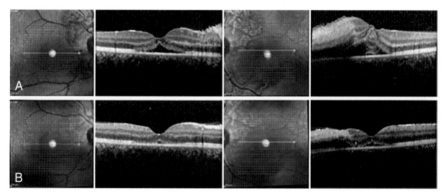

Fig. 45.2 Optical coherence tomography (OCT) B scans of the right eye *(left column)* and left eye *(right column)* at baseline (A) show central subretinal fluid (SRF) in both eyes. Hyperreflective thickening in the inner retinal layer and hyperreflective bands in the inner nuclear layer correspond to cotton wool spots (CWS) and paracentral acute middle maculopathy, respectively. The OCT B scans of the right eye *(left column)* and left eye *(right column)* at follow-up (B) show resolved SRF in the right eye, improved SRF in the left eye, and improvement of the CWS in both eyes. There was slight improvement in the visual acuity of the left eye after 10 days with subjective improvement of vision.

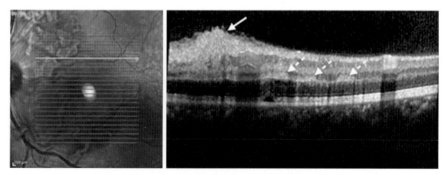

Fig. 45.3 Optical coherence tomography B scan of the left eye at baseline shows a cotton wool spot *(solid arrow)* in the nerve fiber layer and several paracentral acute middle maculopathy or paracentral acute middle maculopathy lesions *(dotted arrows)* in the middle retina.

Assessment

■ This is a case of a 26-year-old healthy male patient with a recent admission for acute pancreatitis who presented with vision loss and peripapillary CWS OU.

Differential Diagnosis

Differential Diagnoses	Etiologies
Purtscher retinopathy	• Trauma (head trauma, long bone fracture or crush injury, chest compression, barotrauma)
Purtscher-like retinopathy (morphologically identical to Purtscher retinopathy but with a nontrauma etiology)	• Pancreatitis (acute + chronic) • Malignancy (pancreatic adenocarcinoma, liquid tumors) • Connective tissue disorders (SLE, scleroderma, dermatomyositis) • Cryoglobulinemia • Hemolytic uremic syndrome/thrombotic thrombocytopenic purpura • Chronic renal failure • Pregnancy complications (preeclampsia, placenta abruptio, HELLP [hemolysis, elevated liver enzymes, and low platelets] syndrome) in women • Embolism (fat, amniotic fluid, air) • Orthopedic surgery • Orbital injections
Medications	Interferon
Local vascular	• Diabetic retinopathy • Incomplete central retinal artery occlusion • Retinal vasculitis

Working Diagnosis

■ Purtscher-like retinopathy secondary to acute pancreatitis.

Diagnostic criteria for Purtscher retinopathy (at least three criteria required for diagnosis)[1]	• CWS (posterior pole) • Retinal hemorrhages (less than 10) • Purtscher flecken • Plausible explanatory etiology • Complementary investigation compatible with the diagnosis

Multimodal Testing and Results

■ Color fundus photography
  ■ Fundus photography showed peripapillary CWS OU (Fig. 45.1). Deeper, gray-white polygonal lesions called Purtscher flecken,[2] which correspond to PAMM lesions with OCT (i.e., inner nuclear layer [INL]) infarcts, can also be identified in Purtscher cases.
  ■ CWS are fluffy, superficial, chalky white lesions along the nerve fiber layer with blurred margins and are located superficial to retinal vessels.
  ■ Additional findings can include macular edema, pseudo–cherry-red spot, intraretinal hemorrhage, and disc edema.[1,3]

- Visual field
  - A central or paracentral scotoma may be identified with Purtscher retinopathy.[4]
- Spectral-domain OCT
  - CWS were present OU (Figs. 45.2 and 45.3) and can be appreciated as areas of hyper-reflective nerve fiber layer thickening and represent inner retinal infarcts.[5]
  - PAMM lesions were present OU (Figs. 45.2 and 45.3) and are hyperreflective, band-like infarcts at the level of the INL (middle retina) that correspond to Purtscher flecken on the fundus examination.[2,5] These leave a legacy of INL thinning in the late phase.
  - Intraretinal fluid and SRF can also be identified with OCT in patients with Purtscher retinopathy (Fig. 45.2).[3]
- Near-infrared reflectance (NIR)
  - NIR images show parafoveal dark-gray lesions corresponding to the PAMM lesions and the Purtscher flecken.[5,6]
- Fluorescein angiography (FA)
  - FA can show retinal capillary nonperfusion and leakage, focal areas of arteriolar occlusion, paravascular staining, and optic disc edema.[4,7,9]
- OCT angiography (OCTA)
  - OCTA can display non perfusion or flow deficit at the level of the superficial (CWS) and deep (PAMM) retinal capillary plexus.[4,7]

Management

- Management consists of treating the inciting cause of Purtscher retinopathy, instituting supportive care, and monitoring for any complications.[3]
- Treatment with high-dose corticosteroid versus observation showed no improvement in visual acuity in one systematic review study of Purtscher retinopathy.[1]
- Visual recovery after Purtscher retinopathy is variable: improvement of visual function without treatment can be seen in the majority of patients, although permanent visual deficits can remain.[8]
- The cause of pancreatitis in this case was heavy alcohol intake. The patient was counseled to discontinue alcohol ingestion and referred for systemic pancreatitis management with an internist.
- Visual acuity remained stable OD (20/30) and improved to 20/60 OS 10 days after presentation and CWS regressed OU. OCT showed improvement of the CWS and SRF in each eye (Fig. 45.2).

Follow-up Care

- There are no previously established guidelines for follow-up.[3]
- Long-term sequelae of Purtscher or Purtscher-like retinopathy include optic atrophy, retinal nerve fiber layer thinning, sheathing of retinal vessels, and inner and middle retinal thinning with OCT. Eyes should be monitored with regular dilated fundus examination and multimodal retinal imaging.[3]

Algorithm 45.1: Algorithm for Peripapillary Cotton Wool Spots

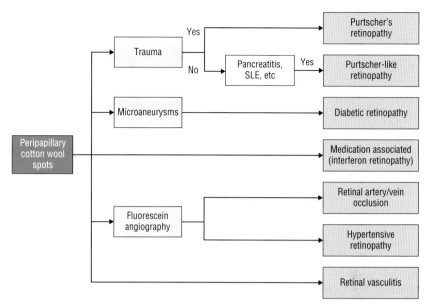

Algorithm 45.1 Algorithm for peripapillary cotton wool spots. *SLE,* Systemic lupus erythematosus.

Key Points

- Consider the causes of Purtscher retinopathy in patients with a peripapillary distribution of CWS.
- Classical etiologies include trauma and pancreatitis, but other causes, such as SLE, interferon, and incomplete central retinal artery occlusion, should also be excluded.
- In Purtscher retinopathy, inner retinal infarcts (i.e., CWS) and middle retinal INL infarcts (i.e., PAMM) both can be identified with examination, fundus photography, and OCT.
- Systemic management of the cause of Purtscher retinopathy is essential. Retinal lesions (i.e., CWS, PAMM) will spontaneously resolve but can leave a legacy of permanent thinning and scotoma.

References

1. Miguel AI, Henriques F, Azevedo LF, Loureiro AJ, Maberley DA. Systematic review of Purtscher's and Purtscher-like retinopathies. *Eye (Lond).* 2013;27(1):1-13.
2. Rahimy E, Kuehlewein L, Sadda SR, Sarraf D. Paracentral acute middle maculopathy: what we knew then and what we know now. *Retina.* 2015;35(10):1921-1930.
3. Tripathy K, Patel BC. Purtscher retinopathy. In: *StatPearls.* StatPearls Publishing; Updated April 3, 2023. Accessed May 13, 2023. Available at: https://www.statpearls.com/point-of-care/28465.
4. Agrawal A, McKibbin MA. Purtscher's and Purtscher-like retinopathies: a review. *Surv Ophthalmol.* 2006;51(2):129-136.
5. Chen X, Rahimy E, Sergott RC, et al. Spectrum of retinal vascular diseases associated with paracentral acute middle maculopathy. *Am J Ophthalmol.* 2015;160(1):26-34.e1.
6. Yu S, Wang F, Pang CE, Yannuzzi LA, Freund KB. Multimodal imaging findings in retinal deep capillary ischemia. *Retina.* 2014;34(4):636-646.
7. Santamaría Álvarez JF, Serret Camps A, Aguayo Alvarez J, García García O. Optic coherence tomography angiography follow-up in a case of Purtscher-like retinopathy due to atypical hemolytic uremic syndrome. *Eur J Ophthalmol.* 2020;30(3):NP14-NP17.
8. Agrawal A, McKibbin M. Purtscher's retinopathy: epidemiology, clinical features and outcome. *Br J Ophthalmol.* 2007;91(11):1456-1459.
9. Gomez-Ulla F, Fente B, Torreiro MG, Salorio MS, Gonzalez F. Choroidal vascular abnormality in Purtscher's retinopathy shown by indocyanine green angiography. *Am J Ophthalmol.* 1996;122(2):261-263.

CHAPTER 46

Unilateral Leukocoria

Mohammad Amr Sabbagh ▪ Michael T. Massengill ▪ George Skopis ▪ Felix Chau

History of Present Illness

A 2-year-old male patient with no medical history presented to clinic with 4 months of an "enlarged, gold right pupil" with some "turning out of the right eye and pain" per the patient's mother.

OCULAR EXAMINATION FINDINGS

Visual acuity was assessed as "fixes and follow" in both eyes. Intraocular pressure was normal to palpation in both eyes. There was a 4+ relative afferent pupillary defect in the right eye. Extraocular movements were full, and the patient was orthophoric with intermittent right eye exotropia.

Anterior segment examination was overall unremarkable, as both eyes exhibited normal adnexa, white and quiet conjunctiva, clear corneas, deep and quiet anterior chambers, and clear lenses. On later examination under anesthesia, neovascularization of the iris of the right eye was present; the left iris was normal.

Dilated funduscopic examination in the right eye revealed leukocoria with diffuse vitreous cells that obscured the view of the optic nerve and macula. Inferiorly, there were snowball-like opacities present. Superiorly, there was a region of subretinal white exudate or possible calcification. The left eye revealed a healthy-appearing optic nerve, well-perfused retinal blood vessels, flat and attached macula, and no abnormalities in the periphery (Fig. 46.1).

IMAGING

B-scan ultrasonography demonstrated numerous vitreous opacities and posterior exudative retinal detachment, along with a hyperechoic mass lesion in the subretinal space. When the gain was decreased to zero dB, there were still opacities present inferiorly, which with higher gain demonstrated posterior shadowing, highly suggestive of calcification. The left eye was normal. A representative B-scan illustrating similar findings is shown in Fig. 46.2.

Magnetic resonance imaging (MRI) of the brain and orbits (with and without contrast) revealed a mildly hyperintense enhancing tissue mass measuring 0.8 cm × 2.2 cm in the posterior third of the right globe and retina with some extension of enhancement into the distal 5 mm of the optic nerve. The tissue exhibited a gradient echo susceptibility, likely secondary to calcification (Fig. 46.3).

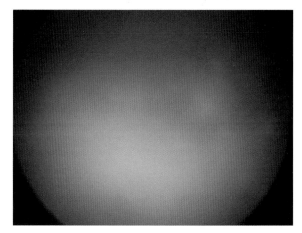

Fig. 46.1 Fundus photograph: extensive vitreous seeds obscuring retinal details.

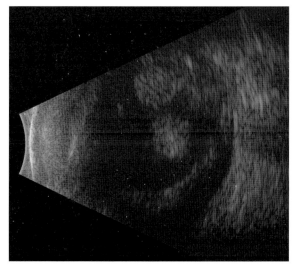

Fig. 46.2 Representative B-scan ophthalmic ultrasound: mass lesion, calcified component with posterior shadowing, exudative retinal detachment, vitreous opacities.

Questions to Ask

- What is the patient's medical history? Specifically, is there any history of inflammatory or infectious conditions? Any history of TORCH (toxoplasmosis, rubella, cytomegalovirus, herpes simplex virus) infections? Trauma?
  - None. Inflammatory or infectious conditions would have more suggestive history and may also be bilateral. Old trauma may present as dehemoglobinized, white vitreous hemorrhage that could mimic cells of inflammation or seeds of retinoblastoma. Congenital infections may also be bilateral.

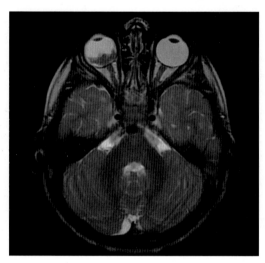

Fig. 46.3 Magnetic resonance imaging brain/orbits, axial scan: right eye with posterior mass lesion, subretinal extension, and optic nerve invasion.

- Does the patient have any systemic signs or symptoms?
  - None. Inflammatory or infectious causes may have more systemic manifestations. TORCH infections, tuberculosis and sarcoidosis, and other alternative diagnoses may present with systemic manifestations, as well as with eye findings. However, these would be unlikely to include an ocular mass lesion resembling retinoblastoma. Only a late presentation of retinoblastoma with metastatic spread would likely have systemic findings beyond the eye.
- Is there a family history of any ocular conditions or systemic malignancies?
  - No eye conditions.
  - Paternal grandfather has a history of non-Hodgkin lymphoma.

Assessment

- This is a 2-year-old male patient with no medical history who presented with leukocoria in his right eye, with examination and imaging findings concerning for retinoblastoma.

Differential Diagnosis

- Cataract
- Coats disease (retinal telangiectasis)
- Familial exudative vitreoretinopathy (FEVR)
- Incontinentia pigmenti
- Myelinated retinal nerve fiber layer
- Persistent fetal vasculature (PFV)
- Retinoblastoma
- Toxocariasis
- Uveitis (infectious and/or inflammatory)
- Old vitreous hemorrhage

Working Diagnosis

- Unilateral nonhereditary retinoblastoma, group E (International Classification of Retinoblastoma)

Multimodal Testing and Results

- Fundus photographs
  - Fundus photographs are useful to document the presence of vitreous seeds and the tumor appearance if visible on examination.
- Ultrasound
  - B-scan ultrasound generally demonstrates a hyperechoic mass with dense opacities and posterior shadowing in the presence of calcifications. Dimensions of the tumor can also be estimated.
- MRI
  - MRI is important both for ocular assessment of retinoblastoma along with any potential extraocular extension. Pineal gland assessment is also important to determine whether pineoblastoma is present.
  - MRI is preferred over computed tomography scan to avoid radiation exposure, which can be particularly harmful in patients with retinoblastoma, especially in the heritable subtype.
  - Our patient's MRI showed possible extension 5 mm into the distal optic nerve.
- Genetic testing
  - Genetic testing was negative, consistent with sporadic, unilateral retinoblastoma.

Management

- Intravenous chemotherapy involves a combination of agents, typically vincristine, etoposide, and carboplatin, in six to nine consecutive cycles and is pursued with germ-line mutation, a positive family history, or invasive disease.[1]
- Intraarterial chemotherapy provides local treatment that can achieve higher drug delivery and may be well suited for unilateral disease but requires special centers for administration. It may also be employed for globe salvage in refractory tumors and even tandem therapy in select cases.[2,3]
- Local treatments with cryotherapy and transpupillary thermotherapy with diode laser can aid in tumor consolidation with the above systemic therapies and for small, focal intraocular seeds.[2]
- Intravitreal chemotherapy may be considered with refractory or recurrent vitreous seed involvement,[4,5] and intracameral injection can be performed to attend to anterior chamber seeding.[2,3]
- Brachytherapy (plaque-radiotherapy) may be used with diffuse anterior segment involvement and in medium-sized chemoresistant tumors that have recurred after systemic therapy.[2,6]
- Enucleation remains an important option especially in group E disease and in other select circumstances, such as realized or suspicion for extraocular extension or after failed salvage therapies.[2]
- External beam radiation can be employed after enucleation with orbital or optic nerve extension or recurrence; however, this increases the risk of secondary malignancies in patients with germline mutations.[2,7]
- Our patient underwent enucleation soon after the initial visit, with pathology confirming a diagnosis of retinoblastoma with extension into the choroid and optic nerve beyond the

lamina cribrosa, though the nerve surgical margin was free of tumor. Per the hematology/oncology service, the patient was considered high risk for systemic metastasis and initiated intravenous chemotherapy (vincristine, carboplatin, etoposide) for a total of six rounds. The patient has since been disease free with no evidence of recurrence.

Follow-up Care

- Patients should be surveilled closely after successful treatment, with high attention paid to local recurrence within 3 years after completion of treatment when risk of disease recurrence is highest, and at least through 7 years of age. Late ocular recurrences are less common but remain possible.[2,8]
- Genetic testing to determine the presence of germline retinoblastoma or mosaicism is important to assess lifetime risk of other malignancies in the patient as well as the need for examinations under anesthesia for surveillance. Family members may also undergo retinoblastoma genetic testing in heritable cases.
- The patient should follow with a pediatric, and later, adult oncologist or cancer survivor clinic for monitoring for secondary malignancies associated with germline mutations in retinoblastoma, which represent a 20% risk. These germline patients are at particular risk of secondary malignancy after external beam radiation, who are at 40% risk.[9-11]

Key Points

- Retinoblastoma can masquerade as other ophthalmic diseases and delay treatment.
- Multiple assessments are integrated simultaneously and in parallel to confirm the diagnosis of retinoblastoma (Fig. 46.4).
- Treatment options are ever evolving and should be selected in conjunction with a knowledgeable ophthalmologist at a facility with access to state-of-the-art resources, such as intraarterial chemotherapy, and in conjunction with a pediatric oncologist.

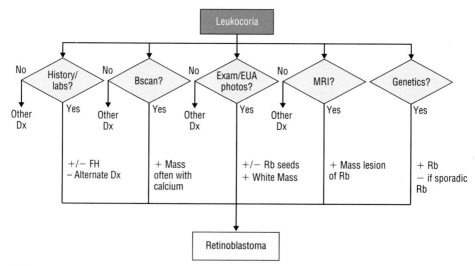

Fig. 46.4 Multiple assessments are integrated simultaneously to reach the diagnosis of retinoblastoma (Rb). *Dx,* Diagnosis; *EUA,* exam under anesthesia; *FH,* family history; *MRI,* magnetic resonance imaging.

- Close surveillance, both by a knowledgeable ophthalmologist for local recurrence and an oncologist for systemic metastasis and secondary malignancies, should follow the completion of treatment.
- Retinoblastoma left untreated is lethal, but survival is improving with advancing knowledge and access to state-of-the-art resources.

References

1. Shields CL, Lally SE, Leahey AM, et al. Targeted retinoblastoma management: when to use intravenous, intra-arterial, periocular, and intravitreal chemotherapy. *Curr Opin Ophthalmol.* 2014;25(5):374-385.
2. Ancona-Lezama D, Dalvin LA, Shields CL. Modern treatment of retinoblastoma: a 2020 review. *Indian J Ophthalmol.* 2020;68(11):2356-2365.
3. Munier FL, Beck-Popovic M, Chantada GL, et al. Conservative management of retinoblastoma: challenging orthodoxy without compromising the state of metastatic grace. "Alive, with good vision and no comorbidity." *Prog Ret Eye Res.* 2019;73:100764.
4. Suzuki S, Kaneko A. Management of intraocular retinoblastoma and ocular prognosis. *Int J Clin Oncol.* 2004;9(1):1-6.
5. Michael DY, Dalvin LA, Welch RJ, Shields CL. Precision intravitreal chemotherapy for localized vitreous seeding of retinoblastoma. *Ocul Oncol Pathol.* 2019;5(4):284-289.
6. Shields CL, Shields JA, De Potter P, et al. Plaque radiotherapy in the management of retinoblastoma: use as a primary and secondary treatment. *Ophthalmology.* 1993;100(2):216-224.
7. Kim JY, Park Y. Treatment of retinoblastoma: the role of external beam radiotherapy. *Yonsei Med J.* 2015;56(6):1478-1491.
8. Shields CL, Honavar SG, Shields JA, Demirci H, Meadows AT, Naduvilath TJ. Factors predictive of recurrence of retinal tumors, vitreous seeds, and subretinal seeds following chemoreduction for retinoblastoma. *Arch Ophthalmol.* 2002;120(4):460-464.
9. Kamihara J, Bourdeaut F, Foulkes WD, et al. Retinoblastoma and neuroblastoma predisposition and surveillance. *Clin Cancer Res.* 2017;23(13):e98-e106.
10. Kleinerman RA, Tucker MA, Tarone RE, et al. Risk of new cancers after radiotherapy in long-term survivors of retinoblastoma: an extended follow-up. *J Clin Oncol.* 2005;23(10):2272-2279.
11. Temming P, Arendt M, Viehmann A, et al. Incidence of second cancers after radiotherapy and systemic chemotherapy in heritable retinoblastoma survivors: a report from the German reference center. *Pediatr Blood Cancer.* 2017;64(1):71-80.

CHAPTER 47

Sudden-Onset Unilateral Vision Loss in a Young Patient With a "Cherry-Red Spot"

Catherine J. Thomas ■ Manjot K. Gill

History of Present Illness

A 48-year-old Asian American woman presented to the emergency department reporting 8 hours of painless loss of vision in her right eye. She denied other associated ocular or neurological symptoms. Her past medical history was notable for well-controlled hypertension and for being a former smoker.

OCULAR EXAMINATION FINDINGS

Visual acuity with correction was hand motions in the right eye and 20/25−2 in the left eye. Intraocular pressures were normal. The external and anterior segment examination was unremarkable. Dilated fundus examination revealed a "cherry-red spot" in the macula and diffuse retinal edema and whitening in the right eye with an area of preserved retina temporal to the disc. Dilated fundus examination of the left eye showed vascular attenuation but was otherwise normal.

IMAGING

Spectral-domain optical coherence tomography (OCT) of the right eye showed an exaggerated foveal contour with diffuse inner retinal edema, marked inner retinal hyperreflectivity, and sparing of the area just temporal to the disc (Fig. 47.1). Fluorescein angiography demonstrated delayed filling and transit times with no evidence of neovascularization.

Questions to Ask

- Does the patient present with other neurological symptoms of stroke?
  - No. However, given the presenting symptoms and examination findings, appropriate workup was performed and included magnetic resonance angiography, computed tomography angiography, and catheter cerebral angiography.
  - Results of imaging studies showed extensive stenosis of the cerebrovascular network with near complete occlusion of the right internal carotid artery with collateral vessel formation. This led to a new diagnosis of Moyamoya disease[1] (Fig. 47.2). The patient subsequently underwent extracranial-intracranial bypass surgery.
- Does the patient have risk factors for embolic conditions, vasculitis, or a hematological/hypercoagulable state?
  - Important vascular risk factors to consider for patients include advancing age, male gender, smoking history, arteriosclerosis, hypertension, diabetes mellitus, and hyperlipidemia.

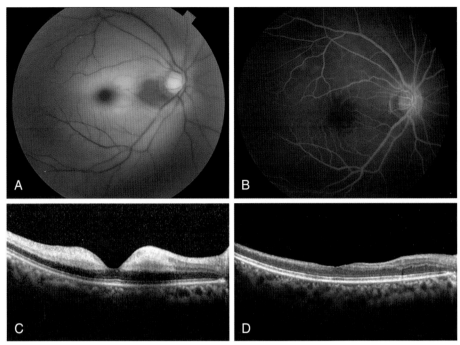

Fig. 47.1 Ophthalmic imaging. (A) Color fundus photograph of the right eye shows classic "cherry-red spot" in the macula and diffuse retinal whitening. There is sparing temporal to the disc with preservation of retinal perfusion. (B) Fluorescein angiogram of the right eye shows reperfusion of the retina. (C) Initial optical coherence tomography (OCT) of the right eye demonstrates inner retinal edema with some sparing nasally in the area corresponding to preserved perfusion temporal to the disc seen in A. (D) OCT of the right eye obtained 2 months after initial presentation demonstrates retinal thinning.

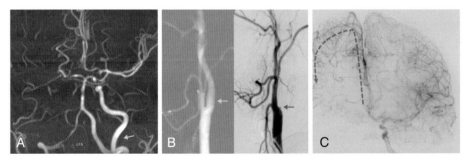

Fig. 47.2 Magnetic resonance angiogram of the brain and catheter cerebral angiogram of the head and neck. (A) Magnetic resonance angiogram of the brain shows complete occlusion of the right internal carotid artery (ICA, *red arrow*) and middle cerebral artery (MCA) along with mild segmental stenosis of the distal left supraclinoid ICA and proximal left MCA. Severe Moyamoya disease was present on the right and mild disease on the left (*green arrow* indicates patent left proximal ICA). (B) Catheter cerebral angiogram of the neck demonstrates complete occlusion of right ICA (right panel, *red arrow*) compared with the nonoccluded left ICA (left panel, *green arrow*). (C) Catheter cerebral angiogram of the head after left ICA injection shows formation of abnormal right-sided collateral arterial supply *(red dotted arrow).*

- Additional diagnostic testing is often warranted and may be tailored to the specific patient.
- Other imaging modalities to consider include transthoracic echocardiography, transesophageal echocardiography, carotid Doppler studies, cerebral angiography, computed tomography of the head, and cerebral magnetic resonance imaging.
- Laboratory tests to consider in younger patients (<50 years) include complete blood cell count, serum chemistries, hemoglobin electrophoresis, prothrombin time, partial thromboplastin time, erythrocyte sedimentation rate, protein C, protein S, antithrombin 3 levels, factor V Leiden, presence of lupus anticoagulant, anticardiolipin antibodies, antinuclear antibodies, antineutrophil cytoplasmic antibodies, angiotensin-converting enzyme, syphilis serology, and serum lipids.
- Does the patient have a history of migraines?
  - Migraines in young people may be associated with retinal vascular occlusions. Proposed mechanisms include increased platelet adhesion, vasoconstriction, and activation of the clotting system.[2]
- Does the patient have a history of trauma?
  - Trauma may give rise to occlusion of the retinal arterial system.
- Does the patient have risk factors for giant cell arteritis?
  - In the appropriate clinical scenario, patients over 50 years of age presenting with acute central retinal artery occlusion (CRAO) should be evaluated for giant cell arteritis including necessary clinical screening questions and laboratory workup. A temporal artery biopsy may also be performed when indicated.

Assessment

- This is a 48-year-old woman with a history of well-controlled hypertension who presented with a CRAO. Extensive workup revealed a diagnosis of Moyamoya disease. Examination and imaging findings were consistent with CRAO with a cherry-red spot in the macula and retinal whitening. The OCT demonstrated inner retinal edema on initial presentation and subsequent retinal thinning on follow-up. The patient underwent craniotomy for external carotid to intracranial anastomosis.

Diagnostic Considerations

- Cardiac valvular disease
- Hereditary and acquired hypercoagulable conditions
- Trauma
- Moyamoya disease
- Vasculitic disorders to consider include giant cell arteritis, Susac syndrome (in cases of multiple branch artery occlusions), systemic lupus erythematosus, polyarteritis nodosa, and granulomatosis with polyangiitis (Wegener granulomatosis)[3]

Differential Diagnosis

- CRAO
- Tay-Sachs disease
- Niemann-Pick disease
- Commotio retinae
- Toxicities: methanol, quinine, carbon monoxide

Working Diagnosis

- CRAO in setting of previously undiagnosed Moyamoya disease

Multimodal Testing and Results

MANAGEMENT

- Immediate stroke evaluation and workup are necessary.
- There is no consensus for treatment for CRAO, though some proposed interventions include:[3]
  - Ocular massage to dislodge embolus
  - Carbogen inhalation
  - Paracentesis and/or topical therapy to lower intraocular pressure
  - Intravenous carbonic anhydrase inhibitors, such as mannitol or acetazolamide
  - Intraarterial thrombolytic therapy
  - Nd:YAG laser embolectomy
- Visual prognosis is poor in the setting of CRAO, except in the presence of a patent cilioretinal artery, where central vision is often spared.[4]
- In the setting of Moyamoya disease, patients require advanced neuroimaging and neurosurgical evaluation.

Follow-up Care

- At 2-month follow-up visit, examination and OCT demonstrated retinal atrophy and thinning (Fig. 47.1D). Vision remained poor at count fingers (CF).
- If patients demonstrate signs of neovascularization, treatment with antivascular endothelial growth factor injections or panretinal photocoagulation should be initiated to prevent further vision loss and complications associated with uncontrolled proliferative disease.

Algorithm 47.1: Cherry-Red Spot Algorithm

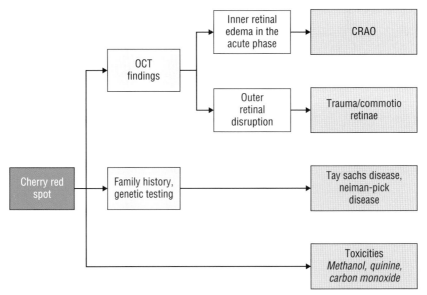

Algorithm 47.1 Cherry-red spot algorithm. *CRAO,* Central retinal artery occlusion; *OCT,* optical coherence tomography.

Key Points

- Occlusion of the CRAO may be due to vascular inflammation, hematological conditions, vasospasm, trauma, or an embolus.
- In the setting of acute vision loss and findings consistent with CRAO, patients should be transferred to a stroke center for immediate evaluation.
- Arteritic CRAO is mostly caused by giant cell arteritis, which should always be ruled out in appropriate clinical scenarios.[3]
- There are no evidence-based treatments for CRAO.
- Moyamoya disease, otherwise known as multiple progressive intracranial occlusion syndrome, is a rare entity of unknown etiology where narrowing or occlusion of the carotid arteries is associated with the development of collateral vascular networks distally.[5]
- Moyamoya disease can affect retinal circulation and should be considered in the differential diagnosis of retinal vascular occlusions in younger patients.

References

1. Rajanala AP, Le HT, Gill MK. Central retinal artery occlusion as initial presentation of Moyamoya disease in a middle-aged woman. *Am J Ophthalmol Case Rep*. 2020;18:100705.
2. Cruysberg JR, Deutman AF. Retinal arterial occlusions in young adults. *Am J Ophthalmol*. 1996;122(1):134.
3. Sim S, Ting D. Diagnosis and management of central retinal artery occlusion. *EyeNet Magazine*. August 2017.
4. Walkden A, Kelly SP. Multimodal imaging of central retinal artery occlusion with retained cilioretinal perfusion. *BMJ Case Rep*. 2016;2016:bcr2016216661.
5. Chace R, Hedges TR III. Retinal artery occlusion due to Moyamoya disease. *J Clin Neuroophthalmol*. 1984;4(1):31-34.

Takayasu Arteritis: Bilateral Progressive Loss of Vision With Aneurysmal Dilatation

Yanliang Li ▪ Monique Munro ▪ Gerardo Ledesma-Gil ▪ William F. Mieler

History of Present Illness

- A 29-year-old female patient presented with a 5-month history of progressive loss of vision in both eyes.
- She also reported red eyes and a foreign body sensation.
- She had no history of previous ophthalmological disorders.
- In the last 2 years, she had been under treatment for vertigo with cinnarizine (antihistamine).

OCULAR EXAMINATION

- Best-corrected visual acuity was 20/1200 in the right eye (OD) and 20/80 in the left eye (OS).
- Her intraocular pressures were 10 mm Hg OD and 8 mm Hg OS.
- Anterior segment examination revealed an afferent pupil defect OD and iris neovascularization OS.
- Dilated fundus examination (Fig. 48.1A, B)
  - Right eye showed disc congestion with surrounding arteriovenous anastomoses, aneurysmal dilatation, distention and tortuosity of central blood vessels, and flame-shaped hemorrhages.
  - Left eye showed increased ramifications and capillarity and white patches.

Imaging

- Fluorescein angiography (FA) (Fig. 48.1C, D)
  - Prolonged arm-to-retina circulation time of 17 seconds
  - Delayed arteriovenous filling time of 30 seconds
  - Reduced choroidal circulation
  - Arteriovenous anastomosis

Questions to Ask: What Would You Do Next?

- Medical history
  - Systemic examination
    - Check systemic blood pressure
    - Decreased brachial artery pulse

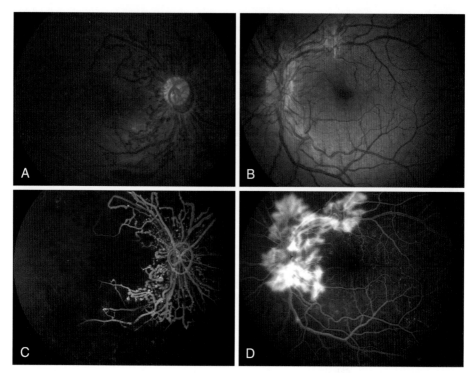

Fig. 48.1 (A) Fundus photograph of the right eye (OD) showing disc edema, peripapillary arteriovenous anastomoses, tortuous vessels, aneurismal dilatation, beading of vessels, increased ramifications and capillarity, and flame-shaped hemorrhages inferiorly. (B) Fundus photograph of the left eye (OS) showing neovascularization, microaneurysms, and retinal nerve fiber layer infarcts. (C) Fluorescein angiography (FA) OD showing arteriovenous shunts and marked neovascularizations. (D) FA OS showing leakage of fluorescein dye.

  - Systemic blood pressure in upper extremities not evaluable
  - Systemic blood pressure in lower limbs: right, 130/90 mm Hg; left, 135/90 mm Hg
- Referral to specialist
  - Blood testing
    - The erythrocyte sedimentation rate was high: 41.
    - Blood chemistry was normal; anti–double-stranded DNA, anticardiolipin antibodies, antinuclear antibodies, antineutrophil cytoplasmic antibodies, fluorescent treponemal antibody absorption, and tuberculosis were negative.

Differential Diagnosis

ASSESSMENT

- Proliferative retinopathies (e.g., diabetes, hypertension)
- Systemic granulomatosis and autoimmune diseases
- Inflammatory aortitis
- Eosinophilic granulomatosis with polyangiitis
- Cerebral aneurysms
- Syphilis
- Fibromuscular dysplasia

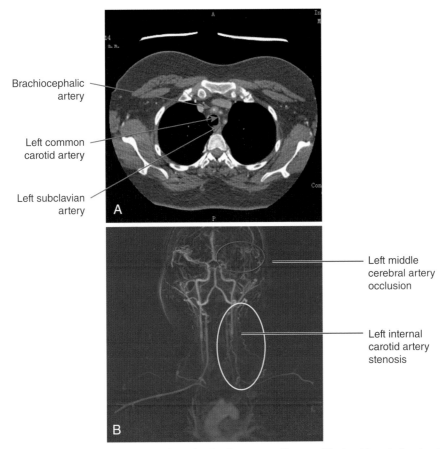

Fig. 48.2 (A) Computed tomography angiography showing narrowed lumens of the brachiocephalic artery, left common carotid artery, and left subclavian artery, indicated by *red arrows* from top to bottom. (B) Magnetic resonance angiography showing occlusion of left middle cerebral artery, indicated by the *red circle,* and long segment stenosis of left internal carotid artery, indicated by the *yellow circle.*

Computed tomography angiography (CTA)/magnetic resonance angiography (MRA)
- CTA (Fig. 48.2)
  - Narrowed lumens of brachiocephalic artery, left common carotid artery, and left subclavian artery
- MRA (Fig. 48.3)
  - Stenosis of internal carotid
  - Occlusion of left middle cerebral artery

Working Diagnosis

- Takayasu arteritis (TA), also known as Takayasu arteritis disease (TKA) bilateral stage 4 (based on the Takayasu Arteritis Classification[1]) and Takayasu retinopathy (according to American College of Rheumatology [ACR] criteria 1990[2]) with ocular ischemic syndrome.

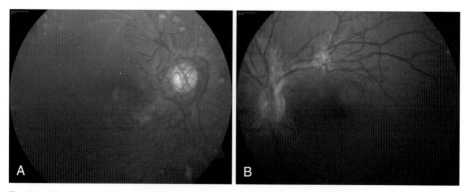

Fig. 48.3 (A) At 1-year follow-up, fundus photograph of the right eye (OD) showing peripapillary arteriovenous anastomoses and obliteration of blood vessels throughout the retina with evidence of panretinal photocoagulation. (B) Fundus photograph OD showing diminished blood vessels throughout the retina inferiorly.

Managment

- Ophthalmic
  - Intravitreal bevacizumab in both eyes
  - Panretinal photocoagulation in both eyes
- Systemic
  - High-dose intravenous corticosteroids methylprednisolone for 3 days, followed by
  - Immunomodulators (azathioprine, prednisolone, methotrexate)

Outcome and Follow-up

At 1-year follow-up, patient's vision was hand motion OD and 20/400 OS because of severe ischemic damage involving the optic nerves and retina. Because of the late stage of Takayasu retinopathy, the patient's visual outcome was limited (Fig. 48.3).

Discussion

TA, is a rare autoimmune disease with chronic granulomatous inflammation mainly involving large arteries,[2] leading to narrowing and possible obliteration. It affects mainly women between the ages of 20 and 40 years and is most commonly seen in Japan, Southeast Asia, India, and Mexico.[3]

Manifestations of TA range from asymptomatic disease to catastrophic neurological impairment. Retinal manifestations are relatively common, with abnormalities reported in up to 35% of patients.[4] There are two classic patterns of retinal involvement in TA: (1) Takayasu retinopathy, a specific manifestation secondary to carotid artery involvement with hypoperfusion of the ophthalmic artery; and (2) hypertensive retinopathy, secondary to chronic systemic hypertension as a sequela to renal artery stenosis. Takayasu retinopathy is characterized by dilatation of retinal veins and occlusion of large arteries, with capillary microaneurysms. In more advanced stages, arteriovenous anastomosis formation and capillary dropout are observed. At the last stage, more serious and sight-threatening complications such as neovascular glaucoma, vitreous hemorrhage, retinal detachment, optic atrophy, and cataract may develop.[5]

FA remains the gold standard for diagnosis.[6] Multimodal imaging, including optical coherence tomography angiography combined with fundus FA, can be a useful tool to evaluate anterior ischemic optic neuropathy and ocular ischemic syndrome in cases of TA.[6] MRA and CTA are more advanced imaging modalities and allow for higher quality and more extensive visualization. Gadolinium- or iodine-enhanced MRA and CTA can help visualize arterial wall thickening, edema, or enhancement in TA, especially in the prestenotic phase.[7]

There are two most common diagnostic criteria for TA, as described by the American College of Rheumatology (ACR) criteria 1990[2] and the modified Ishikawa diagnostic criteria.[8] This patient fulfilled ACR criteria 1, 3, and 6 in addition to two major criteria and three minor criteria of Ishikawa diagnostic criteria. Both are consistent with the diagnosis of Takayasu retinopathy.

The main differential diagnosis for this 29-year-old female patient involved various causes of proliferative retinopathy. However, this patient had no systemic disease history, such as diabetes or hypertension. Alternative differential diagnoses were other causes of large vessel vasculitis, such as inflammatory aortitis due to syphilis, tuberculosis, systemic lupus erythematosus, spondyloarthropathies, and Behcet disease, which were all excluded based on the systemic angiographic feature, a lack of specific features of these diseases, and negative serologies. Fibromuscular dysplasia was also included in the differential, as it can be characterized by resistant hypertension and large vessel vasculitis involving even the retinal vessels. However, angiography did not reveal the classic "beads-on-string" appearance as seen in fibromuscular dysplasia.

Treatment should aim to control disease activity and preserve vascular competence while minimizing long-term side effects. Usually, systemic immunosuppressants are the mainstay of therapy, and glucocorticoids are often the first-line immunosuppressants used. Methotrexate and low-dose aspirin are among the mainstay therapies used to control inflammation.[2] Second-line agents, including cyclophosphamide and azathioprine, can be added if the patient is unresponsive. Interleukin (IL)-6 has been ascertained to be a prominent mediator of the systemic inflammatory response in TKA. Thus IL-6 inhibitors (e.g., tocilizumab, sarilumab, satralizumab) and IL-6 receptor inhibitors (e.g., siltuximab) are potential alternatives in the treatment of TA. When used in combination with corticosteroids, IL-6 blockade allows for a shorter time span of corticosteroid use and reduced relapses; this helps decrease the possibility of corticosteroid-related side effects.[9,10] Li and colleagues[11] found that mycophenolate mofetil may help decrease disease activity and lower corticosteroid dosage in TKA. Tumor necrosis factor alpha (TNF-a) inhibitors (e.g., infliximab, adalimumab) and TNF-a receptor inhibitors (e.g., etanercept) have been shown to be effective in TKA. Comarmond and colleagues[12] reported that anti-TNF–TNF-a therapy in cases of refractory TKA allowed for sustained complete remission in 37% of patients and partial remission in 53.5% of patients. However, 20% of patients experience side effects, and more research is necessary to evaluate the long-term efficacy and safety of anti-TNF–TNF-a therapy.[12] Invasive treatment procedures, including stent placement, endarterectomy, bypass grafts, and angioplasty,[13] are often reserved for cases of severe and symptomatic stenosis or occlusion of the arteries, especially those with progressive ocular ischemia refractory to medication.

Key Points

- TA may involve the eyes with proliferative retinopathy and ocular ischemia.
- Ocular treatment may require anti–vascular endothelial growth factor therapy and possible photocoagulation.
- TA is a systemic autoimmune disease process with granulomatosis inflammation and life-threatening implications.
- Systemic immunosuppressive therapy is oftentimes required.

Algorithm 48.1: Algorithm for Differential Diagnosis and Treatment

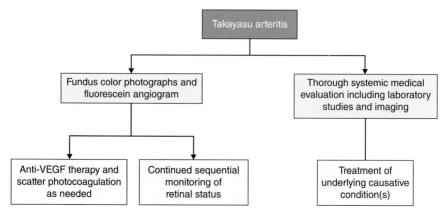

Algorithm 48.1   Algorithm for differential diagnosis and treatment. Key features include the recognition of possible systemic causative factors for the proliferative retinopathy. Although treatment of the ocular findings is required to preserve vision, recognition (and treatment) of the potential life-threatening associations is essential. *anti-VEGF,* anti–vascular endothelial growth factor.

References

1. Uyama M, Asayama K. Retinal vascular changes in Takayasu's disease (pulseless disease), occurrence and evolution of the lesion. In: De Laey JJ, ed. *International Symposium on Fluorescein Angiography Ghent March 28–April 1, 1976.* Dordrecht: Springer Netherlands; 1976:549-554.
2. Arend WP, Michel BA, Bloch DA, et al. The American College of Rheumatology 1990 criteria for the classification of Takayasu arteritis. *Arthritis Rheum.* 1990;33:1129-1134.
3. Serra R, Butrico L, Fugetto F, et al. Updates in pathophysiology, diagnosis and management of Takayasu arteritis. *Ann Vasc Surg.* 2016;35:210-225.
4. Chun Y, Park S, Park I, Chung H, Lee J. The clinical and ocular manifestations of Takayasu arteritis. *Retina.* 2001;21:132-140.
5. Sugiyama K, Ijiri S, Tagawa S, Shimizu K. Takayasu disease on the centenary of its discovery. *Jpn J Ophthalmol.* 2009;53:81-91.
6. Chotard G, Diwo E, Coscas F, Butel N, Saadoun D, Bodaghi B. Fluorescein and OCT angiography features of Takayasu disease. *Ocul Immunol Inflamm.* 2019;27:774-780.
7. Mason JC. Takayasu arteritis: advances in diagnosis and management. *Nat Rev Rheumatol.* 2010;6: 406-415.
8. Sharma BK, Jain S, Suri S, Numano F. Diagnostic criteria for Takayasu arteritis. *Int J Cardiol.* 1996;54(suppl):S141-S147.
9. Kong X, Zhang X, Lv P, et al. Treatment of Takayasu arteritis with the IL-6R antibody tocilizumab vs. cyclophosphamide. *Int J Cardiol.* 2018;266:222-228.
10. Yoshifuji H. Pathophysiology of large vessel vasculitis and utility of interleukin-6 inhibition therapy. *Mod Rheumatol.* 2019;29:287-293.
11. Li J, Yang Y, Zhao J, Li M, Tian X, Zeng X. The efficacy of mycophenolate mofetil for the treatment of Chinese Takayasu's arteritis. *Sci Rep.* 2016;6:38687.
12. Comarmond C, Plaisier E, Dahan K, et al. Anti TNF-α in refractory Takayasu's arteritis: cases series and review of the literature. *Autoimmun Rev.* 2012;11:678-684.
13. Zeng Y, Duan J, Ge G, Zhang M. Therapeutic management of ocular ischemia in Takayasu's Arteritis: a case-based systematic review. *Front Immunol.* 2021;12:791278.

CHAPTER 49

Perifoveal Retinal Whitening and Scotomas in a Sickle Cell Patient

Jennifer I. Lim ■ Daniel W. Wang

History of Present Illness

A 41-year-old man with a history of sickle cell disease presents with a grayish spot in the center of the visual field of his left eye. The onset of symptoms was sudden, and the patient notes no previous episodes. Although the patient notes mild improvement, the symptoms have been persistent for 5 days before the initial presentation. The patient did not have associated ocular pain, flashes, or floaters, and the fellow right eye was unaffected.

OCULAR EXAMINATION FINDINGS

Visual acuities with correction were 20/20 in the right eye and 20/25 in the left eye. Intraocular pressures were 15 mm Hg bilaterally. Pupils were round and reactive without a relative afferent pupillary defect in each eye. External and anterior segment examination were unremarkable. On dilated fundus examination, both optic nerves appeared normal without edema or pallor. The right macula was flat without edema. The left macula had patchy grayish-white perifoveal lesions with a blunted foveal reflex. The vessels of both eyes were slightly attenuated and had a sclerotic appearance peripherally. The peripheral examination of the right eye demonstrated 360 degrees of peripheral laser scars with fibrosis and patches of regressed neovascularization (Fig. 49.1). The peripheral examination of the left eye similarly had peripheral laser scars and signs of regressed neovascularization (Fig. 49.2). There were no salmon patch hemorrhages, sunburst lesions, iridescent spots, retinal or preretinal hemorrhages, or cotton wool spots in either eye.

OPTICAL COHERENCE TOMOGRAPHY

Imaging

Optical coherence tomography (OCT) of the macula of the right eye showed intact retinal layers without edema (Fig. 49.3). The left eye demonstrated patchy perifoveal hyperreflective thickened bands at the level of the inner plexiform layer, inner nuclear layer, and outer plexiform layer, with sparing of the outer nuclear and deeper retinal layers (Fig. 49.4).

Questions to Ask

- Does the patient have any symptoms of giant cell arteritis (GCA)? Although the patient is not of the classic age or gender, GCA may cause retinal ischemia and is a life-threatening condition that must be ruled out.

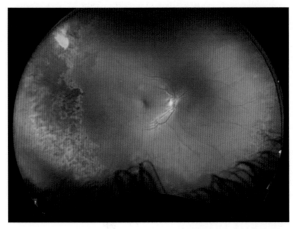

Fig. 49.1 Optos color fundus photograph of the right eye shows attenuation of the peripheral arterioles with whitening seen nasally. There are arteriovenous anastomoses easily seen especially nasally. Note the presence of several clock hours of regressed seafans with fibrosis superotemporally to inferotemporally with adjacent peripheral laser scars.

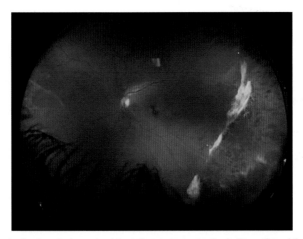

Fig. 49.2 Optos color fundus photograph of the left eye shows marked attenuation of the peripheral arterioles and arteriovenous anastomoses especially nasally. Note the presence of regressed seafans with fibrosis superotemporally. Elsewhere there is marked pigmentation of peripheral laser scars surrounding regressed seafans.

- The patient did not endorse any headache, scalp tenderness, jaw pain, unexplained weight loss, fever, or generalized malaise when asked about these symptoms.
- Does the patient have any major systemic or ocular conditions that could predispose to localized retinal ischemia, such as diabetic retinopathy, hypertension, retinal vein occlusion, or artery occlusion?
  - The patient has a history of sickle cell disease, which may be associated with retinal vascular occlusions. This patient had previous laser retinopexy performed for associated stage 3 proliferative sickle cell retinopathy.

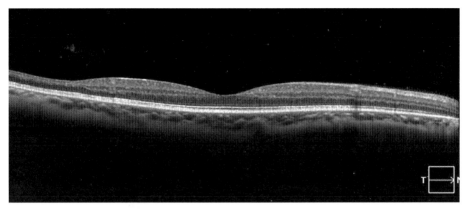

Fig. 49.3 Optical coherence tomography of the macula of the right eye shows marked thinning of the temporal inner retinal layers. The choroid is also thinned.

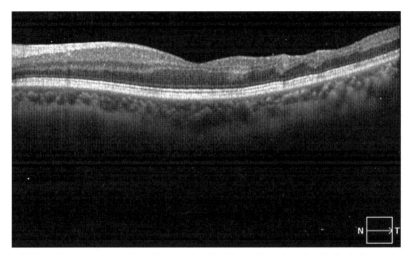

Fig. 49.4 Optical coherence tomography of the macula in the left eye shows irregular thinning in the parafoveal and perifoveal temporal macula. There are perifoveal hyperreflective thickened bands at the level of the inner plexiform layer, inner nuclear layer, and outer plexiform layer with sparing of the outer nuclear and deeper retinal layers.

- Does the patient have any environmental risk factors? It is thought that vasopressors, such as caffeine or medications (e.g., oral contraceptives), or dehydration may precipitate a vaso-occlusive episode.
  - None present
- What is the gender of the patient and age of the patient? Acute macular neuroretinopathy (AMN) is a rare entity that presents similarly and typically affects young, healthy women in their teens to thirties.
  - The patient is a man and is in his early 40s.

Assessment

A 41-year-old man with a history of sickle cell disease presents with paracentral scotoma of the left eye with corresponding hyperreflective lesions of the inner nuclear layer on OCT.

Differential Diagnosis

- Paracentral acute middle maculopathy (PAMM)
- AMN

Working Diagnosis

- PAMM

Multimodal Testing and Results

- Fluorescein angiography (FA)
  - FA demonstrates areas of peripheral capillary dropout in both eyes with areas of re-gressed seafans surrounded by laser scars. Chorioretinal scars are visualized correspond-ing to earlier laser retinopexy. Some leakage is seen in both eyes in areas of regressed seafans. In addition, areas of arteriovenous anastomoses are seen in both eyes. No obvious filling defects or gross abnormalities are noted in the macular region of both eyes (Figs. 49.5 and 49.6).
- Optical coherence tomography angiography (OCTA)
  - OCTA of the right eye demonstrates mild irregularity of the foveal avascular zone but otherwise is unremarkable (Fig. 49.7). The left eye shows a splotchy, irregular vascular pattern with perifoveal vascular flow loss in the superficial capillary plexus, particularly temporally. There is relative preservation of the deep capillary plexus vasculature (Figs. 49.8 and 49.9).
  - OCT and OCTA have proven useful in the assessment of sickle cell retinopathy stage and progression. Thinning in the macular area may show a foveal depression sign clini-cally. On OCT this appears as splaying of the foveal contour.[1] Both OCT and OCTA parameters have been shown to be useful in the assessment of sickle cell retinopathy.[1-3]

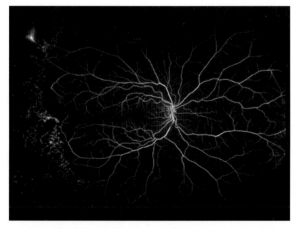

Fig. 49.5 Fluorescein angiography of the right eye shows arteriovenous anastomoses nasally. Note the stain-ing from the laser scars and the area of leakage associated with the neovascularization superotemporally in the periphery. There is also significant ischemia present.

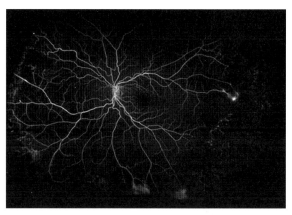

Fig. 49.6 Fluorescein angiography of the left eye shows arteriovenous anastomoses more clearly temporally. Note the staining from the laser scars and the areas of leakage associated with the areas of regressed seafans superotemporally and inferiorly in the periphery. There is also significant ischemia present. No obvious filling defects or gross abnormalities are noted in the macular region.

Management

There is no current treatment for PAMM. The association of PAMM with sickle cell disease, as well as its association with AMN, has been reported.[4] Unlike AMN, which involves the outer nuclear layer and the ellipsoid and interdigitation zones, in PAMM, hyperreflective, thickened bands are seen at the level of the inner plexiform layer, inner nuclear layer, and outer plexiform layer with sparing of the outer nuclear and deeper retinal layers. OCTA is helpful in showing the location of the flow loss, which involves the choriocapillaris in AMN but not in PAMM. In AMN, the deep capillary plexus, but not the superficial, is involved. In PAMM, the superficial and deep capillary plexuses can be involved. Over time, the atrophy of the involved area is seen.

There is generally no treatment, although the use of intraarterial tissue plasminogen activator has been reported in a patient with sickle cell disease and PAMM and an incomplete central retinal artery occlusion[5] with marked loss of central vision. Although full resolution of the scotoma has been reported in that patient, partial resolution of symptoms is more common. Fortunately, our patient experienced resolution of his scotoma and no further episodes over the next year. In patients with sickle cell disease, use of hydroxyurea has been associated with less thinning over time,[2] and one could consider its use for a patient who experienced PAMM or AMN.

Given PAMM's association with multiple vasculopathic conditions, it is important to screen patients for systemic diseases, including retinal vessel occlusions, carotid artery disease, diabetes, hypertension, GCA, or other vasculitides.[6,7] Management should be directed at identifying and minimizing vascular risk factors. In this case transient ischemia related to the patient's sickle cell disease is the etiology.

Follow-up Care

There are no previously established guidelines for follow-up. Follow-up is at the discretion and comfort level of the physician and may be every few weeks or months to document the course of the disease. Our patient was initially followed on a monthly basis until stability and improvement of the observed lesions and symptoms were observed.

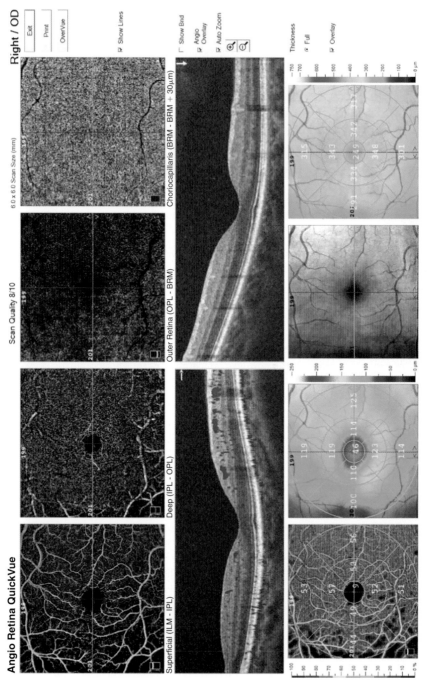

Fig. 49.7 Optical coherence tomography angiography of the right eye demonstrates mild irregularity of the foveal avascular zone. No significant focal loss of the capillary layers is seen.

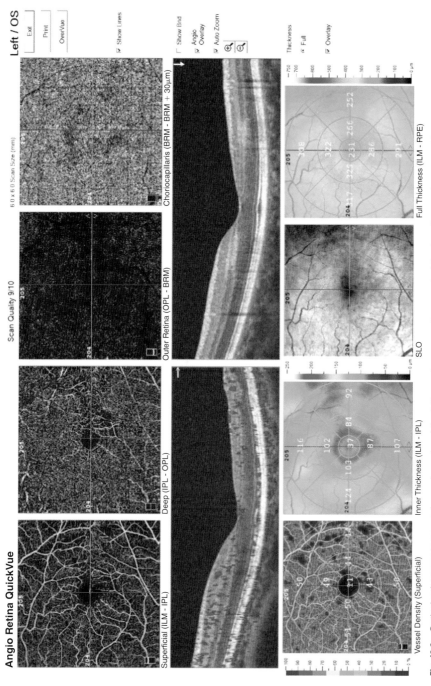

Fig. 49.8 Optical coherence tomography angiography of the left eye shows an enlargement of the foveal avascular zone with perifoveal vascular flow loss in the superficial capillary plexus, particularly temporally. There is some involvement of the deep capillary plexus particularly temporally with intact choriocapillaris.

Angio Retina QuickVue

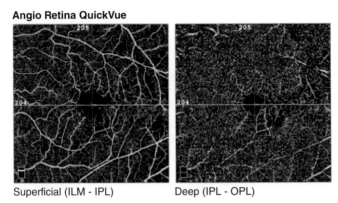

Superficial (ILM - IPL)   Deep (IPL - OPL)

Fig. 49.9   Optical coherence tomography angiography of the left eye loss of the deep capillary plexus particularly temporally.

Algorithm 49.1: Paracentral Acute Middle Maculopathy Algorithm

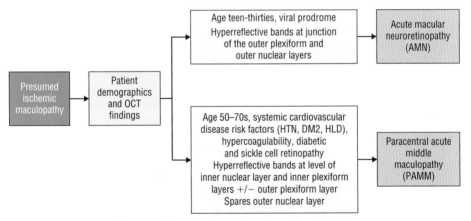

Algorithm 49.1   Paracentral acute middle maculopathy algorithm.

Key Points

- Visual loss with retinal whitening may be due to PAMM
- PAMM lesions result in inner retinal (IPL, INL and OPL) hyperreflective thickened bands on OCT imaging, in contrast to the outer lesions seen with AMN lesions sickle cell patients, due to transient ischemia, may develop PAMM lesions and can sustain vision loss, which usually resolves
- PAMM is associated with multiple vasculopathic conditions and screening for these systemic conditions is indicated if no sysemic cause if known
- OCTA may show associated areas of vascular fow deficits

References

1. Chow CC, Genead MA, Anastasakis A, Chau FY, Fishman GA, Lim JI. Structural and functional correlation in sickle cell retinopathy using spectral-domain optical coherence tomography and scanning laser ophthalmoscope microperimetry. *Am J Ophthalmol*. 2011;152(4):704-711.e2.
2. Lim JI, Niec M, Sun J, Cao D. Longitudinal assessment of retinal thinning in adults with and without sickle cell retinopathy using spectral-domain optical coherence tomography. *JAMA Ophthalmol*. 2021;139(3):330-337.
3. Alam M, Thapa D, Lim JI, Cao D, Yao X. Quantitative characteristics of sickle cell retinopathy in optical coherence tomography angiography. *Biomed Opt Express*. 2017;8(3):1741-1753.
4. Ong SS, Ahmed I, Scott AW. Association of acute macular neuroretinopathy or paracentral acute middle maculopathy with sickle cell disease. *Ophthalmol Retina*. 2021;5(11):1146-1155.
5. Chua MR, Giovinazzo JV, Kaplan RI, et al. Paracentral acute middle maculopathy as a presenting sign of CRAO in sickle cell disease treated with tissue plasminogen activator. *Retin Cases Brief Rep*. 2022;16(5): 553-557.
6. Chen X, Rahimy E, Sergott RC, et al. Spectrum of retinal vascular diseases associated with paracentral acute middle maculopathy. *Am J Ophthalmol*. 2015;160(1):26-34.e21.
7. Rahimy E, Kuehlewein L, Sadda SR, Sarraf D. Paracentral acute middle maculopathy: what we knew then and what we know now. *Retina*. 2015;35(10):1921-1930.

Idiopathic Macular Conditions

CHAPTER 50

A Hypopigmented Lesion in a Baby's Eye

Mark J. Daily

History of Present Illness

A 13-month-old boy is referred to a pediatric ophthalmologist because his mother noticed that his left eye "turns out" intermittently. The child was born full term weighing 8 pounds, 12 ounces. No other physical abnormalities are present, and the child is developing normally. No family members have any ocular abnormalities or history of strabismus.

OCULAR EXAMINATION FINDINGS

Central steady fixation was present in each eye. Motility examination revealed straight eyes and full ocular versions. Cycloplegic refraction was +1.00 sphere bilaterally. Dilated fundus examination showed normal discs, blood vessels, and peripheral retinas. In the left fundus there was a hypopigmented lesion temporal to the fovea (Fig. 50.1).

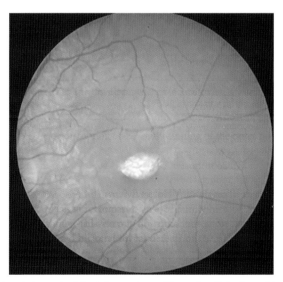

Fig. 50.1 Color fundus photograph of the left eye at age 13 months. Note the pointed, elliptically shaped 1.5-disc-diameter lesion on the temporal edge of the fovea. The lesion is flat and nonpigmented. The underlying choroidal vessels are visible.

IMAGING

Color fundus photographs were taken of each eye. The right eye was normal. The left eye showed a pointed, elliptically shaped 1.5-disc-diameter lesion on the temporal edge of the fovea (Fig 50.1). The lesion was flat and nonpigmented. The underlying choroidal vessels were visible.

Questions to Ask

- Any history of infections during pregnancy? TORCH (toxoplasmosis, rubella, cytomegalovirus, herpes simplex) and Zika viral infections appear as congenital lesions. Some of these harbor more pigmentation and may appear to be more of a scar than simply hypopigmentation.
  - No
- Was there any trauma to the infant during delivery? Rarely chorioretinal lesions can result from trauma.
  - No
- Has the child had any developmental delay? Infectious causes (TORCH) may be associated with various levels of developmental delay.
  - No
- Is there any history of fever or skin lesions?
  - No
- Is the lesion calcified? Calcified lesions increase the concern for TORCH lesions and retinoblastoma.
  - No

Assessment

- A healthy 13-month-old child with an elliptically shaped, pointed, flat, nonpigmented lesion in the left eye adjacent to the fovea.

Differential Diagnosis

- Congenital toxoplasmosis chorioretinal scar
- Traumatic lesion associated with birth
- Congenital hypertrophy of retinal pigment epithelium (hypopigmented)
- Idiopathic lesion—torpedo maculopathy

Working Diagnosis

Torpedo maculopathy

Multimodal Testing

- Fundus photographs of torpedo maculopathy usually show a hypopigmented lesion of 1 to 2 disc diameters with a pointed end toward the fovea and a blunt end on the temporal side. Hyperpigmentation of the border and particularly the temporal end may be present.
- Optical coherence tomography (OCT) of the lesion may show (1) attenuation of the outer layers of the retina and pigment epithelium with transmission into the choroid, or

(2) neurosensory elevation with attenuation of the ellipsoid zone and interdigitation zone.[2]

■ Fluorescein angiography demonstrates a hyperfluorescent window defect of the zone of retinal pigment epithelium (RPE) thinning without late leakage.

Management

Torpedo retinopathy is stable without treatment, but a few reports have shown choroidal neovascularization can occur and threaten central vision.

Gardner syndrome is a subgroup of familial adenomatous polyposis with ocular findings of multiple ellipsoid hypopigmented and hyperpigmented lesions, usually in both eyes. These lesions may resemble a "torpedo" but are usually located outside the macula and may be more pigmented. Any patient with more than one torpedo or lesions outside the temporal macula should be worked up for Gardner syndrome.

Algorithm 50.1: Algorithm for Torpedo Maculopathy

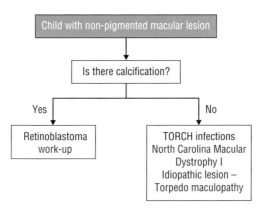

Algorithm 50.1   Algorithm for torpedo maculopathy.

Follow-up

The original examination of this child was at 13 months of age. A follow-up examination 30 years later revealed visual acuities of 20/20 right eye and 20/25 left eye. The patient had two eye muscle surgeries at 4 years and 10 years for intermittent exotropia. Fundus examination showed the torpedo lesion in the same location with more pigmentation on the temporal side (Fig. 50.2), and OCT shows RPE atrophy (Fig. 50.3).

Key Points

■ Torpedo maculopathy is a benign fundus finding, usually in asymptomatic patients.[1,3,4,5]

■ The pathophysiology of the lesion is probably related to embryonic development in late gestation.[6]

■ The fundus lesion is quite characteristic, and an extensive workup is usually not necessary.

■ If multiple lesions are present, one should consider Gardner syndrome.

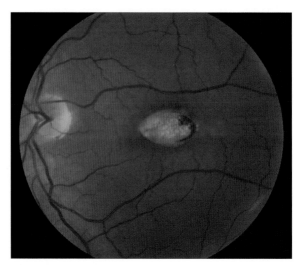

Fig. 50.2 Color fundus photograph of the left eye at age 31 years. Note the torpedo lesion in the same location with more pigmentation on the temporal edge.

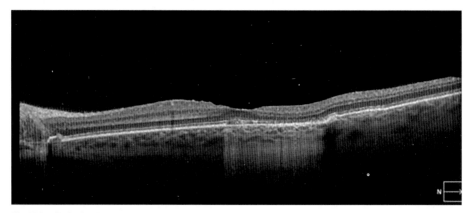

Fig. 50.3 Optical coherence tomography at age 31 years shows loss of the outer retinal layers and retinal pigment epithelium with hypertransmission into the choroid.

References

1. Agarwal A, Gass JDM, Gass JDM. *Gass' Atlas of Macular Diseases*. Edinburgh, Scotland: Elsevier Saunders; 2012:1076-1077.
2. Ali Z, Shields CL, Jasani K, Aslam TM, Balaskas K. Swept-source optical coherence tomography angiography findings in torpedo maculopathy. *Ophthalmic Surg Lasers Imaging Retina.* 2017;48(11):932-935.
3. Daily MJ. Torpedo maculopathy or paramacular spot syndrome. In: *New Dimensions in Retina Symposium*. Chicago, IL: November 7, 1992.
4. Golchet PR, Jampol LM, Mathura Jr JR, Daily MJ. Torpedo maculopathy. *Br J Ophthalmol.* 2010;94:302-306.
5. Rossman RL, Gass JDM. Solitary hypopigmented nevus of the retinal pigment epithelium in the macula. *Arch Ophthalmol.* 1992;110:1762.
6. Shields CL, Guzman JM, Shapiro MD, Fogel LE, Shields JA. Torpedo maculopathy at the site of the fetal bulge. *Arch Ophthalmol.* 2010;128(4):499-501.

CHAPTER 51

Unilateral Painless Vision Loss After a Viral Illness

George Skopis ▓ William F. Mieler

History of Present Illness

A 20-year-old male patient presents with 3 days of experiencing a "black spot" in the center of his vision in the left eye. The patient states that the onset of symptoms was sudden. He denies flashes, floaters, or eye pain. The patient denies any ocular or medical history or any ocular surgical history. One week before the onset of symptoms the patient experienced an upper respiratory tract infection; he has now developed a papular rash on his hands with desquamation on his fingers.

OCULAR EXAMINATION FINDINGS

Best-corrected visual acuity was 20/15 in the right eye and 20/80 in the left eye. Intraocular pressure was normal in both eyes. The anterior segment was normal in both eyes. On dilated fundus examination, the right eye was unremarkable. The left eye showed perifoveal and parafoveal intraretinal hemorrhages with subtle subretinal fluid involving the fovea.

IMAGING

- Fundus photograph: color fundus photograph of the left eye shows intraretinal hemorrhages in the macula with an area of subretinal fluid involving the fovea (Fig. 51.1).
- Optical coherence tomography (OCT): OCT of the left eye shows subretinal fluid with some hyperreflective material at the level of the outer retina and irregularity of the retinal pigment epithelium (RPE) (Fig. 51.2).
- Fundus autofluorescence (FAF): FAF of the left eye shows small areas of hypoautofluorescence correlating to areas of intraretinal hemorrhage and small punctate areas of hyperautofluorescence at the edge of the subretinal fluid location (Fig. 51.3).
- Fluorescein angiogram (FA): FA of the left eye shows multifocal areas of hyperfluorescence at the level of the RPE (Fig. 51.4A) that progresses to hyperfluorescence in a pooling pattern with areas of hypofluorescence due to blockage from the intraretinal hemorrhages (Fig. 51.4B).

Questions to Ask

- Does the patient use any steroid medications? In an otherwise healthy male with macular subretinal fluid, it would be important to ask about steroid medications to investigate the possibility of central serous chorioretinopathy.

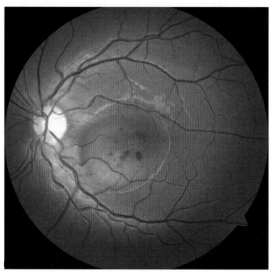

Fig. 51.1 Color fundus photograph of the left eye at initial presentation. Intraretinal hemorrhages adjacent to the area of macular subretinal fluid.

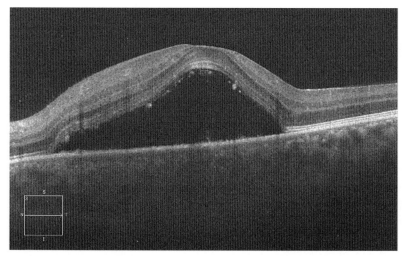

Fig. 51.2 Optical coherence tomography of the left eye at initial presentation. Significant subretinal fluid involving the fovea with hyperreflective material. There is also hyperreflective material at the outer retina and retinal pigment epithelium irregularity.

- Has the patient had a recent upper respiratory tract infection? Preceding viral illness with symptoms of upper respiratory infection has been implicated in multiple disease processes, including white dot syndrome and Vogt-Koyanagi-Harada syndrome, that would be included on the differential diagnosis for this patient.
- Does the patient have a history of sexually transmitted illnesses, or does the patient engage in high-risk sexual practices? Syphilis is a great mimicker and should always be assessed for, especially in a young patient.

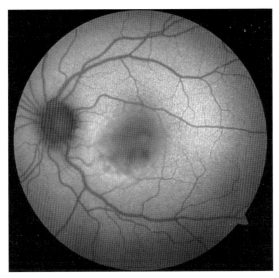

Fig. 51.3   Fundus autofluorescence of the left eye at initial presentation. There is mild hypoautofluorescence in the central macula with faint hyperautofluorescence ring surrounding the area of subretinal fluid.

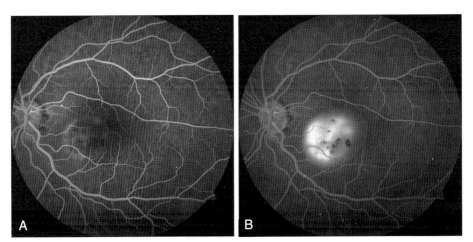

Fig. 51.4   Fluorescein angiogram (FA) of the left eye at initial presentation. (A) FA at 47 seconds showing early hyperfluorescence at multiple points at the level of the retinal pigment epithelium. (B) FA at 6 minutes showing significant hyperfluorescence in pooling pattern.

- What is the patient's refraction? Pathological myopia with choroidal neovascular membrane and subsequent exudation of fluid into the subretinal space can cause this sort of presentation.

Assessment

- The patient is a 20-year-old male patient presenting with acute onset painless vision loss in the left eye with a preceding viral illness that is found to have parafoveal and perifoveal intraretinal hemorrhages with subretinal fluid in the macula.

Differential Diagnosis (see algorithm 51.1 for full algorithm)

- Central serous chorioretinopathy
- Pathological myopia
- Syphilis chorioretinitis
- Harada disease
- Idiopathic choroidal neovascularization
- Acute posterior multifocal placoid pigment epitheliopathy
- Unilateral acute idiopathic maculopathy (UAIM)

Working Diagnosis

- UAIM

Multimodal Testing and Results

- Fundus photographs
  - On fundus examination, patients are found to have neurosensory detachment of the retina in the macula, intraretinal hemorrhages near the neurosensory detachment, and an irregular white/gray thickening to the RPE.[1] A "bull's eye" appearance may occur late in the disease.[1]
- OCT
  - OCT shows fluid accumulation in the subretinal space with hyperreflective material in the subretinal and accumulation in the outer retina with RPE irregularities.[2]
- FAF
  - Early on, FAF shows a mixed pattern of alternative hyperautofluorescence mixed with hypoautofluorescence in the fovea or peripapillary areas.[3] Later in the disease there is more confluent hypoautofluorescence,[3] indicating RPE cell death. The FAF may also show hyperautofluorescent "satellite" lesions that do not appear on near-infrared imaging or fundus photography.[4]
- FA
  - Early FA shows mild subretinal hyperfluorescence, with late stage angiogram showing hyperfluorescence at the level of the RPE and pooling in the subretinal space.[1]

Management

- Patients with UAIM are typically observed because good visual acuity recovery spontaneously occurs.[1-3] Some reports have shown that treatment with oral corticosteroids may hasten visual recovery.[5]
  - Our patient was observed and, over the course of 2 weeks, had significant improvement in visual acuity to 20/20 and improved imaging findings (Figs. 51.5–51.7).
  - At 7 months post initial presentation, OCT imaging shows complete restoration of the ellipsoid zone (Fig. 51.8).
- There is an association between coxsackievirus and development of UAIM.[3,6,7]
  - Our patient was tested for coxsackievirus and had positive serologies as well as the characteristic rash of hand-foot-mouth disease.
  - Testing for coxsackievirus may aid in diagnosis.
- One case report[8] showed that treating a patient with worsened symptoms and examination findings with intravitreal aflibercept led to improved visual acuity.
  - More research needs to be completed before this is recommended for all patients.

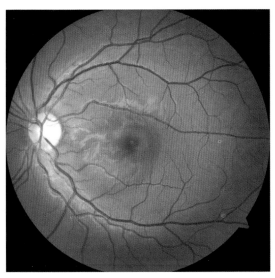

Fig. 51.5 Color fundus photograph of the left eye 2 weeks postinitial presentation. Hemorrhages and subretinal fluid have resolved.

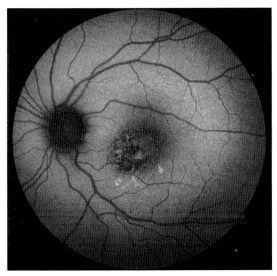

Fig. 51.6 Fundus autofluorescence of the left eye 2 weeks postinitial presentation. Central area of specked hyperautofluorescence and hypoautofluorescence with inferior hyperautofluorescent satellite lesions within previous area of subretinal fluid.

Follow-up Care

- Patients can have profound vision loss; weekly follow-up is advised early on to evaluate for progression of disease.
- Frequent imaging can help identify progression or worsening of the disease process.

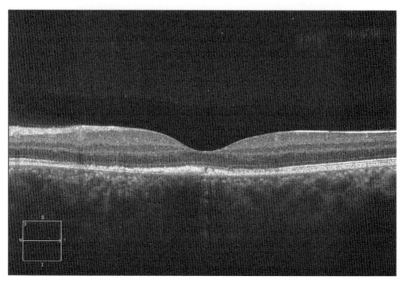

Fig. 51.7 Optical coherence tomography of the left eye 2 weeks postinitial presentation. Subretinal fluid has resolved. There is residual retinal pigment epithelium thickening and attenuated ellipsoid zone.

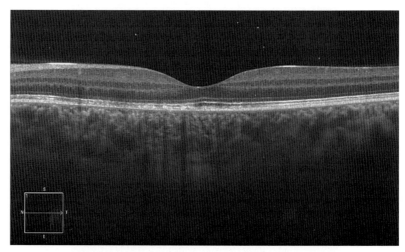

Fig. 51.8 Optical coherence tomography of the left eye 7 months postinitial presentation. There is no subretinal fluid, and there are small persistent areas of retinal pigment epithelium thickening. The ellipsoid zone has reformed.

Algorithm 51.1: Algorithm for Differential Diagnosis of Serous Macular Detachment

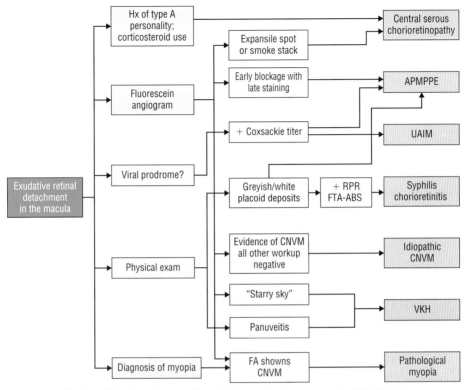

Algorithm 51.1 Algorithm for differential diagnosis of serous macular detachment.

Key Points

- UAIM is thought to be caused primarily by coxsackievirus and to cause significant acute vision loss with usually rapid visual recovery over several weeks.
- Observation is the preferred treatment method.
- Characteristic imaging findings explained above can help lead to accurate diagnosis.

References

1. Yannuzzi LA, Jampol LM, Rabb MF, Sorenson JA, Beyrer C, Wilcox LM. Unilateral acute idiopathic maculopathy. *Retina*. 2012;32:1411-1416.
2. Hughes EH, Hunyor AP, Gorbatov M, Ho I. Acute idiopathic maculopathy with coxsackievirus infection. *Retin Cases Brief Rep*. 2012;6(1):19-21.
3. Jung CS. Multimodality diagnostic imaging in unilateral acute idiopathic maculopathy. *Arch Ophthalmol*. 2012;130(1):50-56.
4. Balaratnasingam C, Lally DR, Tawse KL, et al. A unique posterior segment phenotypic manifestation of coxsackie virus infection. *Retin Cases Brief Rep*. 2016;10(3):278-282.
5. de la Fuente MA. Unilateral acute idiopathic maculopathy: angiography, optical coherence tomography and microperimetry findings. *J Ophthalmic Inflamm Infect*. 2011;1(3):125-127.
6. Beck AP. Is coxsackievirus the cause of unilateral acute idiopathic maculopathy? *Arch Ophthalmol*. 2004;122(1):121-123.
7. Hughes EH. Acute idiopathic maculopathy with coxsackievirus infection. *Retin Cases Brief Rep*. 2012;6(1):19-21.
8. Mylonas G, Prager F, Wetzel B, Malamos P, Deak G, Amon M. Anti-vascular endothelial growth factor for unilateral acute idiopathic maculopathy. *Eur J Ophthalmol*. 2018;28(2):256-258.

CHAPTER 52

Bilateral Presentation of Macular Schisis in a Woman

Nita Valikodath ▩ Jennifer I. Lim

History of Present Illness

We present a case of a 64-year-old woman with an unremarkable medical history referred for an epiretinal membrane of her right eye. She denies blurry vision, floaters, photopsias or flashes, metamorphopsia, or nyctalopia. She denies any history of ocular conditions or ocular surgeries.

OCULAR EXAMINATION FINDINGS

Visual acuity with correction was 20/20 in each eye. Intraocular pressure were normal. Anterior segment examination showed mild nuclear sclerotic cataracts but otherwise was unremarkable. Dilated fundus examination showed radial spoke-like striae of the fovea with a central cyst in the right eye and macular edema of the left eye (Fig. 52.1).

IMAGING

Optical coherence tomography (OCT) showed cyst-like changes in the outer retina in the foveal and parafoveal regions and in the inner retina in the temporal macula in the right eye. OCT of the left eye showed cyst-like changes in the outer retina in the inferior macula (Fig. 52.2).

Questions to Ask

- What is the patient's refractive error? Myopic foveoschisis or myopic traction maculopathy should be considered in the differential diagnosis for retinoschisis.
  - Plano + 0.25 × 153 in the right eye and −0.50 + 0.25 × 009 in the left eye
- Does the patient have a family history of ocular conditions or consanguinity? A family history would be important to ascertain etiologies for retinoschisis such as congenital juvenile X-linked retinoschisis (XLRS), retinitis pigmentosa, or familial internal limiting membrane dystrophy.
  - No
- History of trauma? Trauma has been associated with macular retinoschisis.
  - No
- What medications does the patient take? Medications such as niacin and taxanes can cause cystic macular edema that appears similar to retinoschisis.
  - None

Assessment

- This is a case of a 64-year-old woman with no ocular or surgical history and a negative family history demonstrating bilateral macular schisis of mainly the outer retina on OCT.

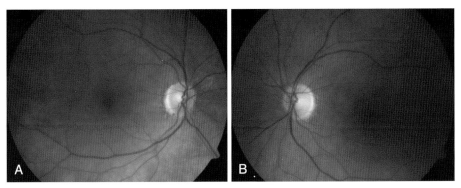

Fig. 52.1 Fundus photograph of the right eye (A) and left eye (B) demonstrating radial spoke-like striae of the fovea.

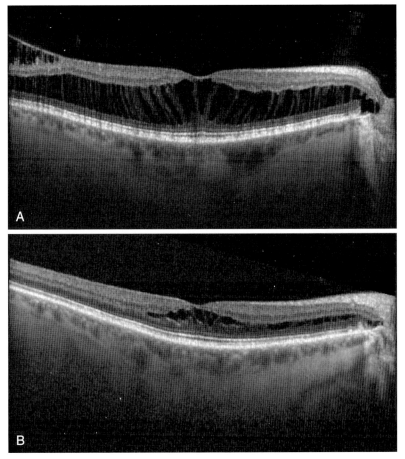

Fig. 52.2 (A) Optical coherence tomography (OCT) of the right eye showing cyst-like changes in the outer retina in the foveal and parafoveal regions and in the inner retina in the temporal macula. (B) OCT of the left eye showing cyst-like changes in the outer retina in the inferior macula.

Differential Diagnosis

- Congenital juvenile X-linked retinoschisis (XLRS)
- Myopic retinoschisis
- Optic pit maculopathy
- Retinitis pigmentosa
- Glaucoma
- Vitreomacular traction
- Degenerative retinoschisis
- Enhanced S-cone syndrome
- Medication associated retinoschisis (niacin, taxanes)
- Familial internal limited membrane dystrophy

Working Diagnosis

- Stellate nonhereditary idiopathic foveomacular retinoschisis (SNIFR)
- Has been described in many studies and can have bilateral or unilateral findings[1,2]

Multimodal Testing and Results

- Fundus photographs
  - On fundus examination, a stellate pattern in the macula is typically visualized, but this may not be present in all patients.[3]
- OCT
  - As mentioned, our patient's OCT showed cyst-like changes in the outer retina in the foveal and parafoveal regions and in the inner retina in the temporal macula in the right eye. OCT of the left eye showed cyst-like changes in the outer retina in the inferior macula.
  - In SNIFR, splitting more commonly involves the outer plexiform layer but can involve the outer nuclear layer as well.[2]
- Electroretinogram (ERG)
  - ERG was obtained, which was normal in both eyes and did not show the characteristic electronegative pattern seen in XLRS (Fig. 52.3).
- Genetic testing
  - This can be obtained to help rule out genetic disorders such as XLRS, retinitis pigmentosa, and enhanced S-cone syndrome. Our patient had a history of good vision her entire life and a negative ERG. In addition, clinical and fundus examination were not suggestive of these hereditary or genetic disorders.
- OCTA
  - A study has shown an avascular schisis cavity in SNIFR, but vascular structures in XLRS.[4]

Management

- Given that this patient was asymptomatic and visual acuity was 20/20 in each eye, the patient was observed.
- General management for SNIFR is typically observation given the relatively good vision in these patients.[5]
- One case report describes the use of dorzolamide, which demonstrated resolution of the schitic changes on OCT and improvement in vision.[6]
- One study reported improved visual and anatomical outcomes after vitrectomy for an outer retinal hole that developed in a patient with SNIFR.[7]

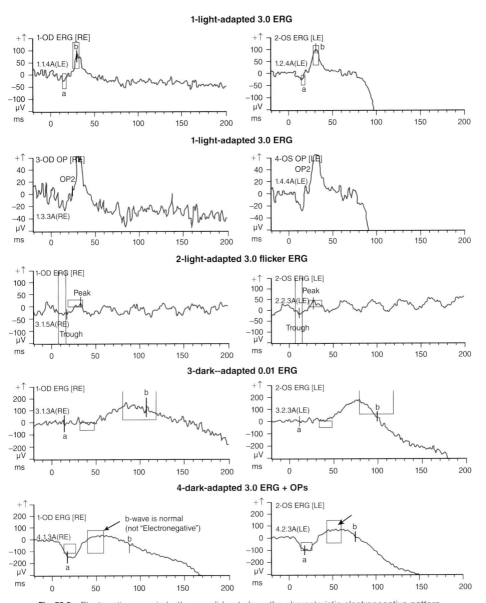

Fig. 52.3 Electroretinogram in both eyes did not show the characteristic electronegative pattern.

Follow-up Care

- There are no previously established guidelines for follow-up.
- Our patient is followed on a biannual basis.
- One study describing unilateral SNIFR with best-corrected visual acuity of 20/20 reports follow-up every 6 months.[5]
- If the patient is symptomatic or demonstrates progression on OCT, more frequent follow-up is indicated.

Algorithm 52.1: Algorithm for Differential Diagnosis of Retinoschisis

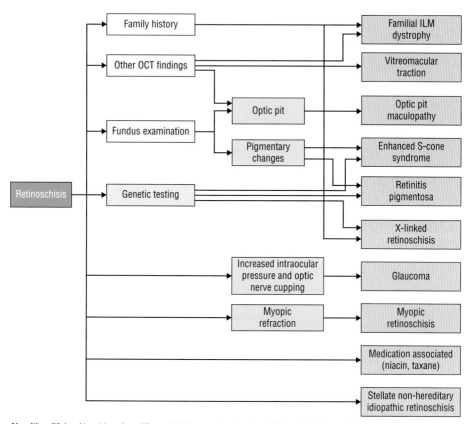

Algorithm 52.1 Algorithm for differential diagnosis of retinoschisis. *ILM,* Internal limiting membrane; *OCT,* optical coherence tomography.

Key Points

- Consider SNIFR in patients with foveomacular retinoschisis with a negative family history, degenerative or acquired etiology.
- Patients tend to have good vision and can be observed.
- Dorzolamide has been reported to improve vision and OCT findings.
- Patients should be followed on a regular basis and at shorter intervals if symptomatic or if there is progression on OCT.

References

1. Agarwal A. Heredodystrophic disorders affecting the pigment epithelium and retina. In Agarwal A, ed. *Gass' Atlas of Macular Diseases.* Vol 1. 5th ed. Elsevier Saunders; 2012. Accessed May 23, 2020.
2. Ober MD, Freund KB, Shah M, et al. Stellate nonhereditary idiopathic foveomacular retinoschisis. *Ophthalmology.* 2014;121(7):1406-1413.

3. Casalino G, Upendran M, Bandello F, Chakravarthy U. Stellate nonhereditary idiopathic foveomacular retinoschisis concomitant to exudative maculopathies. *Eye (Lond)*. 2016;30(5):754-757.
4. Fragiotta S, Leong B, Kaden TR, et al. A proposed mechanism influencing structural patterns in X-linked retinoschisis and stellate nonhereditary idiopathic foveomacular retinoschisis. *Eye*. 2019:33;724-728.
5. Ansel T, Weinberg B, Shenouda-Awad N. *Splitting of differentials: a new type of foveal retinoschisis.* American Academy of Optometry. 1:6.
6. Ajlan RS, Hammamji KS. Stellate nonhereditary idiopathic foveomacular retinoschisis: response to topical dorzolamide therapy. *Retin Cases Brief Rep*. 2019;13(4):364-366.
7. Moraes BRM, Ferreira BFA, Nogueira TM, Nakashima Y, Primiano Júnior HP, Souza EC. Vitrectomy for stellate nonhereditary idiopathic foveomacular retinoschisis associated with outer retinal layer defect. *Retin Cases Brief Rep*. 2022;16(3):289-292.

CHAPTER 53

Bilateral Vitelliform Detachments in a Woman

Meera S. Ramakrishnan ▪ Lawrence A. Yannuzzi

History of Present Illness

We present a case of a 64-year-old woman with history of hypertension, diabetes, and smoking referred for bilateral multifocal neurosensory detachments with vitelliform lesions previously diagnosed as central serous chorioretinopathy (CSC). She reports blurred vision in both eyes for 2 to 3 months. She denies floaters, photopsias or flashes, metamorphopsia, or nyctalopia. She denies any history of ocular conditions or ocular surgeries.

OCULAR EXAMINATION FINDINGS

Visual acuity with correction was 20/40 in each eye. Intraocular pressure was normal. External and anterior segment examinations showed mild nuclear sclerotic cataracts but otherwise were unremarkable. Dilated fundus examination showed multiple symmetrical, variably sized detachments of the neurosensory retina with vitelliform deposits (Fig. 53.1).

IMAGING

Optical coherence tomography (OCT) showed multiple subretinal large serous detachments bilaterally, involving the fovea, with a thick layer of vitelliform material on the outer retinal surface (Fig. 53.2).

Questions to Ask

- Does the patient have a family history of ocular conditions or consanguinity? A family history would be important to ascertain etiologies for vitelliform disorders such as Best disease or pattern dystrophies.
  - No
- Does the patient have a history of cancer? Paraneoplastic syndromes can result in paraneoplastic acute exudative polymorphous vitelliform maculopathy (AEPVM).
  - No
- What medications does the patient take? Medications such as mitogen-activated protein kinase inhibitor (MAPK) and extracellular signal-related kinase 2 (ERK2) inhibitors (usually taken to treat neoplasm) have been associated with multifocal serous or vitelliform retinal detachments. Use of steroids may result in CSC.
  - Amlodipine, metformin, omeprazole, ranitidine, and rosuvastatin. No culprit medications are noted.

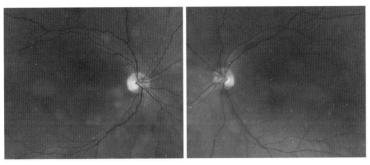

Fig. 53.1 Optos color fundus photographs of the posterior pole of both eyes in a 64-year-old woman reveal multiple serous retinal detachments.

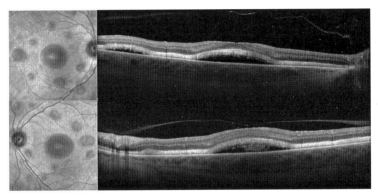

Fig. 53.2 Near infrared of both eyes reveals multiple hyporeflective lesions throughout the macula in both eyes. Corresponding optical coherence tomography scans through these lesions reveal serous detachments of the retina with thick hyperreflective material layering along the ellipsoid zone.

Assessment

This is a case of a 64-year-old woman with no ocular or surgical history and a negative family history demonstrating bilateral symmetrical vitelliform retinal detachments on OCT.

Differential Diagnosis

- Best disease
- Multifocal vitelliform dystrophy
- Sjögren-Larsson syndrome
- Pattern dystrophies
- Age-related macular degeneration (AMD)
- Pseudoxanthoma elasticum
- Vitreomacular traction (VMT) syndrome
- Macular telangiectasia type 2
- CSC
- Idiopathic AEPVM
- Paraneoplastic syndromes
- MAPK inhibitor retinopathy

Working Diagnosis

Idiopathic AEPVM

Multimodal Testing and Results

- Fundus photographs
  - On fundus examination, early findings include multiple bilateral symmetrical well-defined serious retinal detachments, which vary in size (polymorphous). They appear bleb-like, are multiple (at least five per eye), and with foveal involvement.[1]
  - Numerous small bleb-like lesions can also develop in a honeycomb distribution along the vascular arcades. This is less common.[2]
  - Over time, vitelliform material can accumulate within the serous detachments. The vitelliform material frequently precipitates to form menisci, so-called pseudohypopyon lesions. The vitelliform lesions can be present for months to years and may eventually resolve or progress to retinal pigment epithelium changes.
- OCT
  - Our patient has no drusen, no thickening of the choroidal layer, and no abnormal vitreous adhesion to suggest other etiologies like AMD, CSC, and VMT.
  - Multiple large and small dome-shaped retinal detachments with hyporeflective subretinal fluid are seen in AEPVM.[10] When vitelliform deposits accumulate, there is a thick hyperreflective material layering on the outer retinal surface.
  - After resolution of the deposits, the ellipsoid layer largely remains intact, explaining the restoration of good vision in most patients.
  - Intraretinal cysts can be present in the earlier stages when subretinal fluid is present.
- Fundus autofluorescence (FAF)
  - The vitelliform deposits shows characteristic intense hyperautofluorescence.[3]
  - FAF is one of the key diagnostic tests for idiopathic AEPVM. The intense autofluorescence is due to lipofuscin-rich vitelliform deposits, which may be due to phagocytized photoreceptor outer segments.[4]
- Fluorescein angiography (FA)
  - The vitelliform material is hypofluorescent due to blockage. The optic nerve and vasculature are normal, without signs of inflammation or increased permeability.
  - The cystic changes on OCT do not show leakage on FA.
- Electrophysiologic tests
  - Electroretinogram (ERG) is largely normal or may have slightly abnormal results on multifocal ERG.
  - Electrooculogram can be abnormal in half of patients, similar to bestrophinopathies.[1,5]
- Genetic testing
  - This can be obtained to help rule out genetic disorders such as bestrophinopathy or pattern dystrophy from mutations in *BEST1* or *peripherin/RDS*.[1,6]
- OCTA
  - Choroidal neovascularization may sometimes complicate the course and can be identified on OCTA.

Management

- The patient was referred to her internist for age-appropriate cancer screening, which also included a full body skin examination to rule out cutaneous melanoma. Given her history of smoking, she also underwent chest computed tomography. Workup was negative for any malignancy.

- The patient's visual acuity remained 20/40, without any secondary changes of choroidal neovascularization (CNV) or atrophy.
- General management for idiopathic AEPVM is typically observation given the high likelihood of spontaneous resolution and relatively preserved good vision in these patients, though electrophysiological abnormalities may persist.[7]
- However, given significant overlap of clinical presentation with Best disease and paraneoplastic AEPVM, age-appropriate cancer screening should be performed.[8,9]
- Patients with early onset (age <20 years) and abnormal electrophysiologic tests should also be considered for genetic testing.
- One case of secondary CNV was treated with a single intravitreal injection of triamcinolone acetonide.[1]

Follow-up Care

- There are no previously established guidelines for follow-up.
- Our patient is followed on a biannual basis to monitor the evolution from serous subretinal fluid, to vitelliform deposits, to resolution, which could occur over months to years.
- If the patient is symptomatic or demonstrates progression on OCT, more frequent follow-up is indicated.

Algorithm 53.1: Differential Diagnosis for Vitelliform Detachments

Algorithm for DDx for vitelliform detachments

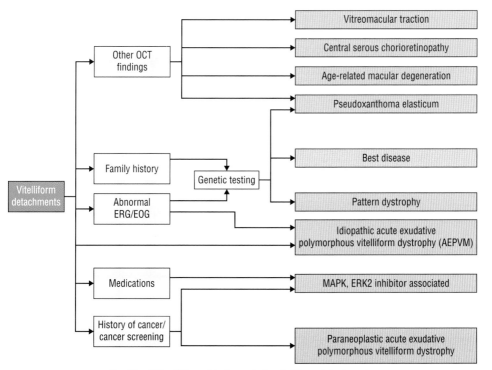

Algorithm 53.1 Differential diagnosis for vitelliform detachments.

Key Points

- Consider idiopathic AEPVM in patients with bilateral vitelliform detachments with a negative family history or a degenerative or secondary etiology.
- Genetic testing and most importantly age-appropriate cancer screening is highly recommended.
- Patients tend to maintain good vision and can be observed.
- Patients should be followed on a regular basis and at shorter intervals if symptomatic or if they have progression on OCT.

References

1. Barbazetto I, Dansingani KK, Dolz-Marco R, et al. Idiopathic acute exudative polymorphous vitelliform maculopathy: clinical spectrum and multimodal imaging characteristics. *Ophthalmology.* 2018;125(1):75-88.
2. Gass JD, Cuang EL, Granek H. Acute exudative polymorphous vitelliform maculopathy. *Trans Am Ophthalmol Soc.* 1988;86:354-366.
3. Vaclavik V, Ooi KG, Bird AC, et al. Autofluorescence findings in acute exudative polymorphous vitelliform maculopathy. *Arch Ophthalmol.* 2007;125:274-277.
4. Spaide RF. Autofluorescence from the outer retina and subretinal space: hypothesis and review. *Retina.* 2008;28:5-35.
5. Gerth C, Zawadzki RJ, Werner JS, Heon E. Detailed analysis of retinal function and morphology in a patient with autosomal recessive bestrophinopathy (ARB). *Doc Ophthalmol.* 2009;118:239-246.
6. Fung AT, Yzer S, Goldberg N, et al. New *BEST1* mutations in autosomal recessive bestrophinopathy. *Ophthalmology.* 2005;112:825-833.
7. Kozma P, Locke KG, Wang YZ, et al. Persistent cone dysfunction in acute exudative polymorphous vitelliform maculopathy. *Retina.* 2007;27:109-113.
8. Modi KK, Roth DB, Green SN. Acute exudative polymorphous vitelliform maculopathy in a young man: a case report. *Retin Cases Brief Rep.* 2014;8:200-204.
9. Francis JH, Habib L, Abramson DH, et al. Clinical and morphologic characteristics of MEK inhibitor-associated retinopathy: differences from central serous chorioretinopathy. *Ophthalmology.* 2017;124(12):1788-1798.
10. Brasil OF, Vianna RN, Moraes RT. Optical coherence tomography findings of the acute exudative polymorphous vitelliform maculopathy. *Ophthalmic Surg Lasers Imaging.* 2010;9:1-2.

CHAPTER 54

Hypopigmented Subretinal Lesion in an Elderly Man

Michael T. Andreoli

History of Present Illness

A 65-year-old man with an unremarkable past medical history was referred for concern of intraocular lymphoma. He denies visual symptoms in either eye.

OCULAR EXAMINATION FINDINGS

Visual acuity was 20/25. Intraocular pressure was normal. External and anterior segment examination showed pseudophakia in each eye. Dilated fundus examination showed a yellow circinate lesion superotemporally in the right eye (Fig. 54.1). No vitreous cell or haze was present.

IMAGING

Fundus autofluorescence showed a target-shaped ring of hyperautofluorescence over the lesion (Fig. 54.2). Optical coherence tomography (OCT) revealed a dramatic elevation, without expansion of the choroid, in the area (Fig. 54.3). B scan ultrasound demonstrated a focal hyperechoic lesion with significant posterior shadowing in the choroid or sclera (Fig. 54.4).

Questions to Ask

- Has the patient had a history of malignancy? Metastatic lesions can be solitary or multifocal and can be yellow or creamy in color.
  - No
- Is there associated vitreous haze or cells? Primary vitreoretinal lymphoma commonly demonstrates prominent vitreous haze or cells.
  - No
- Are there any known electrolyte abnormalities? Sclerochoroidal calcifications may be secondary to systemic electrolyte abnormalities.
  - No
- Does the patient have any known parathyroid or kidney problems? Sclerochoroidal calcifications may be associated with parathyroid or kidney conditions.
  - No

Assessment

- This is a case of a 65-year-old man with no pertinent medical history and with a yellow circinate lesion in the superotemporal near periphery that shows hyperautofluorescence and shadowing on ultrasound.

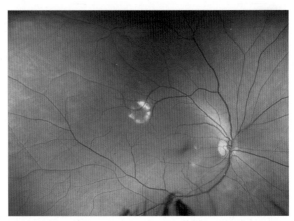

Fig. 54.1 Fundus photography: widefield Optos fundus photography demonstrates a deep, yellow circinate lesion in the superotemporal near periphery.

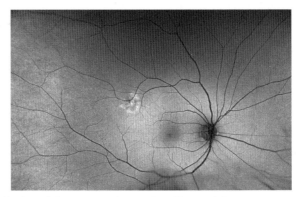

Fig. 54.2 Fundus autofluorescence shows a ring of hyperautofluorescence over the lesion.

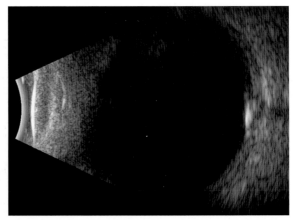

Fig. 54.3 Ultrasound: B scan shows a hyperechoic lesion at the level of the choroid or sclera with posterior shadowing.

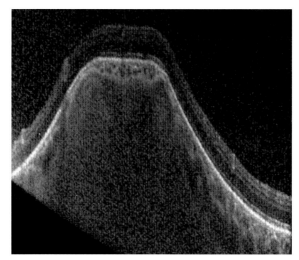

Fig. 54.4 Optical coherence tomography shows a mountain-like protrusion at the level of the sclera, without expansion of the overlying choroid.

Differential Diagnosis

- Sclerochoroidal calcification
- Presumed solitary circumscribed retinal astrocytic proliferation
- Choroidal osteoma
- Focal scleral nodule
- Primary vitreoretinal lymphoma
- Choroidal neovascular membrane

Working Diagnosis

- Sclerochoroidal calcification

Multimodal Testing and Results

- Fundus photography
  - On fundus examination, a hypopigmented arc-shaped or circinate lesion in the supero-temporal, or less commonly inferotemporal, near periphery is typical. Findings are usually identified in patients over the age of 55 years. In some cases, the lesions can be quite large (Fig. 54.5) and cover a large area.[1,2]
- OCT
  - OCT may show subtle or striking anterior protrusion of the sclera in the area, without an apparent choroidal mass.[1]
- Fundus autofluorescence
  - FAF commonly reveals hyperautofluorescence or isoautofluorescence over the lesion.

Management

- Given the benign nature of sclerochoroidal calcifications, no treatment is indicated. Most lesions are idiopathic, but up to 20% may be secondary to electrolyte abnormalities.[3]

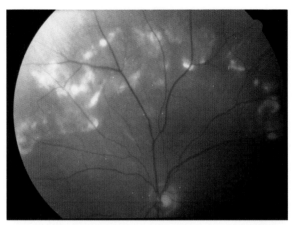

Fig. 54.5 Fundus photograph of the left eye taken in 1986, showing multiple, scattered, and yellowish solid choroidal plaques. Note the irregular geographical outlines and variable sizes. Fundus appearance was unchanged 2 years later. (Reproduced with permission from *JAMA Ophthalmology*.)

A medical history focused on known metabolic imbalances or diuretic use, followed by a workup for hyperparathyroidism, Gitelman syndrome, Bartter syndrome, and renal disease, is prudent.[3]

Follow-up Care

- Surveillance is recommended to monitor for development of choroidal neovascularization.

Algorithm 54.1: Algorithm for Sclerochoroidal Calcification

Sclerochoroidal calcification

- Hypopigmented deep subretinal lesion → superotemporal or inferotemporal location → shadowing or calcium or ultrasound → choroidal process on OCT → consider osteoma

Primarily scleral findings on OCT → consider sclerochoroidal calcification

Other location → prominent calcification → consider choroidal osteoma

→ Vitreous cells/haze or subretinal deposits → consider primary vitreoretinal lymphoma

→ Dome-shaped indentation of choroid on OCT → focal scleral nodule

→ Overlying subretinal fluid or retinal edema → consider fluorescein angiogram to assess for choroidal neovascularization

Algorithm 54.1 Algorithm for sclerochoroidal calcification.

Key Points

■ Sclerochoroidal calcification is a relatively uncommon finding, most often seen as an arcuate or circinate hypopigmented lesion in the superotemporal near periphery.[4,5]

■ Ultrasound or OCT can be used to confirm the diagnosis.

■ Systemic questioning and possible laboratory workup should be considered at time of diagnosis.

References

1. Hasanreisoglu M, Saktanasate J, Shields PW, Shields CL. Classification of sclerochoroidal calcification based on enhanced depth imaging optical coherence tomography "mountain-like" features. *Retina*. 2015;35(7):1407-1414.
2. Schachat AP, Robertson DM, Mieler WF, et al. Sclerochoroidal calcification. *Arch Ophthalmol*. 1992;110(2):196-199.
3. Shields CL, Hasanreisoglu M, Saktanasate J, Shields PW, Seibel I, Shields JA. Sclerochoroidal calcification: clinical features, outcomes, and relationship with hypercalcemia and parathyroid adenoma in 179 eyes. *Retina*. 2015;35(3):547-554.
4. Sivalingam A, Shields CL, Shields JA, et al. Idiopathic sclerochoroidal calcification. *Ophthalmology*. 1991;98(5):720-724.
5. Lim JI, Goldberg MF. Idiopathic sclerochoroidal calcification. *Arch Ophthalmol*. 1989;107(8):1122-1123.

CHAPTER 55

Jello-like Circles in My Vision

Mark J. Daily

History of Present Illness

A 20-year-old female college senior student presented with a chief report of "Jello-like" circles in her vision for 6 months, which began during a semester abroad in Madrid, Spain.

Six months ago the patient awoke with blurry circles in her central vision in both eyes. A few days before this, she had a flu-like illness with mild fever and muscle aches, which resolved without treatment. The circles have persisted unchanged since they first appeared. She was otherwise healthy and was on oral contraceptive medication.

She was examined by an ophthalmologist and neurologist in Spain. The ocular examination was reported as normal with vision of 20/20 in each eye. An extensive workup was undertaken including complete blood cell count, sedimentation rate, C-reactive protein, sodium, potassium, chloride, magnesium, iron, calcium, phosphorous, glucose, urea, uric acid, blood urea nitrogen, bilirubin, alkaline phosphatase, cholesterol, triglycerides, high- and low-density lipoprotein, vitamin B_{12}, folic acid, serum proteins, rheumatoid factor, antinuclear antibodies, fluorescent treponemal antibody absorption, HIV, toxoplasmosis titer, Epstein-Barr titer, vitamin D, thyroid-stimulating hormone, and cortisol levels. Imaging included magnetic resonance imaging (MRI) of head and brain and MRI angiography of head and brain.

All the laboratory tests were normal or negative, and the MRI showed "multiple pin-point hyper-intense images of the cerebral hemispheres compatible with ischemic lesions of microangiography as a first possibility or demyelinating or postvaccination or postinfectious disease." The MRI angiogram was normal.

The patient was prescribed lamotrigine, a medication used to treat seizures and bipolar disorders, and a mineral supplement.

OCULAR EXAMINATION FINDINGS

Visual acuity without correction was 20/20 in each eye. Pupils were 4 mm and equally reactive. Motility was full, and fields were full to confrontation. External and anterior segment examinations were normal, and intraocular pressures were 16 mmHg. The dilated fundus examination showed mild macular abnormalities in each eye (Figs. 55.1 and 55.2). The margins of the right optic nerve were slightly blurred compared with the left optic nerve. The remainder of the fundus examination was normal. The patient drew semicircular patterns of visual abnormalities on Amsler grid testing of each eye (Figs. 55.3 and 55.4).

IMAGING

- Color fundus photographs: Subtle mottling of the pigment epithelium is visible in each macula (Figs. 55.1 and 55.2). Fluorescein angiography was normal in both eyes, with no staining of the right optic disc.

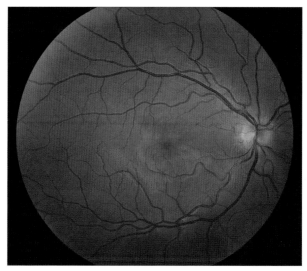

Fig. 55.1   Color photograph of right eye showing slight alteration of macular pigment.

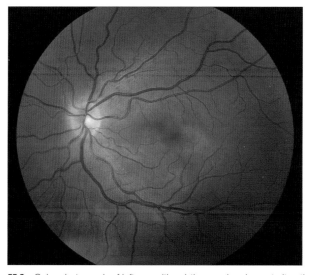

Fig. 55.2   Color photograph of left eye with subtle macular pigment alteration.

- Optical coherence tomography (OCT) testing revealed a dramatic circular alteration of the reflectance in the near-infrared spectroscopy photographs of each eye (Figs. 55.5 and 55.6). In the areas of the hyporeflectance, there was thinning and alteration of the outer nuclear layers and photoreceptors in the OCT image. A review of the OCT images taken 6 months before in Spain also showed outer layer retinal disruption (Figs. 55.7 and 55.8).

BERNELL M-R-M GRID TEST RECORDING CHART
(Maculopathy-Retinopathy-Metamorphopsia)
Use For
M-R-M Grid Test Book, 553M Slide and Amsler Grid Test
RE

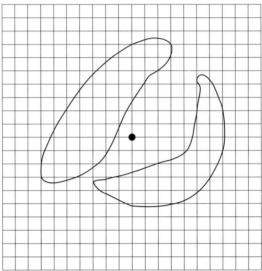

Fig. 55.3   Amsler grid drawing by the patient (right eye).

BERNELL M-R-M GRID TEST RECORDING CHART
(Maculopathy-Retinopathy-Metamorphopsia)
Use For
M-R-M Grid Test Book, 553M Slide and Amsler Grid Test
LE

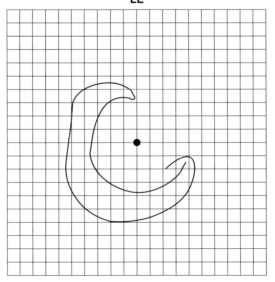

Fig. 55.4   Amsler grid drawing by the patient (left eye).

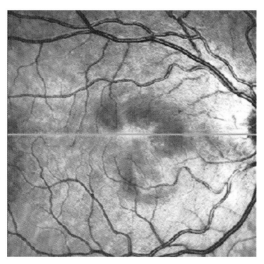

Fig. 55.5   Near-infrared image of right macula.

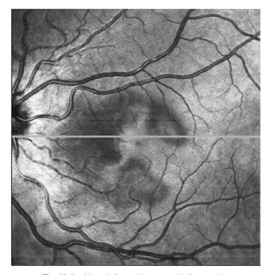

Fig. 55.6   Near-infrared image of left macula.

Assessment

A 19-year-old healthy woman presents with a 6-month history of persistent scotomas in each eye, with dramatic changes on near-infrared OCT images and outer layer retinal disruption. An extensive medical workup was negative.

Differential Diagnosis

- Central serous retinopathy
- Multiple evanescent white-dot syndrome
- Acute posterior multifocal placoid pigment epitheliopathy
- Optic neuritis

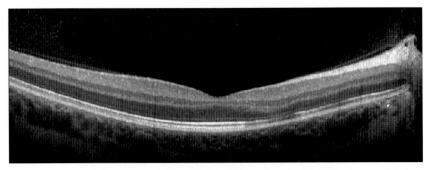

Fig. 55.7 Optical coherence tomography of the right eye with parafoveal outer nuclear layer and photoreceptor disruption.

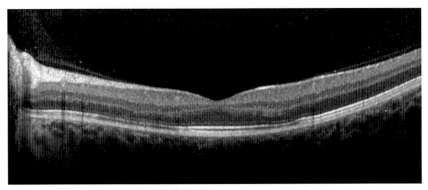

Fig. 55.8 Optical coherence tomography of the left eye with outer layer disruption on both sides of foveal depression.

Working Diagnosis

Acute macular neuroretinopathy

Multimodal Testing and Results

- Fundus photographs: In this case there was a very subtle alteration of the pigment epithelium 6 months after onset, but often no changes can be visualized in the acute phase. On red-free photographs, parafoveal gray areas corresponding to the scotomas may be visible.
- Fluorescein angiography: This test is usually normal.
- OCT: The most helpful test is the near-infrared images taken by OCT. Outer retinal disruption is usually visible on the OCT slices[3,4] (Figs. 55.7 and 55.8).

Management

- No treatment has been shown to be helpful. The scotomas can persist, sometimes for years, although patients seem to be able to function well despite the defects.
- Having the patient draw the scotomas on an Amsler grid can be very helpful to identify the scotomas, which may be hard for the patient to verbalize.

Algorithm 55.1: Algorithm for Evaluation of Scotoma

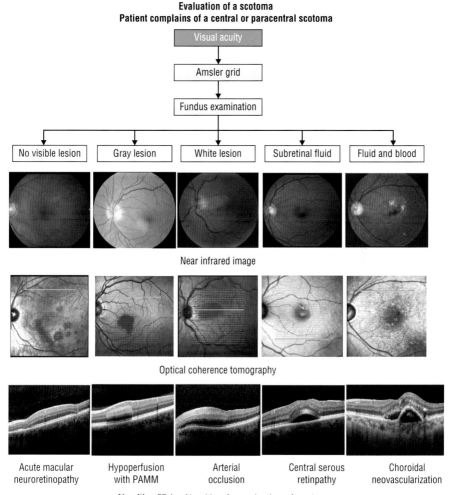

Algorithm 55.1   Algorithm for evaluation of scotoma.

Follow up

The patient continued to notice the scotomas for over a year, but said that they became "less bothersome" and she functioned normally.

Key Points

- Acute macular neuroretinopathy[1,2] should be in the differential when the patient is young, healthy, and quite specific about a clearly delineated central scotoma. Typically, the patient can readily draw this area on an Amsler grid.
- The near-infrared image on the OCT is the most helpful test.[5]
- There is no treatment for persistent scotomas.

References

1. Bos PJ, Deutman AF. Acute macular neuroretinopathy. *Am J Ophthalmol*. 1975;80:573-584.
2. Bhavsar KV, Rahimy E, Joseph A, Freund KB, Sarraf D, Cunningham Jr ET. Acute macular neuroreti-nopathy: a comprehensive review of the literature. *Surv Ophthalomol*. 2016;61:538-565.
3. Vance KK, Spaide RF, Freund KB, Wiznia R, Cooney MJ. Outer retinal abnormalities in acute macular neuroretinopathy. *Retina*. 2011;31:441-445.
4. Fawzi AA, Pappuru RR, Sarraf D, et al. Acute macular neuroretinopathy: long-term insights revealed by multimodal imaging. *Retina*. 2012;32:1500-1513.
5. Kerrison J, Pollock S, Biousse V. Coffee and doughnut maculopathy: a cause of acute central ring scotomas. *Br J Ophthalmol*. 2000;84:158-164.

Toxic/Secondary

CHAPTER 56

Bilateral Maculopathy in a Middle-Aged Woman With Interstitial Cystitis

Néda Abraham ◾ Meira Fogel-Levin ◾ SriniVas Sadda ◾ David Sarraf

History of Present Illness

A 59-year-old woman presented with a 4-year history of decreased vision and progressive nyctalopia. Past medical history was remarkable for depression, chronic fatigue, fibromyalgia and interstitial cystitis (IC).

OCULAR EXAMINATION FINDINGS

Snellen visual acuities were 20/20 in the right eye (OD) and 20/30 in the left eye (OS). Intraocular pressures were normal. External and anterior segment examinations were within normal limits in both eyes (OU). Dilated fundus examination showed retinal pigment epithelium (RPE) mottling and RPE clumps in the perifoveal region OU.

IMAGING

- Ultrawide-field (UWF) fundus photography (California, Optos) demonstrated pericentral RPE mottling OU with a normal peripheral retina OU (Fig. 56.1A, B).
- Spectralis multicolor photography (Heidelberg Engineering, Inc.) and near-infrared reflectance (NIR) showed punctate perifoveal hyperreflective lesions OU (Fig. 56.2A–D).
- Fundus autofluorescence (FAF) 55 degrees (Fig. 56.3) and UWF FAF (Fig. 56.1C, D) illustrated a speckled network of hyperautofluorescent and hypoautofluorescent lesions centered around the fovea OU. These lesions corresponded to focal areas of RPE thickening evident on cross-sectional spectral domain optical coherence tomography (OCT) and en face OCT OU.
- OCT angiography excluded macular neovascularization (Fig. 56.4).

Questions to Ask

- Does the patient have any family history of age-related macular degeneration (AMD) or pattern dystrophy? AMD and pattern dystrophy can be associated with RPE alterations in the perifoveal region.
  - No

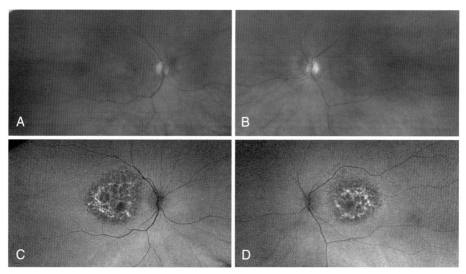

Fig. 56.1   Ultrawide-field (UWF) color (A and B) and autofluorescent (C and D) imaging of a 59-year-old patient with interstitial cystitis and pentosan polysulfate exposure (cumulative dosage 1606 g). Color UWF (A and B) demonstrates retinal pigment epithelial alterations in the macula in both eyes (OU). UWF autofluorescence (C and D) shows a speckled pattern of hyper- and hypoautofluorescence centered around the fovea with normal peripheral retina OU.

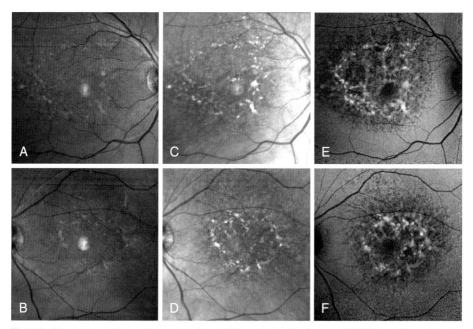

Fig. 56.2   Spectralis multicolor photography (A and B), near-infrared reflectance (NIR) (C and D), and fundus autofluorescence (E and F) for the right and left eyes in the same patient with pentosan-associated maculopathy. Multicolor and NIR images show a symmetrical pattern of hyperreflective lesions centered around the fovea in each eye. Fundus autofluorescence (30-degree) shows a speckled network of hyper- and hypoautofluorescent lesions centered on the fovea in both eyes. Focal areas of hypoautofluorescent retinal pigment epithelial atrophy are also noted in each eye.

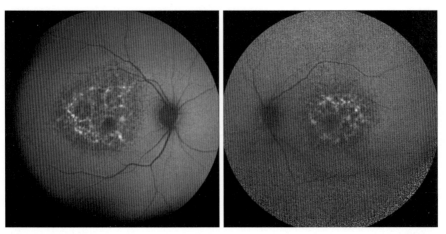

Fig. 56.3 Fundus autofluorescence images (55-degree) show a speckled network of hyper- and hypoauto-fluorescent lesions centered on the fovea in both eyes.

- Does the patient have a family or personal history of diabetes mellitus or hearing loss? Maternally inherited diabetes and deafness syndrome (MIDD) can present with RPE mottling centered on the fovea.
  - No
- Has the patient been treated with pentosan polysulfate sodium (PPS)?
  - Yes. She was treated with PPS (Elmiron; Janssen Pharmaceuticals, Titusville, NJ) for IC at a dosage of 100 mg twice a day for 22 years for a cumulative dose of 1606 grams. PPS was discontinued in December 2019.

Assessment

- A 59-year-old woman receiving PPS to treat IC for 22 years (cumulative dose 1606 g) presented with progressive nyctalopia, vision loss, and bilateral maculopathy. Multimodal retinal imaging showed a speckled pattern of symmetrical RPE abnormalities centered on the fovea with NIR and FAF OU and corresponding hyperreflective areas of RPE thickening by OCT.

Differential Diagnosis

- Age-related macular degeneration (AMD)
- Macular dystrophy (i.e., pattern dystrophy)
- Mitochondrial syndrome (i.e., maternally inherited diabetes and deafness syndrome [MIDD])
- Pachychoroid disease (i.e., pachychoroid pigment epitheliopathy)

Working Diagnosis

- PPS-associated maculopathy

Multimodal Imaging

- Fundus color photos
  - RPE mottling centered on the fovea can be identified with macular examination.

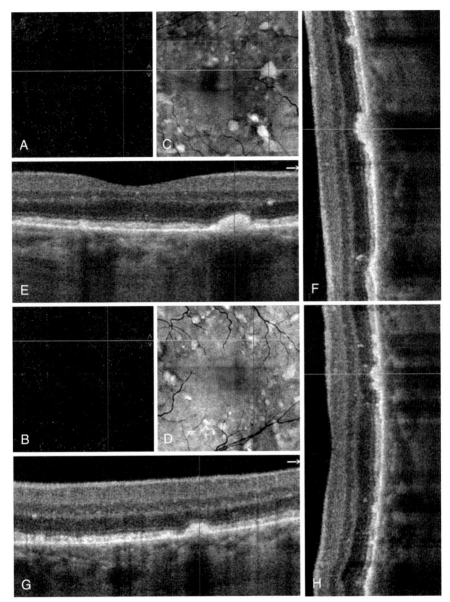

Fig. 56.4 En face (3 x 3 mm) optical coherence tomography (OCT) angiography (A and B), centered on the fovea, and corresponding en face OCT (C and D) and OCT B-scans (E–H) from the right and left eyes. Note the absence of macular neovascularization with en face OCT angiography (outer retina slab) in each eye (A and B). En face OCT (C and D), segmented at the retinal pigment epithelium, and cross-sectional OCT B-scans (E–H) show the characteristic hyperreflective RPE lesions associated with pentosan polysulfate sodium maculopathy that are differentiated from macular drusen.

- Fundus autofluorescence
    - The 30-degree, 55-degree, and UWF FAF illustrate a speckled pattern of hyperauto-fluorescence and hypoautofluorescence symmetrically centered on the fovea (and in more severe cases also centered around the disc) OU.
- B-scan OCT
    - Cross-sectional OCT shows multifocal hyperreflective areas of RPE thickening that are morphologically different from macular drusen.[1-6]
- En face OCT
    - Perifoveal hyperreflective deposits corresponding to the areas of RPE thickening visible on cross-sectional OCT can be appreciated with en face OCT.
- OCT angiography (OCTA)
    - OCTA should be performed to rule out macular neovascularization (MNV), which can complicate PPS maculopathy.[3,4,6] MNV was excluded in our case.

Management

- Discontinue PPS treatment in consultation with primary care physician.
- Follow up in 9 to 12 months with OCT and FAF to assess for possible progression of macular disease and also perform OCTA to exclude MNV.
- Recommend self-testing with Amsler grids to help detect macular neovascularization early.

Follow-up Care

- There are no previously established guidelines for follow-up.
- Recent studies have demonstrated that PPS maculopathy can continue to progress years after discontinuing the medication.[7] Progression can be monitored with sequential FAF and OCT. More severe forms of PPS toxicity can be associated with extensive macular atrophy and more severe vision loss.[3,6]
- MNV can complicate PPS associated maculopathy.[4] MNV precautions with Amsler grid monitoring are essential for the patient. If any symptoms of metamorphopsia and/or distortion with Amsler grid testing develop, patients should return urgently for retinal examination and imaging, including OCTA, to rule out MNV. Anti–vascular endothelial growth factor injection therapy should be initiated at the earliest possible detection of MNV.

Key Points

- Multimodal retinal imaging is essential in patients with PPS exposure to screen for macular toxicity and to detect the early signs of PPS-associated maculopathy.
- Multimodal retinal imaging screening is critical, as patients with PPS macular toxicity may initially be asymptomatic with excellent visual acuity. More severe cases may be associated with vision loss and macular atrophy.
- Patients should be followed at shorter intervals when reaching PPS cumulative dosages of more than 1000 g. The prevalence of PPS-associated maculopathy is 15%, but this increases to 40% in those with cumulative doses greater than 1000 g and 55% in those with cumulative doses greater than 1500 g.[2,3,6]

Algorithm 56.1: Algorithm for Bilateral Maculopathy With Perifoveal Retinal Pigment Epithelium *(RPE)* Mottling

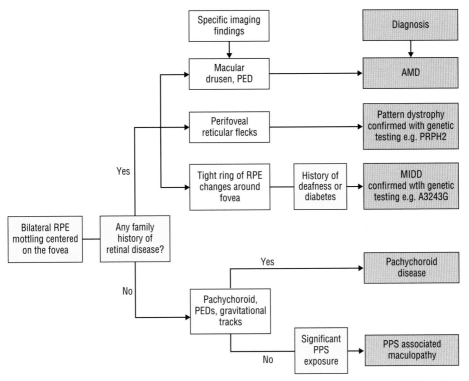

Algorithm 56.1   Algorithm for bilateral maculopathy with perifoveal retinal pigment epithelium *(RPE)* mottling. *AMD,* age-related macular degeneration; *MIDD,* maternally inherited diabetes and deafness syndrome; *PED,* pigment epithelial detachment; *PPS,* pentosan polysulfate sodium.

References

1. Pearce WA, Chen R, Jain N. Pigmentary maculopathy associated with chronic exposure to pentosan polysulfate sodium. *Ophthalmology.* 2018;125(11):1793-1802.
2. Hanif AM, Armenti ST, Taylor SC, et al. Phenotypic spectrum of pentosan polysulfate sodium-associated maculopathy: a multi-center study. *JAMA Ophthalmol.* 2019;137(11):1275-1282.
3. Wang D, Au A, Gunnemann F, et al. Pentosan-associated maculopathy: prevalence, screening guidelines, and spectrum of findings based on prospective multimodal analysis. *Can J Ophthalmol.* 2020;55(2):116-125.
4. Mishra K, Patel TP, Singh MS. Choroidal neovascularization associated with pentosan polysulfate toxicity. *Ophthalmol Retina.* 2020;4(1):111-113.
5. Lindeke-Myers A, Hanif AM, Jain N. Pentosan polysulfate maculopathy. *Surv Ophthalmol.* 2022;67(1):83-96.
6. Wang D, Velaga SB, Grondin C, et al. Pentosan polysulfate maculopathy: prevalence, spectrum of disease, and choroidal imaging analysis based on prospective screening. *Am J Ophthalmol.* 2021;227:125-138.
7. Abou-Jaoude MM, Davis AM, Fraser CE, et al. New insights into pentosan polysulfate maculopathy. *Ophthalmic Surg Lasers Imaging Retina.* 2021;52(1):13-22.

CHAPTER 57

Bilateral Chronic Photopsias in a Woman

J.D. Wilgucki ▓ Jennifer I. Lim

History of Present Illness

A 65-year-old woman with a history of non–small cell lung cancer (NSCLS) with metastasis to the brain presented with visual disturbances in both eyes. She describes the vision changes as "television static or sparkles" that had been present for the past 5 years with recent improvement. She denies any loss of vision, trauma, or history of eye surgery/procedures. She does confirm mild nyctalopia, although she denies any family history of retinal degeneration or macular degeneration.

OCULAR EXAMINATION FINDINGS

At her initial presentation, best corrected visual acuities were 20/20 in each eye, intraocular pressures were normal (13 right eye and 15 left eye), and trace nuclear sclerosis was present. Dilated fundus examination of each eye showed a clear vitreous, healthy optic nerve, sharp foveal reflex, and absence of retinal hemorrhage, cotton wool spots, macular edema, drusen, or retinal or choroidal metastases (Fig. 57.1).

IMAGING

A spectral domain optical coherence tomography (OCT) scan (Fig. 57.2) demonstrated parafoveal outer retinal attenuation in both eyes. A concurrent OCT angiogram (OCTA) (Fig. 57.3) showed no abnormalities.

Questions to Ask

■ Does the patient have a family history of ocular conditions or consanguinity? A family history would be important to ascertain etiologies for retinal dystrophies such as cone dystrophy and rod-cone dystrophy, as well as macular degeneration.
  ■ No.
■ What is the current status of the patient's cancer? Is it in remission? Does the patient have recent neurological imaging and up-to-date systemic screening? Given her history of systemic/metastatic cancer, it is important to understand the patient's current medical status and to have documentation of neuroimaging.
  ■ The patient's cancer was in remission. Recent screening magnetic resonance imaging, positron emission tomography, and computed tomography scans showed no evidence of recurrence in the lung.

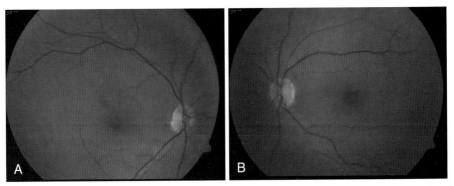

Fig. 57.1 Color fundus photographs of the right (A) and left (B) eyes show normal optic nerves, sharp foveal reflexes, and absence of retinal hemorrhage, cotton wool spots, drusen, or retinal or choroidal metastases.

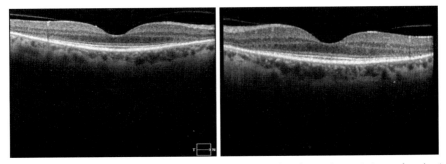

Fig. 57.2 Spectral domain optical coherence tomography scans of each eye demonstrate parafoveal outer retinal attenuation. Note loss of the outer nuclear layer and ellipsoid layers in each eye.

- What past or current cancer treatment is the patient undergoing? What medications does the patient take? There are multiple different chemotherapeutic regiments that are associated with retinal toxicity, such as mitogen-activated protein kinase (MEK) inhibitors, alkylating agents, checkpoint inhibitors, and anaplastic lymphoma kinase (ALK) inhibitors.
  - She had been taking multiple different chemotherapeutic regiments with ALK inhibitors. The patient was currently taking crizotinib for 4 years, followed by ceritinib for 3 years and most recently switched to alectinib. She noted that once she had switched to alectinib, her visual disturbances improved.

Assessment

- This is a case of a 65-year-old woman with a history of metastatic NSCLC on multiple chemotherapeutic agents demonstrating chronic photopsias and parafoveal outer retinal attenuation on OCT.

Differential Diagnosis

- Medication-induced retinal toxicity
- Cancer-associated retinopathy

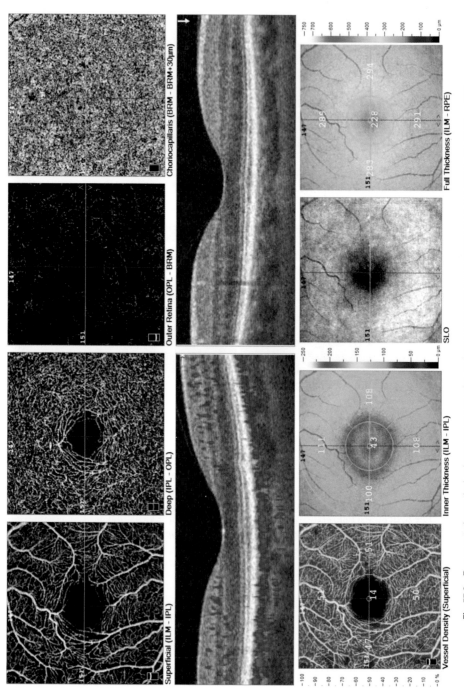

Fig. 57.3 Representative optical coherence tomography angiogram appears normal in the right eye. There are no flow voids.

Superficial (ILM - IPL)

Deep (IPL - OPL)

Outer Retina (OPL - BRM)

Choriocapillaris (BRM - BRM+30µm)

Vessel Density (Superficial)

Inner Thickness (ILM - IPL)

SLO

Full Thickness (ILM - RPE)

- Cone dystrophy
- Rod and cone dystrophy
- Central areolar choroidal dystrophy
- Age-related macular degeneration
- Retinal metastasis

Working Diagnosis

- Retinal toxicity associated with ALK inhibitor use

Multimodal Testing and Results

- Fundus photographs
  - Fundus examination was normal in our patient. There is no documented standard presentation for ALK inhibitor retinal toxicity.
- OCT
  - This patient's OCT demonstrated parafoveal outer retinal attenuation specific to the ellipsoid zone in both eyes. There is limited data on ALK inhibitor retinal toxicity. Outer retinal attenuation is a common nonspecific finding in medication-induced retinal toxicity and retinal dystrophies.
- Electroretinogram (ERG)
  - An ERG was obtained given the patient's history of metastatic lung cancer and target anticancer agents. The ERG showed a mixed rod/cone diminished response, specifically a diminished b-wave in dark-adapted state (Fig. 57.4). ALK inhibitors have been shown to affect the signaling process of retinal ganglion cells creating a functional disturbance possibly leading to visual disorders. Furthermore, a study found crizotinib decreased the b-wave amplitude during dark adaption.[1-3]
- OCTA
  - Our patient had a normal OCTA. There is no data in literature documenting OCTA changes in ALK inhibitor–related retinal toxicity.

Management

- After discussing the OCT and ERG findings, the patient's subjective symptoms, and her remission status with her oncologist, it was decided to discontinue the ALK inhibitor treatment.
- The patient was followed every 3 to 4 months, and her symptoms continued to abate.
- One year after her initial presentation, she expressed near complete resolution of her symptoms, and a follow-up ERG showed normalization (Fig. 57.5).
- Two years later, the patient's vision has remained stable, and the OCT has remained unchanged with no improvement in the outer retinal changes and no restoration of the ellipsoid zone. She continues to be in remission.

Follow-up Care

- There are no previously established guidelines for follow-up.
- Our patient is followed every 6 months.

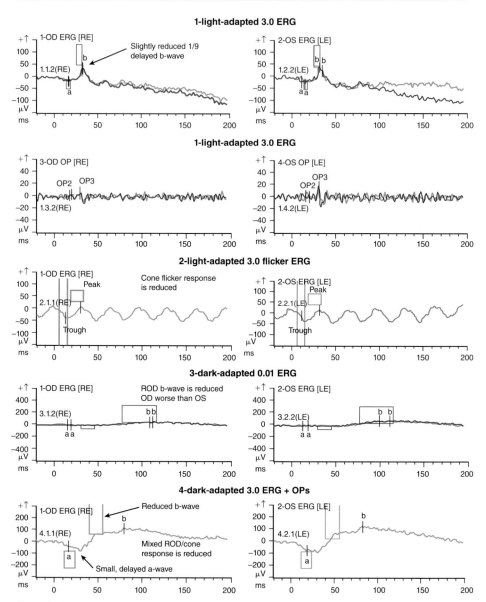

Fig. 57.4 Electroretinogram (ERG) taken while the patient was taking the ALK inhibitor. The right eye responses are shown on the left half of the figure, and the right eye responses are shown on the right half. Note the light-adapted ERG shows a slightly reduced and delayed b-wave in the right eye and normal response in the left eye. The cone flicker responses are also reduced in both eyes. The dark-adapted rod response shows a reduced b-wave, more so in the right eye than in the left eye. The dark-adapted mixed rod/cone response is reduced in the right eye and within the lower limit of normal in the left eye. (Note: The *green and red boxes* depict the normal ranges.)

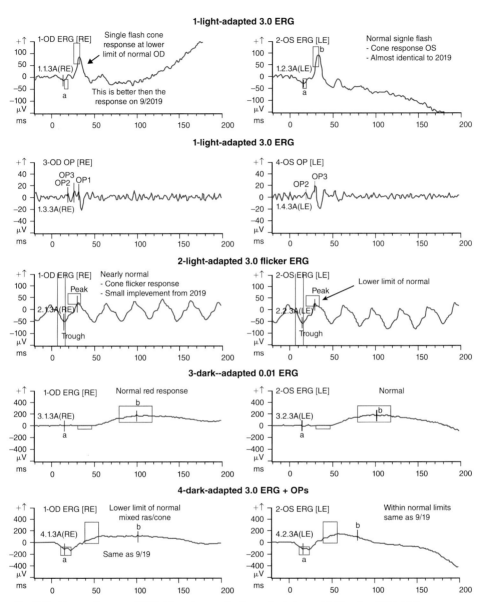

Fig. 57.5 Electroretinogram (ERG) taken 1 year after the patient stopped taking the ALK inhibitor now appears normal. The right eye responses are shown on the left half of the figure, and the right eye responses are shown on the right half. Note the light-adapted ERG shows the response is now at the lower limit of normal in the right eye and is normal in the left eye. The cone flicker responses are now at the lower limit of normal in each eye. The dark-adapted rod responses are normal in both eyes. The dark-adapted mixed rod/cone response is now at the lower limit of normal in the right eye and within normal in the left eye. (Note: The *green and red boxes* depict the normal ranges.)

Key Points

- Consider retinal medication toxicity in patients with nonspecific visual reports and a history of known retinal toxic agents.[4-9]
- Despite ALK inhibitor–induced retinal toxicity, the patient's vision remains excellent with nonspecific visual reports.
- ALK inhibitor–induced retinal toxicity shows documented ERG changes that improve with cessation of the ALK inhibitor.
- Patients should be followed on a regular basis and at shorter intervals based on clinical findings.

Algorithm 57.1: Chronic Photopsias

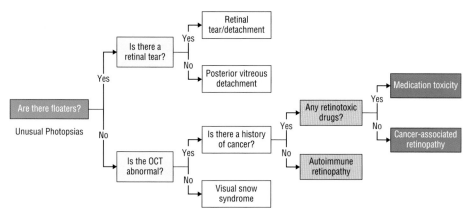

Algorithm 57.1   Chronic photopsias.

References

1. Kwak EL, Bang YJ, Camidge DR, et al. Anaplastic lymphoma kinase inhibition in non-small-cell lung cancer. *N Engl J Med.* 2010;363(18):1693-1703.
2. Ishii T, Iwasawa S, Kurimoto R, Maeda A, Takiguchi Y, Kaneda M. Crizotinib-induced abnormal signal processing in the retina. *PLoS One.* 2015;10(8):e0135521.
3. Liu CN, Mathialagan N, Lappin P, et al. Crizotinib reduces the rate of dark adaptation in the rat retina independent of ALK inhibition. *Toxicol Sci.* 2015;143(1):116-125.
4. Camidge DR, Bang YJ, Kwak EL, et al. Activity and safety of crizotinib in patients with ALK-positive non-small-cell lung cancer: updated results from a phase 1 study. *Lancet Oncol.* 2012;13:1011-1019.
5. Shaw AT, Kim DW, Nakagawa K, et al. Crizotinib versus chemotherapy in advanced ALK-positive lung cancer. *N Engl J Med.* 2013;368:2385-2394.
6. Solomon BJ, Mok T, Kim DW, et al. First-line crizotinib versus chemotherapy in ALK-positive lung cancer. *N Engl J Med.* 2014;371:2167-2177.
7. Chelala E, Hoyek S, Arej N, et al. Ocular and orbital side effects of ALK inhibitors: a review article. *Future Oncol.* 2019;15(16):1939-1945.
8. Fu C, Gombos DS, Lee J, et al. Ocular toxicities associated with targeted anticancer agents: an analysis of clinical data with management suggestions. *Oncotarget.* 2017;8(35):58709-58727. Erratum in: *Oncotarget.* 2019;10(9):1011-1013.
9. Jusufbegovic D, Triozzi PL, Singh AD. Targeted therapy and their ocular complications. In: Singh A, Damato B, eds. *Clinical Ophthalmic Oncology.* Berlin, Heidelberg: Springer; 2014.

CHAPTER 58

Bilateral Serous Retinal Detachments in a Man With Metastatic Melanoma

Irmak Karaca ■ Quan Dong Nguyen ■ Diana V. Do ■
Hashem Ghoraba ■ Chris Or

History of Present Illness

A 46-year-old man with the diagnosis of T2a superficial spreading metastatic melanoma presented with blurry vision and photophobia in both eyes for 1 week. His history was unremarkable for ocular diseases or surgeries. Six weeks before his visual reports, he had started on ipilimumab (3 mg/kg) chemotherapy for his metastatic disease. His vision was worse after the third and most recent cycle of ipilimumab.

OCULAR EXAMINATION FINDINGS

At the initial examination, visual acuity (VA) was 20/100 in both eyes. There were fine, non-granulomatous keratic precipitates bilaterally. Dilated fundus examination showed multiple pockets of serous retinal detachments (RDs) in the macula.

IMAGING

Initial evaluation with fundus photography, autofluorescence, and spectral-domain optical coherence tomography (OCT) (Figs. 58.1 and 58.2) revealed bilateral serous RD in the macula. Fluorescein angiography (FA) demonstrated mild pooling of dye in the areas corresponding to serous RD, along with normal vasculature and absence of active leakage bilaterally. OCT of both eyes showed serous RD involving the fovea with irregular retinal pigment epithelium (RPE).

Questions to Ask

- Does the patient have any risk factors for serous RD? Does the patient have a history of systemic diseases such as hypertension or renal failure? Bilateral serous RD (exudative RD) can be seen in patients with uncontrolled high blood pressure and renal failure.
  - No.
- Does the patient use any medications that could lead to serous RD? Medications like mitogen-activated protein kinase inhibitors can cause drug-related exudative RD bilaterally.
  - Yes. The patient was started on ipilimumab for the metastatic melanoma.

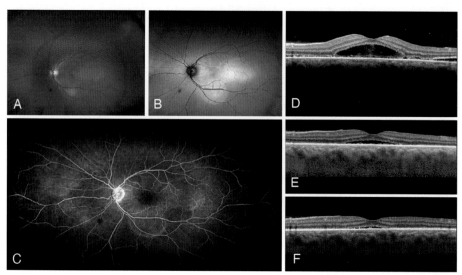

Fig. 58.1 (A) Color wide-field fundus photograph of the left eye shows multiple pockets of serous retinal detachment (RD) at the macula. (B) Fundus autofluorescence image of the left eye shows presence of hyperautofluorescent areas corresponding to the serous RD in the macula. (C) Fluorescein angiography of the left eye shows normal vasculature and absence of leakage of the optic disc or macula. There is mild pooling of dye in the areas corresponding to the serous RD. (D) Spectral-domain optical coherence tomography (OCT) of the left eye at initial presentation shows large serous RD involving the fovea. There is irregularity of the retinal pigment epithelium. (E) OCT of the left eye performed at 1-week follow-up visit (on no treatment for the ocular disease) shows marked decrease in the subretinal fluid. (F) OCT performed at 2-week follow-up visit (on no treatment for the ocular disease) shows near-complete resolution of serous RD with only residual subretinal fluid.

Assessment

This is a case of a 46-year-old man with a T2a superficial spreading metastatic melanoma demonstrating bilateral serous RD after the third infusion of ipilimumab chemotherapy.

Differential Diagnosis

1. Idiopathic
   - Coats disease
   - Central serous chorioretinopathy
   - Uveal effusion syndrome
2. Congenital
   - Nanophthalmos
   - Optic nerve colobomas (morning glory syndrome)
   - Familial exudative vitreoretinopathy
3. Neoplastic
   - Choroidal melanoma
   - Choroidal nevus
   - Choroidal hemangioma
   - Choroidal metastasis
   - Retinoblastoma
   - Primary intraocular lymphoma

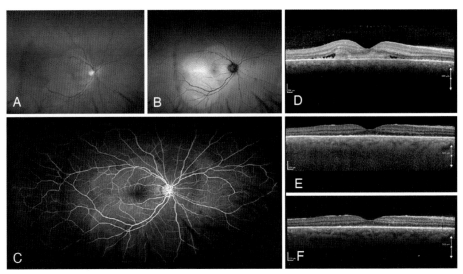

Fig. 58.2 (A) Color wide-field fundus photograph of the right eye shows multiple pockets of serous retinal detachment (RD). (B) Fundus autofluorescence image shows hyperautofluorescent areas in the areas of serous RDs. (C) Fluorescein angiography image at the peak phase shows mild pooling of dye extending beyond the inferior arcade. There is no evidence of active leakage. (D) Spectral-domain optical coherence tomography (OCT) of the right eye at the time of initial presentation shows serous RD involving the fovea with subretinal hyperreflective deposits. Retinal pigment epithelium appears irregular. (E) OCT performed at 1-week follow-up visit shows marked decrease in the subretinal fluid and the hyperreflective material. (F) OCT performed at 2-week follow-up visit (on no treatment for the ocular disease) shows complete resolution of the serous RD.

4. Iatrogenic
   - Panretinal photocoagulation
   - Scleral buckle
   - Hemorrhagic choroidal detachment
   - After retinal detachment surgery
5. Inflammatory
   - Scleritis
   - Orbital cellulitis
   - Orbital pseudotumor
6. Uveitis associated
   - Infectious
     - Syphilis
     - Toxoplasma chorioretinitis
     - Cytomegalovirus retinitis
     - Herpes zoster ophthalmicus
   - Autoimmune
     - Vogt-Koyanagi-Harada (VKH) disease
     - Sympathetic ophthalmia
7. Vascular factors and systemic causes
   - Age-related macular degeneration
   - Preeclampsia/eclampsia in pregnancy
   - Hypertensive retinopathy

- Chronic renal failure
- Congestive heart failure
- Diabetic retinopathy
- Sarcoidosis
- Inflammatory bowel disease
- Disseminated intravascular coagulation
- Hyperviscosity
- Immunoglobulin A nephropathy
- Polyarteritis nodosa
- Wegener granulomatosis
- Rheumatoid arthritis
- Systemic lupus erythematosus
- Carotid-cavernous fistula

Working Diagnosis

- Ipilimumab-associated retinopathy presenting with bilateral serous RD

Ipilimumab is a humanized monoclonal antibody against cytotoxic T-cell associated antigen 4 (CTLA-4) that enhances immune response against tumors by inhibition of CTLA-4–mediated T-cell suppression. Therefore immune-related adverse events can be observed, particularly in the skin and gastrointestinal tract. Overall, ocular side effects are rare (about 1.3% of ipilimumab-treated patients) but include anterior uveitis,[1,2] optic neuropathy,[3] Graves-like disease,[4] orbital inflammation,[2] and VKH-like syndrome.[5-7]

Bilateral, severe hypertensive fibrinous anterior uveitis, mild disc edema, choroidal folds, and choroidal lesions on indocyanine green angiography constituting a VKH-like picture have been related to ipilimumab use.[6] A granulomatous panuveitis, with vitritis and choroiditis simulating VKH disease, has been previously described to be associated with ipilimumab chemotherapy.[7] One study reported bilateral serous RD without overt inflammatory signs in a patient with aural lentiginous melanoma during ipilimumab treatment.[8] A rare case of bilateral choroidal neovascular membranes was also documented in a man taking ipilimumab for metastatic melanoma.[9]

Multimodal Testing and Results

- Fundus photography
  - Wide-angle colored fundus photographs showed bilateral multiple pockets of serous macular RD.
  - In one case, at 1 year after completing ipilimumab chemotherapy, a "sunset-glow" fundus appearance developed and mimicked the classic late stage of VKH syndrome.[5]
- Autofluorescence
  - Fundus autofluorescence showed the presence of hyperautofluorescent areas corresponding to the serous RD areas.
- FA
  - FA showed mild pooling in the areas corresponding to serous RD, with no active leakage bilaterally, similar to an earlier study.[8] Acute presentation with bilateral vitritis, choroiditis, and serous RD similar to VKH disease may demonstrate multiple areas of pinpoint leakage at the level of RPE.[7]

- OCT
  - At initial presentation, OCT in the right eye demonstrated serous RD involving the fovea with subretinal hyperreflective deposits. OCT of the left eye similarly indicated large serous RD involving the fovea. RPE appeared irregular in both eyes.
  - At 1-week follow-up, both eyes showed marked reduction in the subretinal fluid, and the right eye revealed decreased hyperreflective material. OCT performed at 2-week follow-up indicated complete and near-complete resolution of the serous RD in right and left eyes, respectively.

Management

- At 1-week follow-up, VA improved to 20/60 in the right eye and 20/40 in the left eye. Bilateral serous RD resolved spontaneously after cessation of ipilimumab.
- Given the spontaneous resolution of the subretinal fluid, the patient was observed without any treatment or intervention. The subsequent dose of chemotherapy was withheld until the resolution of ocular findings.
- Currently, there are no established treatment guidelines for this condition, and management of these patients demands close cooperation with the oncologist.
- One case with severe hypertensive anterior uveitis, disc edema, and VKH-like presentation secondary to ipilimumab chemotherapy was controlled with topical prednisolone acetate and systemic prednisone (1 mg/kg), which was slowly tapered, in addition to antiglaucoma drugs. Ipilimumab therapy was discontinued because of ocular inflammation in agreement with the oncologists.[6]
- In one study, bilateral multifocal serous RD without signs of inflammation was managed with the addition of oral dexamethasone (4 mg daily) to the initial regimen of 1 month of topical prednisolone acetate.[8]
- One patient with suggestive signs of VKH disease related to ipilimumab chemotherapy was initiated on high-dose intravenous corticosteroids for 3 days followed by oral corticosteroids. Three weeks after the presentation, the patient's serous RD totally resolved, and oral corticosteroid was tapered to discontinuation in 4 weeks.[7]

Follow-up Care

- There are no established guidelines for follow-up.
- If the patient demonstrates persistence or progression of subretinal fluid, more frequent and longer follow-up with more intensive treatment, including topical and systemic steroids, should be considered.

Algorithm 58.1: Exudative Retinal Detachment Workup, Systemic Associations, and Fundus Examination Findings

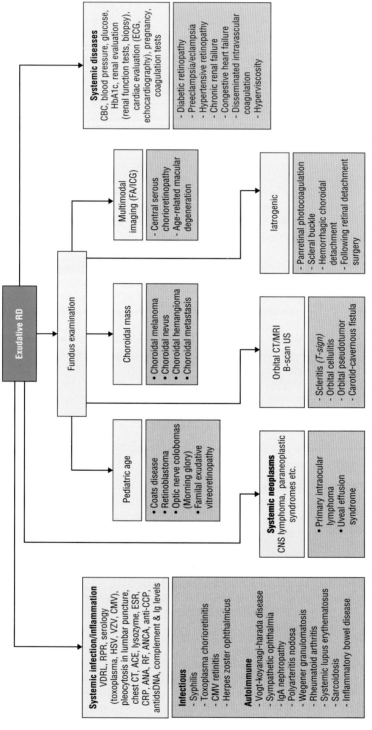

Algorithm 58.1 Exudative retinal detachment workup, systemic associations, and fundus examination findings.

Algorithm 58.2: Algorithm of Exudative Retinal Detachment Differential Diagnoses

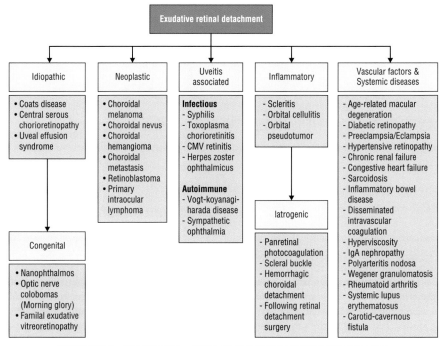

Algorithm 58.2 Algorithm of exudative retinal detachment differential diagnoses.

Key Points

- Consider drug-related causes in the differential diagnosis of bilateral serous RD, particularly in patients with cancer using systemic chemotherapeutics.
- Patients with ipilimumab-associated retinopathy can have resolution of their serous RD upon stopping ipilimumab. In severe cases, topical and systemic corticosteroids might help decrease serous RD.
- Patients particularly receiving novel anticancer drugs should be closely monitored both before and after the chemotherapy in terms of possible ocular adverse effects.

References

1. Robinson MR, Chan CC, Yang JC, et al. Cytotoxic T lymphocyte–associated antigen 4 blockade in patients with metastatic melanoma: a new cause of uveitis. *J Immunother.* 2004;27:478-479.
2. Papavasileiou E, Prasad S, Freitag SK, et al. Ipilimumab-induced ocular and orbital inflammation—a case series and review of the literature. *Ocul Immunol Inflamm.* 2016;24(2):140-146.
3. Yeh OL, Francis CE. Ipilimumab-associated bilateral optic neuropathy. *J Neuroophthalmol.* 2015;35:144-147.
4. Borodic G, Hinkle DM, Cia Y. Drug-induced Graves disease from CTLA-4 receptor suppression. *Ophthalmic Plast Reconstr Surg.* 2011;27:e87-e88.
5. Crosson JN, Laird PW, Debiec M, et al. Vogt-Koyanagi-Harada-like syndrome after CTLA-4 inhibition with ipilimumab for metastatic melanoma. *J Immunother.* 2015;38:80-84.
6. Fierz FC, Meier F, Caloupka K, Böni C. Intraocular inflammation associated with new therapies for cutaneous melanoma—case series and review. *Klin Monbl Augenheilkd.* 2016;233(4):540-544.
7. Wong RK, Lee JK, Huang JJ. Bilateral drug (ipilimumab)-induced vitritis, choroiditis, and serous retinal detachments suggestive of Vogt-Koyanagi-Harada syndrome. *Retin Cases Brief Rep.* 2012;6(4):423-426.
8. Mantopoulos D, Kendra KL, Letson AD, Cebulla CM. Bilateral choroidopathy and serous retinal detachments during ipilimumab treatment for cutaneous melanoma. *JAMA Ophthalmol.* 2015;133:965-967.
9. Modjtahedi BS, Maibach H, Park S. Multifocal bilateral choroidal neovascularization in a patient on ipilimumab for metastatic melanoma. *Cutan Ocul Toxicol.* 2013;32(4):341-343.

CHAPTER 59

Bilateral Blurred Vision and Eye Redness With Bacillary and Serous Retinal Detachments

Karl N. Becker ▪ Robert A. Hyde ▪ Pooja Bhat

History of Present Illness

A 34-year-old woman with history of cutaneous melanoma (stage 3 lesion excised 8 months before presentation) on her leg was referred by an outside ophthalmologist for further evaluation. She reports that her vision became blurry about 1 week before presentation and that her eyes started being red at the same time. She has had mild pain with eye movements but no photophobia. She reports flashes of light that started 4 days before presentation and floaters 3 days before presentation.

OCULAR EXAMINATION FINDINGS

At her initial presentation, visual acuity was count fingers at 3 feet in the right eye and 20/400 in the left eye. The left eye had constricted fields to confrontation, but pupils were noted to be normal with no afferent pupillary defect. Both eyes showed inferior keratic precipitates, 2+ cell and 1+ flare, and iris nodules. Dilated ophthalmoscopy revealed bilateral rare, pigmented cells in the vitreous, bilateral hyperemic optic discs with mildly blurred margins, and bilateral macular subretinal fluid (SRF), choroidal folds, and scattered yellow subretinal deposits. The right eye had a bullous serous detachment of the inferior retina, and the left eye had multiple focal areas of SRF (Fig. 59.1).

Questions to Ask (Fig. 59.2)

■ Does the patient have systemic symptoms such as headache or tinnitus or have signs of vitiligo or poliosis? Evaluation for signs of Vogt-Koyanagi-Harada (VKH) syndrome is important.
   ■ She reports only a mild headache a few times per week, unchanged recently.
■ What is the current status of the patient's cancer? Is it in remission? Does the patient have a recent neurological imaging study and up-to-date systemic screening? With a history of systemic/metastatic cancer it is important to understand the patient's current medical status and to have documentation of normal neuroimaging.
   ■ The cancer was evaluated and treated within the past year. She had a systemic workup that included both positron emission tomography/computed tomography and magnetic resonance imaging brain scans that were both negative.

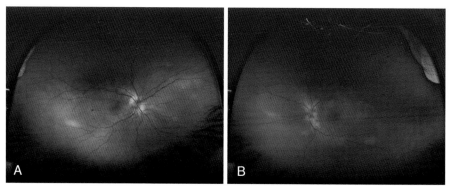

Fig. 59.1 Color wide-field images of the right (A) and left (B) eyes. Images show optic discs were hyperemic with mildly blurred margins, maculae with subretinal fluid, choroidal folds, and scattered yellow subretinal deposits. (A) Inferior bullous serous detachment of the inferior retina. (B) Multiple focal areas of subretinal fluid.

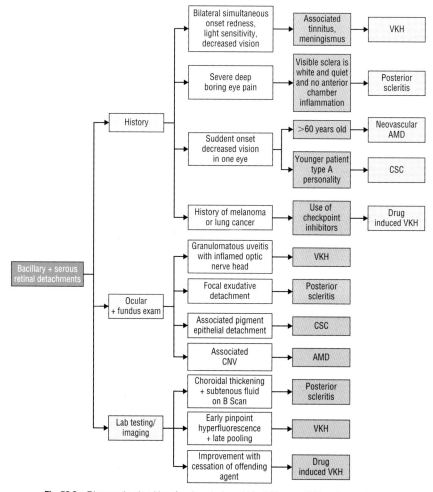

Fig. 59.2 Diagnostic algorithm for drug-induced Vogt-Koyanagi-Harada syndrome.

- What past or current treatment is the patient receiving for treatment of the melanoma? What medications does the patient take? There are multiple different chemotherapeutic regiments that are associated with retinal toxicity and ocular inflammation, such as mitogen-activated protein kinase (MEK) inhibitors, checkpoint inhibitors, alkylating agents, and anaplastic lymphoma kinase inhibitors.
  - She had been taking MEK inhibitors (dabrafenib and trametinib) for about 6 months before onset of symptoms.

Assessment

This is a case of a 34-year-old woman with history of cutaneous melanoma and taking MEK inhibitors with bilateral panuveitis, serous and bacillary retinal detachments, and decreased vision.

Differential Diagnosis

- VKH syndrome
- Medication-induced retinal toxicity
- Central serous chorioretinopathy
- Tuberculosis choroiditis
- Panuveitis related to dabrafenib and trametinib
- Syphilis

Working Diagnosis

Panuveitis related to dabrafenib and trametinib

Multimodal Testing and Results

- Optical coherence tomography (OCT) (Fig. 59.3)
  - Multiple bacillary detachments with hyper- and hyporeflective collections under the neurosensory retina in each macula, as well as loss of normal choroidal vascular architecture.
- Fundus autofluorescence
  - Multiple hyperautofluorescent round overlapping lesions involving the entire macula in each eye correlating with the areas of bacillary retinal detachment. Smaller round areas of increased hyperautofluoresence are noted within the larger lesions.

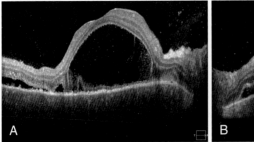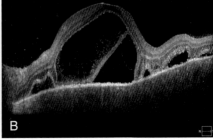

Fig. 59.3 Optical coherence tomography single-line images of the right (A) and left eyes (B) demonstrate multiple bacillary detachments with hyper- and hyporeflective collections under the neurosensory retina in each macula, as well as loss of normal choroidal vascular architecture.

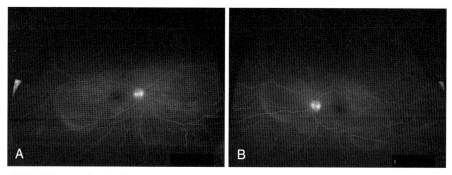

Fig. 59.4 Mid-phase fundus fluorescein angiogram images of the right (A) and left (B) eyes. Both eyes demonstrate optic disc leakage with staining of the areas of serous retinal detachment.

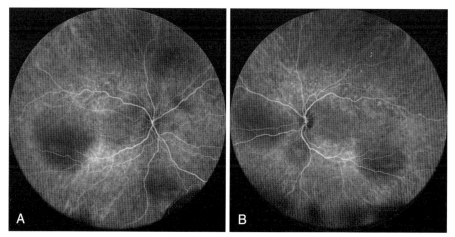

Fig. 59.5 Late indocyanine green angiography images showing hypocyanescent lesions corresponding to the areas of serous retinal detachment in the right (A) and left eyes (B).

- Fluorescein angiography (Fig. 59.4)
  - Optic disc leakage in each eye with staining of the documented areas of bacillary detachment as described earlier.
- Indocyanine green angiography (Fig. 59.5)
  - Hypocyanescence of the aforementioned described lesions.

Management

- The case was discussed with the patient's oncologist, including retinal findings and ocular inflammation. The patient had no evidence of metastatic melanoma, had clean margins on excision, and had only been placed on MEK inhibitors to decrease the chance of melanoma recurrence. Because of the severe ocular disease, her oncologist agreed to hold the MEK inhibitors.
- After confirming negative syphilis and tuberculosis serologies, the patient was started on oral prednisone 1 mg/kg/day in an effort to expedite the improvement of her inflammatory lesions.

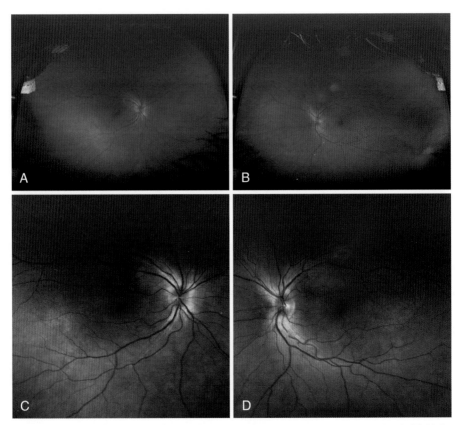

Fig. 59.6 Color wide-field images of the right (A) and left (B) eyes after resolution of the subretinal fluid. Persistent disc hyperemia and mottling of the retinal pigment epithelial cells is noted in a higher magnification image of both eyes (C and D).

Follow-up Care

- The patient was followed on a weekly basis until steady improvement of vision and SRF on OCT was noted.
- After cessation of MEK inhibitors, resolution of the SRF was noted in the right eye at 6 weeks and in the left eye at 3 weeks (Figs. 59.6 and 59.7).
- Oral prednisone was tapered over 3 months.

Key Points

- MEK inhibitors can cause a VKH-like syndrome.[1]
- Consider medication toxicity and drug-induced uveitis in patients with visual reports and a history of known insulting agents.[1-4]
- A VHK-like inflammatory syndrome is one of the many presentations of MEK inhibitor–related ocular toxicity.[1,3]
- Bacillary retinal detachments can be seen in VKH and VKH-like syndromes.[1,4]

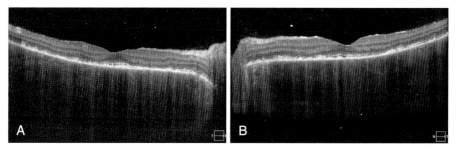

Fig. 59.7 Optical coherence tomography single-line images of the right (A) and left eyes (B) demonstrate resolution of the bacillary detachments.

References

1. Draganova D, Kerger J, Caspers L, Willermain F. Severe bilateral panuveitis during melanoma treatment by dabrafenib and trametinib. *J Ophthalmic Inflamm Infect.* 2015;5:17.
2. Sarny S, Neumayer M, Kofler J, El-Sabrawi Y. Ocular toxicity due to trametinib and dabrafenib. *BMC Ophthalmol.* 2017;17:146.
3. Francis JH, Habib L, Abramson DH, et al. Clinical and morphologic characteristics of MEK inhibitor–associated retinopathy: differences from central serous chorioretinopathy. *Ophthalmology.* 2017; 124(12):1788-1798.
4. Cicinelli MV, Giuffré C, Marchese A, et al. The bacillary detachment in posterior segment ocular diseases. *Ophthalmol Retina.* 2020;4(4):454-456.

CHAPTER 60

Bilateral Decreased Vision in a Middle-Aged Man With Optical Coherence Tomography Findings of Foveal Ellipsoid Disruption

Sudip D. Thakar ▪ Catherine J. Thomas ▪ Manjot K. Gill

History of Present Illness

We present a case of a 43-year-old HIV-positive man who was well controlled on highly active antiretroviral therapy (HAART) therapy and referred for an 8-month history of bilateral progressive blurry vision. He had no ocular or pertinent family history.

OCULAR EXAMINATION FINDINGS

Visual acuities with correction were 20/40 and 20/50 in the right and left eyes, respectively. Intraocular pressures were normal. The external and anterior segment examinations were unremarkable. Dilated fundus examination did not reveal any obvious pathology (Fig. 60.1).

IMAGING

Spectral-domain optical coherence tomography (OCT) of each eye showed a focal, foveal defect of the outer retina involving the ellipsoid zone (EZ) (Fig. 60.2). Autofluorescence (AF), near-infrared reflectance (NIR), and fluorescein angiography (FA) were unremarkable.

Questions to Ask

- Does the patient have a family history of retinal or macular dystrophies?
  - No
    - Pattern dystrophy, specifically adult-onset foveomacular dystrophy (AOFMD), can appear similar to poppers maculopathy. AOFMD can present with yellowish subfoveal lesions on examination. On OCT, there is subfoveal material at the level of retinal pigment epithelium (RPE) (Fig. 60.3). This is in contrast to poppers maculopathy, in which the defect occurs at the EZ.
- Does the patient have a history of retinal disease?
  - No
    - Macular telangiectasia type 2 can present with crystals on examination. OCT may reveal foveal inner and outer retinal loss leading to cavitation (Fig. 60.4). Fluorescein angiography shows foveal telangiectatic vessels that leak.

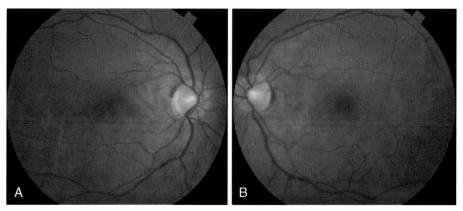

Fig. 60.1 Color fundus photographs of right (A) and left eyes (B) show normal appearing macula.

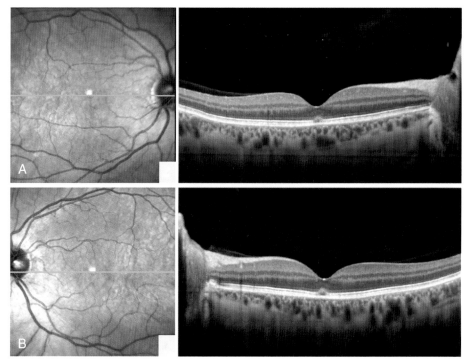

Fig. 60.2 Near-infrared reflectance and spectral-domain optical coherence tomography of right (A) and left eyes (B) show foveal outer retinal defect involving the ellipsoid zone.

- Does the patient have a history of sungazing, eclipse viewing, welding, or laser pointer use?
    - No
        - Photochemical injury from sungazing can cause focal, central disruption of EZ and retinal pigment epithelium (RPE) on OCT.
        - Photothermal injury from laser pointers similarly can cause disruption of retinal layers and may appear bilaterally symmetrical if both eyes are involved.

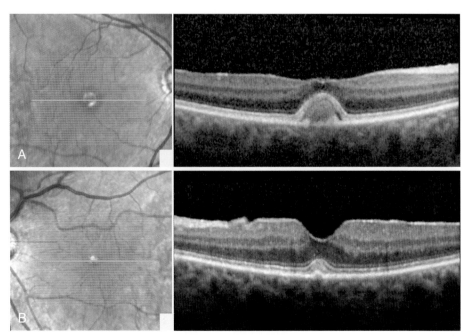

Fig. 60.3 Near-infrared reflectance and spectral-domain optical coherence tomography of right (A) and left eyes (B) show subfoveal vitelliform lesion.

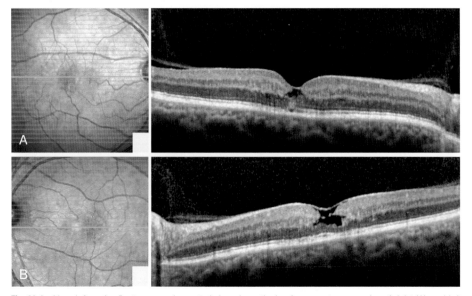

Fig. 60.4 Near-infrared reflectance and spectral-domain optical coherence tomography of right (A) and left eyes (B) show internal limiting membrane draping over cystoid spaces in macular telangiectasia Type 2. There is also inner retinal loss and outer retinal disruption in both eyes.

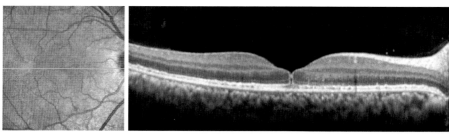

Fig. 60.5 Near-infrared reflectance and spectral-domain optical coherence tomography of right eye demonstrating irregularity and disruption of the ellipsoid zone in a patient with blunt trauma after a paintball injury. The foveal contour is also exaggerated with early full-thickness dehiscence.

- Does the patient have a history of trauma?
  - No
    - Trauma may give rise to structural changes on OCT at any level depending on the type of injury and the retinal layers involved.
    - Specifically, commotio retinae refers to retinal whitening in the posterior pole with disruption or loss of photoreceptor outer segments (Fig. 60.5).
- Does the patient have a history of drug abuse?
  - Yes. Regular use of "poppers" for the past 4 years.
    - Poppers belong to the group of alkyl nitrite compounds and are inhaled recreationally for their psychoactive effects.[1] They are commonly used by men having sex with men for euphoric and myorelaxant effects.[1]
    - The use of poppers has been linked to disruption of central photoreceptors and subsequent visual reports including decreased visual acuity, central scotoma, and distortion.[2]
- Does the patient take any other medications?
  - Yes. HAART, escitalopram, and aripiprazole.
    - Although not taken by this patient, tamoxifen can cause crystalline retinopathy with OCT findings of central EZ loss and cavitation.
- Is there any history of recent viral illness, use of epinephrine or caffeine, hypotension, or hematological disorders?
  - No
    - These are risk factors for development of acute macular neuroretinopathy (AMN). In females, oral contraceptive use is also a risk factor.
    - On NIR, wedge-shaped or petaloid lesions are often seen. The OCT findings characteristic of AMN include disruption of EZ and thinning of the outer nuclear layer (Fig. 60.6).

Assessment

- This is a case of a 43-year-old man whose HIV infection was controlled on HAART therapy and was without significant past ocular or family history. Social history was notable for poppers usage. Although his examination did not show obvious pathology, spectral-domain OCT demonstrated bilateral foveal defects of the EZ.

Differential Diagnosis

- Poppers maculopathy
- AOFMD

- Photic retinopathy (includes solar or eclipse retinopathy, exposure to other bright lights including light microscopes and welding arc flashes)
- Laser pointer retinal injury
- Macular telangiectasia type 2
- Tamoxifen toxicity
- Trauma
- AMN
- Macular degeneration

Working Diagnosis

- Poppers or alkyl nitrate maculopathy
  - History of poppers use with characteristic bilateral disruption of foveal EZ on OCT

Multimodal Testing and Results

- Fundus photographs
  - No obvious irregularities were detected in our patient (Fig. 60.1).
  - Fundus examination may demonstrate subtle irregularities or a yellowish lesion within the fovea.[2,3]
- AF
  - Normal in both eyes
- OCT
  - As described earlier, our patient's OCT demonstrated focal, foveal defects of the outer retina involving the EZ (Fig. 60.2).
  - Disruption of the foveal cone EZ is most characteristic of poppers maculopathy.[2,4]
- FA
  - Normal in both eyes

Management

- Recommended immediate discontinuation of poppers.
- The prognosis of poppers maculopathy is unclear given the lack of long-term follow-up in the literature. One study reported one out of three patients with visual acuity improvement at follow-up.[5]

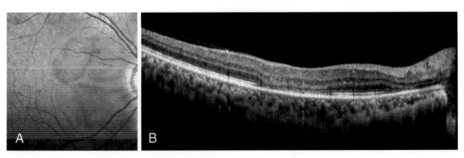

Fig. 60.6 (A) Near-infrared reflectance of the right eye showing perifoveal wedge shaped defects in acute macular neuroretinitis. (B) Optical coherence tomography of the right eye showing corresponding outer nuclear layer thinning and disruption of the ellipsoid zone.

Follow-up Care

- A 2-month follow-up was recommended in our patient. Unfortunately, he was noncompliant.
- If the patient demonstrates progression on OCT, closer monitoring, as well as alternative diagnoses, should be considered.

Algorithm 60.1: Algorithm Representing Optical Coherence Tomography *(OCT)* Finding of Foveal Outer-Retinal Disruption Including A Differential With Some Distinguishing Characteristics

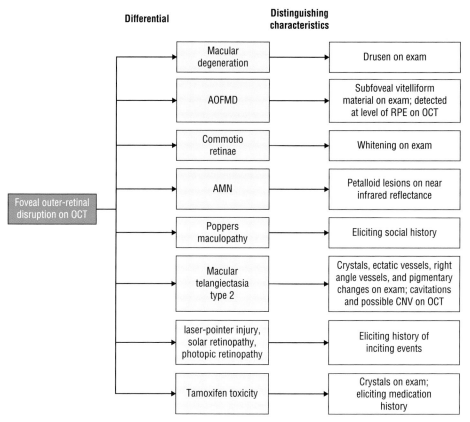

Algorithm 60.1 Algorithm representing optical coherence tomography *(OCT)* finding of foveal outer-retinal disruption including a differential with some distinguishing characteristics. *AMN,* Acute macular neuroretinopathy; *AOFMD,* adult-onset foveomacular dystrophy; *CNV,* choroidal neovascularization; *RPE,* retinal pigment epithelium.

Key Points

- The differential for foveal outer retinal disruption on OCT should include AOFMD, solar or eclipse retinopathy and other photic retinopathies (including welder's maculopathy, light microscope toxicity), laser pointer injury, poppers maculopathy, macular telangiectasia type 2, tamoxifen toxicity, trauma, AMN, or macular degeneration.
- History is critical in identifying the underlying cause. It is important to elicit a social history with attention to poppers when presented with a patient without ocular history with bilateral foveal changes on OCT.
- Immediate discontinuation of poppers is recommended.

References

1. Davies AJ, Borschmann R, Kelly SP, et al. The prevalence of visual symptoms in poppers users: a global survey. *BMJ Open Ophthalmol*. 2016;1:1-6.
2. Davies AJ, Kelly SP, Naylor SG, et al. Adverse ophthalmic reaction in poppers users: case series of "poppers maculopathy". *Eye (Lond)*. 2012;26(11):1479-1486.
3. Docherty G, Eslami M, O'Donnell H. "Poppers maculopathy": a case report and literature review. *Can J Ophthalmol*. 2018;53(4):e154-e156.
4. Mentes J, Batioglu F. Multimodal imaging of a patient with poppers maculopathy. *GMS Ophthalmol Cases*. 2020;10:Doc16.
5. Pahlitzsch M, Mai C, Joussen AM, Bergholz R. Poppers maculopathy: complete restitution of macular changes in OCT after drug abstinence. *Semin Ophthalmol*. 2016;31(5):479-484.

CHAPTER 61

Bilateral Central Scotoma With Macular Pigmentary Changes in a Young Man

Ivy Zhu ▦ Andrew W. Francis

History of Present Illness

A 13-year-old boy was referred by an outside ophthalmologist for bilateral reduced central vision for 3 months. The vision loss was painless, constant, and symmetrical. The patient denied any recent trauma. Medical history was significant for multiple psychiatric conditions including attention deficit hyperactivity disorder, depression, generalized anxiety disorder, and posttraumatic stress disorder.

OCULAR EXAM FINDINGS

On examination, best-corrected visual acuity was 20/50 in the right eye and 20/60 in the left eye. Intraocular pressures, pupils, confrontational visual fields, and extraocular motility were within normal limits. The anterior segment examination was unremarkable. Dilated fundus examination revealed yellow-gray mottled lesions of the fovea in both eyes (Fig. 61.1).

IMAGING

Optical coherence tomography (OCT) and fluorescein angiogram (FA) were obtained. OCT of both eyes showed outer retinal loss with hyperreflective bands extending from the retinal pigment epithelium (RPE), consistent with pigment migration (Fig. 61.2). FA showed hypofluorescence with surrounding hyperfluorescence of the central lesions, consistent with pigment staining (Fig. 61.3).

Questions to Ask

- Did the patient have any family history of known eye conditions?
  - The patient was adopted with his biological sister, who had no known medical or ocular problems. Other family history was unknown.
- Did the patient have any other systemic conditions?
  - Besides the known psychiatric history, the patient denied any other medical problems in the review of systems.
- Did the patient have access to a laser pointer?
  - The patient's parents reported that he did have access to a laser pointer purchased online and often self-isolated in his room playing with the laser.

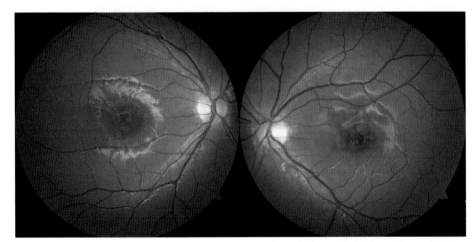

Fig. 61.1 Color fundus photograph of the right and left eyes demonstrating similar hyperpigmented foveal changes in an otherwise unremarkable posterior segment.

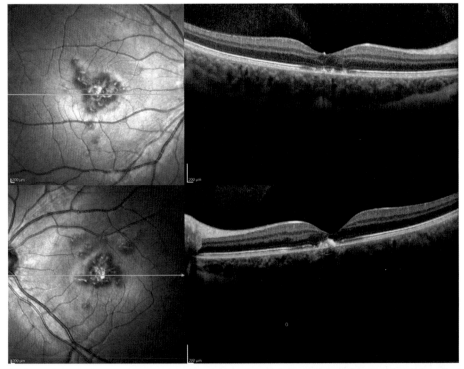

Fig. 61.2 Optical coherence tomography of the right *(top)* and left *(bottom)* eyes demonstrating outer retinal disruption with associated retinal pigment epithelium irregularities and hyperreflective bands.

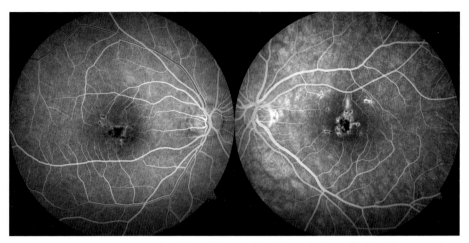

Fig. 61.3 Fluorescein angiogram of the right and left eyes. The right eye is pictured in the early venous phase demonstrating central blockage with peripheral staining. The left eye is pictured in the late venous phase and has similar findings to the right eye. Note the bright vertical linear streak superior to the fovea in the left eye.

- Had the patient ever stared into the laser pointer?
  - The patient adamantly denied self-harm, though his parents stated that it was highly possible.

Assessment

- A 13-year-old man without known family history of ocular problems reported subacute onset of bilateral, symmetrical, painless vision loss and was found to have central macular pigment mottling in the setting of prior exposure to a laser pointer.

Differential Diagnosis

- Hereditary macular dystrophy, including Stargardt disease
- Solar retinopathy
- Drug-induced toxicity
- Trauma
- Multifocal choroiditis
- Ocular histoplasmosis syndrome
- Placoid retinopathy
- Laser-induced maculopathy

Working Diagnosis

- The sudden onset, lack of family history, and exposure to a laser pointer in a young patient with an extensive psychiatric history strongly suggest laser pointer–induced maculopathy.

Multimodal Testing and Results

- Color fundus photographs reveal foveal pigmentary changes. The fovea is often affected in these patients due to fixation on the laser light source.

- FA demonstrates blockage and staining associated with the foveal pigment mottling. Fluorescein can be helpful in clearly delineating the outline of the pigment clumps. A key diagnostic clue in this and other cases of laser-induced maculopathy is often the presence of vertical linear lesions, which are thought to occur because of a reflexive Bell phenomenon. In the left eye (Fig. 61.3), there is a vertical linear lesion superior to the fovea that is better visualized compared with the fundus photograph.
- OCT through these lesions shows RPE irregularities with intraretinal migration. This can be a useful imaging modality to monitor the patient and observe for any evidence of subsequent choroidal neovascularization.
- Electroretinogram (ERG) can be performed in cases of diagnostic uncertainty when a macular dystrophy is also suspected. In these situations, the full field ERG is normal because the pathology is limited to a small area of the macula only.

Management

- There currently exists no standard of care in treating retinal damage associated with laser-induced maculopathy.
- The severity of damage varies with duration of exposure, device output power, and laser wavelength. Blue laser light is thought to be the most damaging wavelength because of its ready absorption by foveal xanthophyll pigment and melanin.
- In most cases, providers have observed these lesions with spontaneous mild visual recovery noted by some.
- There are a few case reports of improvement with systemic administration of corticosteroids (e.g., 1 mg/kg of oral prednisone), but it is unclear whether these patients would have spontaneously improved without intervention.
- Sequelae such as full-thickness macular hole, epiretinal membrane, and premacular hemorrhage can develop and are usually managed with the standard of care for these conditions (e.g., surgical intervention such as pars plana vitrectomy).
- It is critical to ensure the laser pointer is removed from the patient's possession and appropriate psychiatric care is established to prevent further self-harm in cases of intentional injury.

Follow-up Care

- After initial injury, patients should be followed closely (e.g., monthly) to monitor for worsening and/or continued insults.
- Once stability has been established, follow-up can be slowly extended.

Algorithm 61.1: Algorithm Representing the Differential Diagnosis of Central Macular Pigmentary Changes

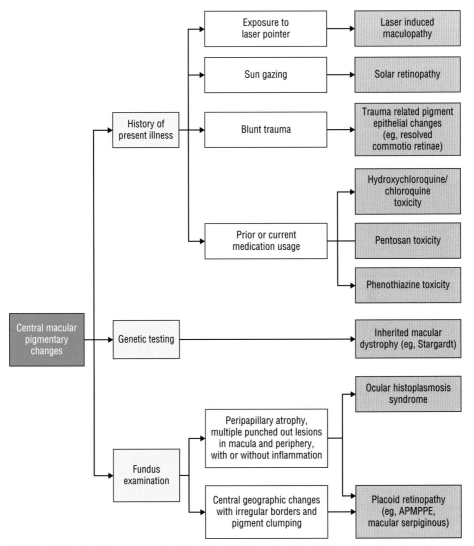

Algorithm 61.1 Algorithm representing the differential diagnosis of central macular pigmentary changes. *APMPPE,* Acute posterior multifocal placoid pigment epitheliopathy.

Key Points

- Provider suspicion of laser maculopathy should be high in situations of sudden central vision loss in a young person associated with macular pigment mottling and no family history of vision loss.
- Patients and their guardians should be questioned explicitly about use of or exposure to lasers.
- This condition classically presents in young men with a history of psychiatric problems, though accidental injury may also occur. In cases of intentional self-harm, patients may initially deny laser exposure.

- Fundus examination typically reveals pigmentary yellow or gray mottling. Vertical linear streaks have been described, resulting from a Bell reflex, and can be particularly helpful in making this diagnosis.
- Additional multimodal imaging can also be useful, including FA, which well demarcates the pigment mottling, and OCT, which reveals vertical hyperreflective bands.
- No standard of care in management currently exists, though some cases have been reported of improvement after systemic corticosteroid administration. However, the role of steroids is unclear, as spontaneous improvement has also been reported.
- Appropriate referral of these patients for psychiatric care and counseling is critical to address any underlying behavioral concerns and prevent further self-harm.

References

Luttrull JK, Hallisey J. Laser pointer-induced macular injury. *Am J Ophthalmol.* 1999;127(1):95-96.

Torp-Pedersen T, Welinder L, Justesen B, et al. Laser pointer maculopathy—on the rise? *Acta Ophthalmol.* 2018;96(7):749-754.

Alsulaiman SM, Alrushood AA, Almasaud J, et al. High-power handheld blue laser-induced maculopathy: the results of the King Khaled Eye Specialist Hospital Collaborative Retina Study Group. *Ophthalmology.* 2014;121(2):566-572.

Chen X, Dajani OAW, Alibhai AY, et al. Long-term visual recovery in bilateral handheld laser pointer-induced maculopathy. *Retin Cases Brief Rep.* 2021;15(5):536-539.

Bhavsar KV, Wilson D, Margolis R, et al. Multimodal imaging in handheld laser-induced maculopathy. *Am J Ophthalmol.* 2015;159(2):227-231.

Raoof N, O'Hagan J, Pawlowska N, et al. "Toy" laser macular burns in children: 12-month update. *Eye (Lond).* 2016;30(3):492-496.

Neoplastic/Infiltrative

CHAPTER 62

Unilateral Exudative Retinal Detachment in an Elderly Woman

Angela S. Li ■ Irmak Karaca ■ Diana V. Do

History of Present Illness

A 74-year-old woman presented with a progressive decline in vision in both eyes over the past 2 weeks. She denies presence of or any changes in floaters, flashes of lights, curtain defect, eye pain, or any recent illnesses. She did not have any history of ocular diseases or surgeries.

OCULAR EXAMINATION FINDINGS

Visual acuities were 20/50 in the right eye and 20/30 in the left eye. Intraocular pressures were 13 mm Hg and 14 mm Hg in right and left eyes, respectively. Slit lamp examination showed moderate cataracts (2+ nuclear sclerosis, 3+ cortical) in both eyes. Fundus examination (limited by cataracts) revealed cotton wool spots (CWS) nasal to the optic disc and on the vascular arcades bilaterally. In the right eye, elevation of the macula, flame-shaped hemorrhages, and CWS were also documented (Fig. 62.1A, B).

IMAGING

At presentation, wide-angle fundus photography showed CWS nasal to the optic disc and around the superior and inferior vascular arcades in both eyes. There were flame-shaped hemorrhages, as well as a preretinal hemorrhage in the superonasal periphery of the right eye. Optical coherence tomography (OCT) of the right eye showed serous retinal detachment (RD) in the macula, and the left eye demonstrated focal thickening of retinal nerve fiber layer temporal to the optic disc corresponding to a large CWS with no evidence of subretinal fluid (Fig. 62.1C, D). Fluorescein angiography (FA) showed hypo- and hyperfluorescent retinal pigment epithelium (RPE) changes (suggestive of leopard spot retinopathy) at the posterior pole, which is more prominent in the superior macula, along with diffuse, mild peripheral leakage from the capillaries in the right eye. However, there was no vascular leakage in the macula to explain subretinal fluid (Fig. 62.2). A similar pattern of leakage was seen in the left eye. B-scan of the right eye was unremarkable except for a slightly thickened choroid.

Questions to Ask

■ Does the patient have any history of diabetes mellitus or hypertension? CWS and flame-shaped hemorrhages can be seen in diabetic retinopathy or hypertensive retinopathy.

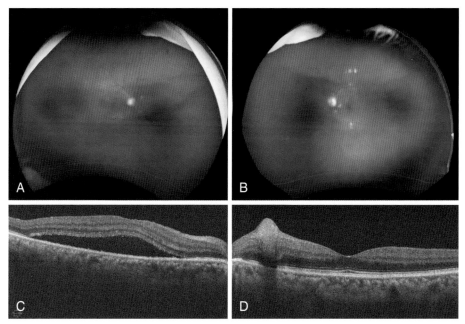

Fig. 62.1 Wide-angle fundus photography and spectral-domain optical coherence tomography (OCT) at the initial presentation. (A and B) Wide-angle fundus photographs of both eyes show bilateral diffuse cotton wool spots (CWS) in the posterior pole. Flame-shaped hemorrhages in the superior macula and inferonasal periphery of the optic disc are present in the right eye. (C) OCT of the right eye shows a serous retinal detachment in the macula. (D) OCT of the left eye demonstrates focal thickening of the retinal nerve fiber layer temporal to the optic nerve; this corresponds to a large CWS with no evidence of subretinal fluid.

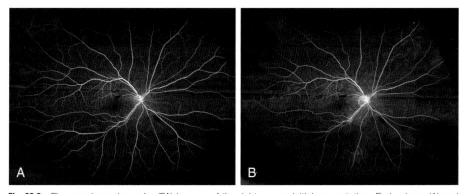

Fig. 62.2 Fluorescein angiography (FA) images of the right eye on initial presentation. Early-phase (A) and late-phase (B) FA of the right eye shows hypo- and hyperfluorescent retinal pigment epithelium changes (suggestive of leopard spot retinopathy) at the posterior pole, more prominently in the superior macula, along with diffuse mild peripheral leakage from the capillaries. There is notably no vascular leakage in the macula.

- The patient had a history of hypertension that was well controlled with amlodipine, and most recent blood pressures were around 130/80 mm Hg.
  - She also had prediabetes with a most recent hemoglobin A1C of 6.0%.
- Does the patient have any travel history or potential exposures to infectious agents? Is there any history of autoimmune diseases? Both infectious and inflammatory causes can be associated with serous RD.
  - The patient denied any recent travel or exposure to pets or animals.
  - She did have a self-reported history of rheumatoid arthritis for which she was not on any medication and was asymptomatic.
- What medications does the patient currently take? For instance, steroids are known to be a risk factor for central serous chorioretinopathy.
  - The patient only takes amlodipine for hypertension and did not have any history of steroid use or other medications.
  - The patient did state she was experiencing recent stressors as the sole breadwinner for her family.

Assessment

- This is the case of a 74-year-old woman with well-controlled hypertension, prediabetes, and no ocular history who presented with unilateral serous RD in the right eye.

Differential Diagnosis

- Vascular
  - Exudative age-related macular degeneration
  - Polypoidal choroidal vasculopathy
  - Hypertensive retinopathy
  - Diabetic retinopathy
- Inflammatory or infectious
  - Vogt-Koyanagi-Harada disease
  - Posterior scleritis
  - Inflammatory diseases of the choroid (white dot syndromes)
  - Ocular histoplasmosis
  - Lupus choroidopathy
- Neoplastic
  - Choroidal melanoma
  - Choroidal metastases from leukemia or lymphoma
- Other causes
  - Central serous chorioretinopathy
  - Optic disc pit

Working Diagnosis

Because of high suspicion for systemic causes of the patient's serous RD, blood work was done immediately, which included a complete blood cell count (CBC), comprehensive metabolic panel (CMP), inflammatory markers (erythrocyte sedimentation rate [ESR], C-reactive protein [CRP], rheumatoid factor, antinuclear antibodies (ANA), antineutrophil cytoplasmic antibodies, angiotensin-converting enzyme, and lysozyme), and infectious studies (QuantiFERON, treponemal studies, and Lyme assay). CBC showed 200 white blood cells/μL with large number of blasts. The patient was diagnosed with B-cell acute lymphoblastic leukemia (ALL) with central nervous system (CNS) involvement. Thus her serous RD was attributed to the initial presentation of acute leukemia, and CWS and retinal hemorrhages were the manifestations of leukemic retinopathy.

Multimodal Testing and Results

- Fundus photographs
  - Retinopathy in leukemia can be a result of direct neoplastic infiltration or secondary causes such as anemia, thrombocytopenia, or hyperviscosity. Hemorrhages can occur at all levels of the retina and are usually located in the posterior pole. White-centered hemorrhages (known as Roth spots) are particularly suggestive of a systemic disorder.[1] Other findings seen on fundus photography may include venous dilation and tortuosity, microaneurysms, or CWS.[2]
- OCT
  - OCT of the right eye showed serous RD in the macula. OCT can easily detect serous RD even if the subretinal fluid may not be apparent on a fundus examination or color fundus photography. OCT may also show thickening of the nerve fiber layer indicative of nerve fiber layer infarction and swelling.[3]
- FA
  - FA is useful to determine whether the serous RD is related to vascular leakage, which is the case in neovascular/exudative age-related macular degeneration, diabetic retinopathy, retinal vasculitis, and other retinal vascular pathologies. Signs of retinal vasculitis on FA should warrant an infectious workup but do not exclude the possibility of malignancy, particularly if an opportunistic infection is identified as a cause.[4] In the present case, FA did not show any vascular leakage in the macula that could have explained the subretinal fluid, thus raising the suspicion for systemic causes.
- Laboratory testing
  - Laboratory testing can be helpful in cases with serous RD to assess for systemic diseases. CBC and CMP are useful initial blood tests, and additional studies for infectious (tuberculosis, syphilis, and Lyme disease) and inflammatory (ESR/CRP) markers along with autoantibodies like rheumatoid factor and ANA might aid in the diagnosis.[5]
- Cranioorbital imaging
  - Once the patient was diagnosed with leukemia, orbital magnetic resonance imaging showed an enhancement of the right optic nerve likely due to leukemic infiltration.

Management and Follow-up Care

- After laboratory test results, the patient was immediately notified and asked to go to the emergency department for direct hospital admission. She was hospitalized for a month, during which she was diagnosed as having B-cell ALL with CNS involvement. She was initiated on chemotherapy by the oncology team and initially followed by a retina specialist every 1 to 2 months. Her serous RD and retinal hemorrhages completely resolved 6 months after the initiation of chemotherapy (Fig. 62.3).
- The management of serous RD linked to systemic diseases generally includes the treatment of underlying disease.

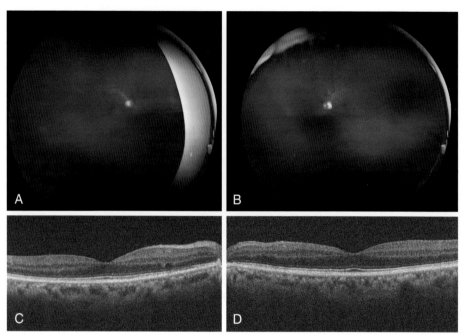

Fig. 62.3 Wide-angle fundus photography and OCT obtained 6 months after the initial presentation. (A and B) Wide-angle fundus photographs of both eyes show resolution of bilateral cotton wool spots (CWS) and flame-shaped hemorrhages. (C and D) OCT demonstrates the resolution of serous retinal detachment (right eye) and CWS (left eye) after treatment of the underlying malignancy.

Algorithm 62.1: Algorithm Showing Differential Diagnosis for Unilateral Serous Retinal Detachment

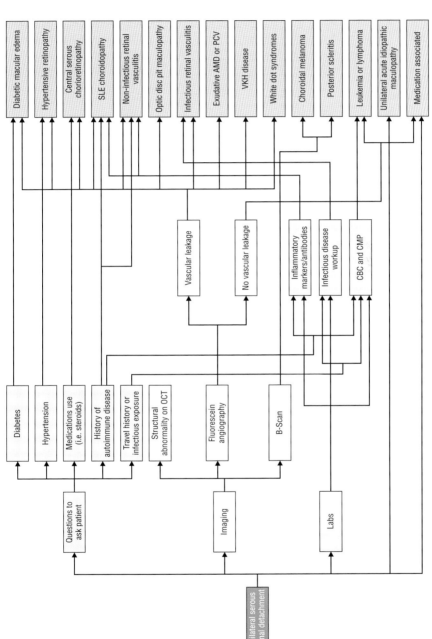

Algorithm 62.1   Algorithm showing differential diagnosis for unilateral serous retinal detachment. *AMD*, Age-related macular degeneration; *CBC*, complete blood cell count; *CMP*, comprehensive metabolic panel; *OCT*, optical coherence tomography; *PCV*, polypoidal choroidal vasculopathy; *SLE*, systemic lupus erythematosus; *VKH*, Vogt-Koyanagi-Harada disease.

Key Points

- Serous macular detachment could develop as a result of systemic diseases. In select cases, it may be the initial finding of undiagnosed leukemia.[1,6] Therefore considering a broad differential diagnosis is important, particularly in a patient with no ocular history. Proper laboratory evaluation is needed to elucidate the diagnosis.
- Serous macular detachments typically resolve as the underlying condition is treated.

References

1. Jackson N, Reddy SC, Hishamuddin M, Low HC. Retinal findings in adult leukaemia: correlation with leukocytosis. *Clin Lab Haematol.* 1996;18(2):105-109.
2. Schachat AP, Markowitz JA, Guyer DR, Burke PJ, Karp JE, Graham ML. Ophthalmic manifestations of leukemia. *Arch Ophthalmol.* 1989;107(5):697-700.
3. Sharma T, Grewal J, Gupta S, Murray PI. Ophthalmic manifestations of acute leukaemias: the ophthalmologist's role. *Eye (Lond).* 2004;18(7):663-672.
4. Talcott KE, Garg RJ, Garg SJ. Ophthalmic manifestations of leukemia. *Curr Opin Ophthalmol.* 2016;27(6):545-551.
5. Hassanpoor N, Niyousha MR. Acute lymphoblastic leukemia presenting as acute Vogt-Koyanagi-Harada syndrome. *Case Rep Ophthalmol.* 2020;11(2):481-485.
6. Rosenthal AR. Ocular manifestations of leukemia: a review. *Ophthalmology.* 1983;90(8):899-905.

CHAPTER 63

Perifoveal Calcified Lesion in Young Girl Patient

Sayena Jabbehdari ▦ William F. Mieler

History of Present Illness

An otherwise healthy 5-year-old female patient was referred to our retina division for a lesion that was noted temporal to the macula in the right eye. According to the patient's mother, the patient had been visually asymptomatic. There was no medical history of trauma, cancer, infectious, inflammatory, or autoimmune conditions. Her past surgical history and family history were unremarkable. She had no known drug allergies and was not taking any medications. Reviews of systems were also unremarkable.

Questions to Ask

- What is the ocular examination's result?
- What is the result of spectral-domain optical coherence tomography (SD-OCT) and B-scan?

Assessment

On ocular examination, the best-corrected visual acuity was 20/30 in both eyes without any elements of amblyopia. Extraocular movements were intact, and the pupils were round and reactive, without any relative afferent pupillary defect. Anterior and posterior segment examination was unremarkable. Vitreous cavity was quiet. Fundus examination revealed a yellowish-orange oval choroidal lesion temporal to the macula in the right eye, approximately 3.5 mm in maximum diameter, with well-delineated margins (Fig. 63.1). No feeder vessels were observed, and no cells were seen in the vitreous cavity.

Differential Diagnosis

The differential diagnosis for lesions in the choroid containing calcium includes choroidal osteoma, retinoblastoma, choroidal calcified granuloma, astrocytic hamartoma (astrocytoma), idiopathic sclerochoroidal calcification, and retinal intraocular foreign body.

- Flowcharting (see Fig. 63.2)

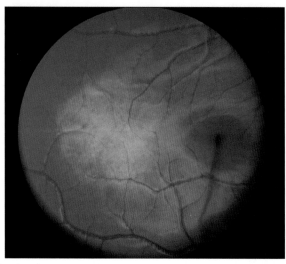

Fig. 63.1   Color fundus photograph: a yellowish-orange oval choroidal lesion temporal to the fovea of the right eye.

Algorithm 63.1: Algorithm for Calcified Choroidal Lesion in a Young Girl.ar Histoplasmosis Syndrome

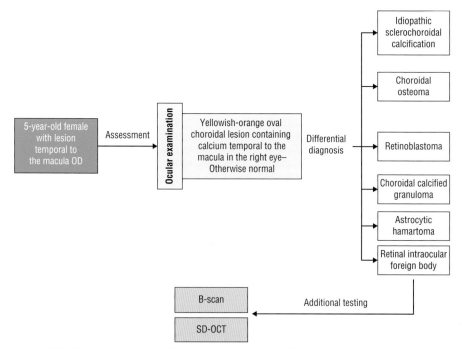

Algorithm 63.1   Algorithm for Calcified Choroidal Lesion in a Young Girl.ar histoplasmosis syndrome.

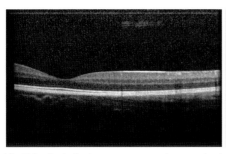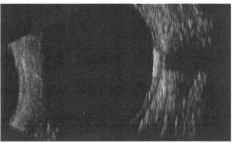

Fig. 63.2 Optical coherence tomography: no subretinal fluid or choroidal neovascularization. Echography: flat lesion containing calcification with high-intensity echoes from the inner surface of the lesion and posterior shadowing.

- Multimodal testing and results: less and more severe variations and working diagnosis
  - Ultrasound B-scan assessment showed a flat choroidal lesion containing calcification suggested by high-intensity echoes with posterior shadowing. OCT imaging did not reveal any evidence of subretinal fluid or choroidal neovascularization (CNV) (Fig. 63.2). The fellow eye was normal. An examination under anesthesia showed no additional abnormalities. Given the clinical findings, the patient was diagnosed with a choroidal osteoma, and observation was recommended.
  - Choroidal osteoma is a benign, rare, and classically unilateral tumor that can cause vision-threatening complications after tumor growth, decalcification, and through development of CNV.[1,2] Eyes with extrafoveal choroidal osteoma often maintain good visual acuity, but those osteomas affecting the macula can produce significant visual loss. This may be caused by retinal pigment epithelial and photoreceptor atrophy, the presence of serous subretinal fluid, and/or development of CNV associated with the lesion.[1,2]
  - Although photodynamic therapy (PDT) has been reported to be effective in achieving regression of the mass in some cases,[3] decalcification may be complicated by secondary CNV, necessitating close monitoring in these patients.

Management

The osteoma in our patient remained stable for the next 11 months, during which time the child had been assessed every 3 to 4 months. At 11 months, the lesion showed evidence of enlargement in the basal dimensions, with progression toward the center of the fovea. Visual acuity was stable at 20/30 in both eyes, yet there was concern regarding the growth of the lesion. At that point, treatment of the tumor with PDT was recommended in an attempt to induce decalcification and reduce the chances of further progression through the fovea. The treatment was carried out under general anesthesia, which was administrated via endotracheal intubation. The patient was briefly placed in a sitting position and her face was turned toward the laser. An 83-second laser spot at 689 nm (50 J/cm^2), coupled with intravenous verteporfin (6 mg/m^2) was performed. The treatment was well tolerated. Two-week follow-up did not show any changes in fundus findings, and visual acuity remained stable at 20/30 in both eyes.

However, 2 months later the patient demonstrated reduced visual acuity of 20/200 in the right eye with no subjective visual reports. Fundus examination revealed a new intraretinal hemorrhage along the nasal border of the lesion involving the macular region. Although the size of the osteoma itself was stable, a new ring of pigmentary change at the nasal aspect of the lesion was noted (Fig. 63.3). The presence of CNV was confirmed with fluorescein angiography (FA) obtained under anesthesia.

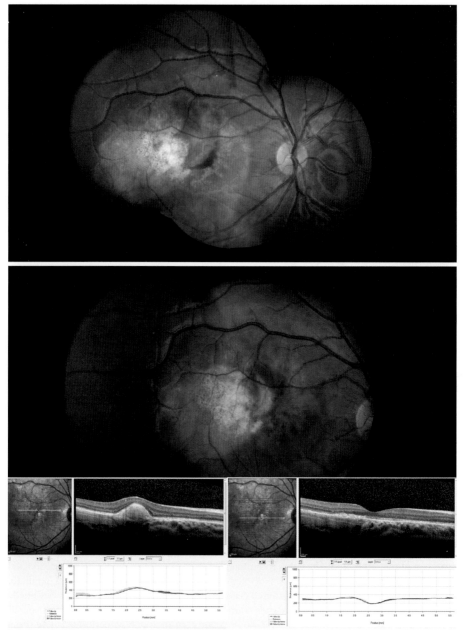

Fig. 63.3 Hemorrhage and ring of pigmentary changes in choroidal neovascularization along the nasal border of the lesion, enveloping the macular region. Color fundus photograph: choroidal neovascularization after being treated with four intravitreal injections of bevacizumab. Optical coherence tomography: no residual subretinal/intraretinal fluid. Pigment epithelial detachment superior to the fovea.

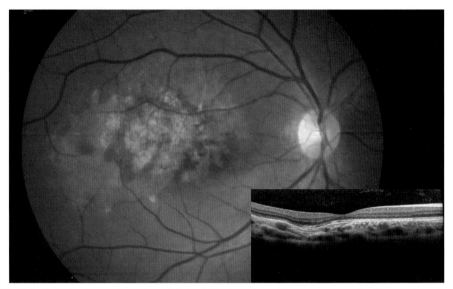

Fig. 63.4 Color fundus photograph: partial decalcification of choroidal osteoma invading the macula region. Optical coherence tomography: restoration of a normal foveal contour with mild focal choroidal excavation temporal to the foveola. No subretinal fluid or any other signs of active neovascularization.

Intravitreal anti–vascular endothelial growth factor (anti-VEGF) treatment was recommended, and bevacizumab (0.05 mL of 1.25 mg) was administered at the time of the FA. After the initial treatment, three additional bevacizumab injections were administered spaced 6 weeks apart over the next 4 months, resulting in regression of the CNV with improvement in visual function back to 20/20 in the right eye at 6 months posttreatment (Fig. 63.4).

CNV secondary to choroidal osteoma can be successfully treated with anti-VEGF injections.[4,5]

There have been reported cases of laser-induced and PDT-induced CNV in choroidal hemangioma,[6,7] but there is no report on PDT-induced CNV in a choroidal osteoma. However, it has been reported that reperfusion after PDT occurs typically 6 to 12 weeks after a single treatment.[8] Decalcification produced by the PDT may lead to disruption of the RPE and thinning or loss of the Bruch membrane and choriocapillaris, which can contribute to the development of CNV.[1,5]

CNV can be seen generally in osteoma patients. The absence of CNV before PDT and over prolonged follow-up visits in our patient make the diagnosis of CNV due to reperfusion more probable. Despite the initial development of CNV, the patient has done remarkably during the 7 years of follow-up posttreatment.

Follow-up

The patient was seen every 4 to 6 months, and at final follow-up after 9 years, there was no evidence of new CNV growth or change in the lesion size. Eventually, the osteoma decalcified along the temporal border of the fovea, with resultant mild macular pigment mottling and atrophy without fluid or hemorrhage. Follow-up OCT imaging (and echography) confirmed restoration of a normal foveal contour with mild temporal focal choroidal excavation, without evidence of significant calcification and or active CNV. Best corrected visual acuity stabilized at 20/40 in the right eye.

Algorithm 63.2: Algorithm Showing Management of Choroidal Osteoma

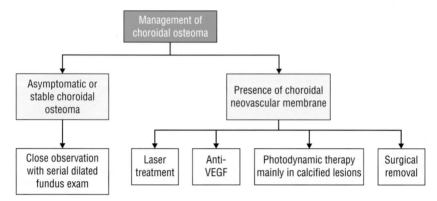

Algorithm 63.2   Algorithm showing management of choroidal osteoma. *Anti-VEGF,* Anti–vascular endothelial growth factor.

Key Points

- PDT has been reported as a successful approach in inducing choroidal osteoma decalcification and stabilization.
- Although it may be an effective treatment to prevent tumor growth toward the foveola in extrafoveal osteomas, decalcification may be complicated by secondary CNV, necessitating close monitoring in these patients.

References

1. Shields CL, Sun H, Demirci H, Shields JA. Factors predictive of tumor growth, tumor decalcification, choroidal neovascularization, and visual outcomes in 74 eyes with choroidal osteoma. *Arch Ophthalmol.* 2005;123:1658-1666.
2. Mizota A, Tanabe R, Adachi-Usami E. Rapid enlargement of choroidal osteoma in a 3-year old girl. *Arch Ophthalmol.* 1998;116:1128-1129.
3. Shields CL, Materin MA, Mehta S, et al. Regression of extrafoveal choroidal osteoma following photodynamic therapy. *Arch Ophthalmol.* 2008;126:135-137.
4. Song WK, Koh HJ, Kwon DW, et al. Intravitreal bevacizumab for choroidal neovascularization secondary to choroidal osteoma. *Acta Ophthalmol.* 2009;87:100-101.
5. Shields CL, Perez B, Materin MA, et al. Optical coherence tomography of choroidal osteoma in 22 cases: evidence for photoreceptor atrophy over the decalcified portion of the tumor. *Ophthalmology.* 2007;114:53-58.
6. Laovirojjanakul W, Sanguansak T, Yospaiboon Y, et al. Laser-induced choroidal neovascularizations: clinical study of 3 cases. *Case Rep Ophthalmol.* 2017;8:429-435.
7. Nagesha CK, Walinjkar JA, Khetan V. Choroidal neovascular membrane in a treated choroidal hemangioma. *Indian J Ophthalmol.* 2016;64:606-608.
8. Miller JW, Schmidt-Erfurth U, Sickenberg M, et al. Photodynamic therapy with verteporfin for choroidal neovascularization caused by age-related macular degeneration: results of a single treatment in a phase 1 and 2 study. *Arch Ophthalmol.* 1999;117(9):1161-1173.

CHAPTER 64

Bilateral Vitreous Floaters

Jose(ph) Serafin Pulido ▪ Carol Shields

History of Present Illness

A 62-year-old man noted floaters in both eyes for a few months. He described some headaches as well. He had been in good health otherwise and previously underwent cataract surgery with intraocular lens implantation 4 years ago in both eyes.

OCULAR EXAMINATION FINDINGS

Visual acuity with correction was 20/20 in both eyes. Intraocular pressure was normal. External and anterior segment examination showed posterior chamber lens implant with cells in the anterior vitreous (Fig. 64.1A, B). Dilated fundus examination revealed cells in the vitreous of both eyes.

IMAGING

Optical coherence tomography (OCT) showed cells on the surface of the retina in both eyes and no cystoid macula edema (CME) (Fig. 64.2).

Questions to Ask

- Is the patient immunocompromised?
  - No, but if he were younger, then the odds of being immunocompromised would be higher.
- Has the patient had chronic lymphocytic leukemia (CLL)?
  - No. CLL carries a chance of Richter transformation, which is associated with diffuse large B-cell lymphoma (DLBCL).

Assessment

- This is a case of a 62-year-old man with headaches and cells in the vitreous of both eyes and no cystoid macular edema.

Differential Diagnosis

- Bilateral endogenous endophthalmitis
- Tuberculosis
- Syphilis
- Birdshot chorioretinitis
- Vitreoretinal lymphoma (VRL)

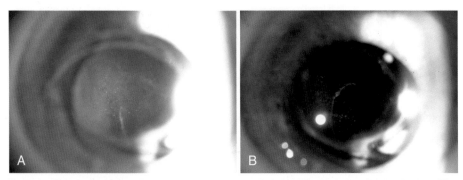

Fig. 64.1 (A) Note the large cells in the anterior vitreous right behind the posterior chamber implant. (B) A posterior capsulotomy, behind which are still vitreous strands with cells attached to the fibrous strands.

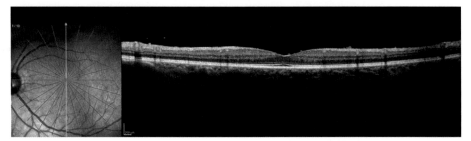

Fig. 64.2 Optical coherence tomography showing cells on the surface of the retina and extending into the vitreous.

- Intermediate uveitis
- Whipple disease

Working Diagnosis

- VRL. The presence of vitreous cells in the absence of macular edema should increase the probability of VRL. Most commonly, VRL is bilateral, and the chance of central nervous system (CNS) involvement is greater with bilateral cases. Careful determination is needed to be sure that unilateral disease is truly present.[1]

Multimodal Testing and Results

- Ultrasonography
  - Ultrasonography shows cells in the vitreous, and there can be cells in the Berger space by ultrasound biomicroscopy (Fig. 64.3).
- Fundus photographs
  - On fundus examination, with VRL, there can be cells in the vitreous and/or cells under the retinal pigment epithelium (RPE), or under the retina (Fig. 64.4, Fig. 64.5).
- OCT
  - Besides cells in the vitreous, there can be subretinal infiltrates and/or sub-RPE cells (Fig. 64.6). If there is no CME and there are vitreous cells, that can be a sign of VRL, but CME can rarely be present with VRL.[2]

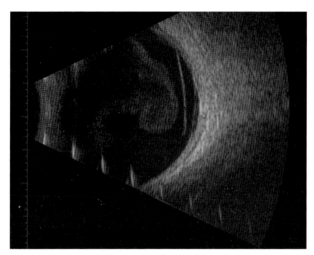

Fig. 64.3 Ultrasonography showing a posterior vitreous detachment, in which cells are present.

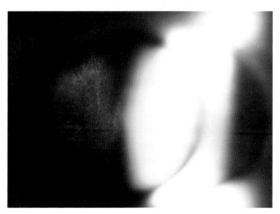

Fig. 64.4 A case of vitreoretinal lymphoma in a phakic eye with extensive cells in the anterior vitreous.

- Magnetic resonance imaging (MRI) of the brain
  - MRI is required in every case of suspected VRL, and if negative, it should still be done every 3 to 4 months until the diagnosis has been ruled out (Fig. 64.7).
- Positron emission tomography (PET) scan of the body
  - PET should be done the first time that VRL has been diagnosed to make sure that it is not secondary to DLBCL from elsewhere. Most cases of VRL are DLBCL either associated with CNS lymphoma or that might then develop CNS lymphoma. Some are secondary to DLBCL in other locations in the body, including the testes. Rarely, VRL can be secondary to T-cell lymphoma. Those are commonly associated with CME.
- Laboratory testing
  - The most important variant for DLBCL is those with positive MYD88 variants, especially the MYD88 L265P variant found in 80% of cases of VRL DLBCL, so polymerase chain reaction techniques to evaluate for this variant is 80% sensitive and very specific.[3-5] Histopathology is still helpful, especially when immunostaining is done, because DLBCL is CD20 positive. The use of flow cytology is probably not

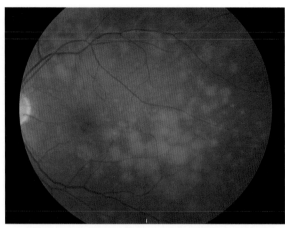

Fig. 64.5 Fundus photograph shows that there are multiple subretinal aggregates of vitreoretinal lymphoma cells.

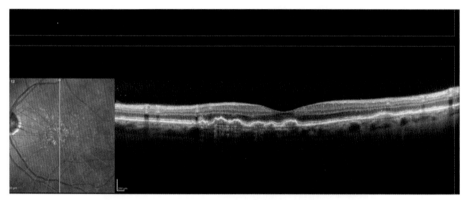

Fig. 64.6 Optical coherence tomography shows subretinal pigment epithelial conglomerates.

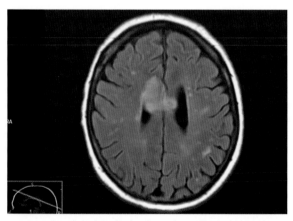

Fig. 64.7 Magnetic resonance imaging of the brain of a patient with vitreoretinal lymphoma at the time the patient was first seen. A central nervous system biopsy should be done.

very helpful because the cells are lost, and usually many are required. If there are enough pathology cells in the brain, it is better to do pathology there. If there are only cells in the eye, then preoperative discussions should be held with an ocular pathologist as to what is the best method to make the diagnosis. Again, flow cytology is usually not worthwhile. Likewise, doing a chorioretinal biopsy is typically not worthwhile because the VRL cells are separated by the Bruch membrane from the choroid and there are inflammatory T cells in the choroid that can obfuscate the diagnosis. Doing a retinal, vitreous, or sub-RPE biopsy is reasonable if it is preoperatively determined that there are not enough cells in the vitreous and there are sufficient cells in the subretinal space.[6]

Management

- The brain MRI revealed a CNS mass. Biopsy of the brain mass showed the presence of DLBCL (Fig. 64.6).
- The patient was treated systemically and also received multiple intravitreal methotrexate and intravitreal rituximab injections and was followed carefully for many months.

Follow-up Care

- Patients need to be followed carefully for both intraocular and CNS recurrences.[7,8] If MYD88 is mutated, then treatments that are targeted to this mutation and pathway become important treatment options.

Algorithm

For related algorithms, see Algorithms 64.1 and 64.2.

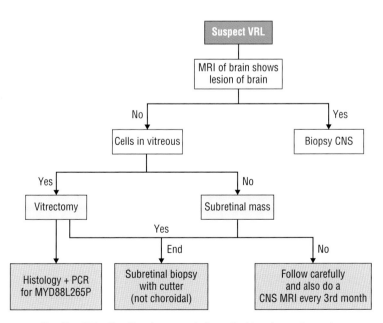

Algorithm 64.1   Algorithm for suspect vitreoretinal lymphoma diagnosis.

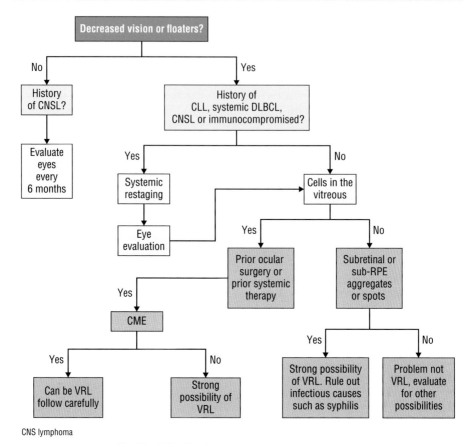

Algorithm 64.2   Algorithm for decreased vision or floaters.

Key Points

■ VRL is a great masquerader and has to be considered in cases of patients that have atypical findings of vitritis and/or subretinal lesions and infectious causes including syphilis. Other noninfectious uveitis conditions should also be considered.

■ If CME is not present and there are vitreous cells, then this should be a *red flag* that the patient could have VRL (Fig. 64.8).

■ Biopsy is required to make the diagnosis. If there is no evidence of CNS disease, then careful determination as to what and how to biopsy is needed.

■ MYD88 is an important protein that is mutated in many cases of VRL and is also a good marker for disease.

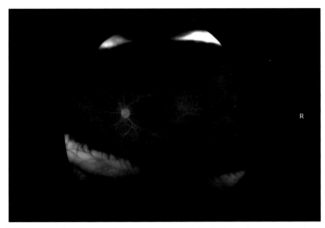

Fig. 64.8 Wide-field fluorescein angiography showing no macular leakage in a case of vitreoretinal lymphoma and no prior surgery.

References

1. Dalvin LA, Pulido JS, Shields CL, et al. Vitreoretinal lymphoma: central nervous system lymphoma risk with unilateral or bilateral ocular tumour: a multicentre collaboration. *Eye (Lond)*. 2023;37(1):54-61.
2. Carreras E, Salomão DR, Nadal J, et al. Macular edema is a rare finding in untreated vitreoretinal lymphoma: small case series and review of the literature. *Int J Retina Vitreous*. 2017;3:15.
3. Raja H, Salomão DR, Viswanatha DS, Pulido JS. Prevalence of MYD88 L265P mutation in histologically proven, diffuse large B-cell vitreoretinal lymphoma. *Retina*. 2016;36(3):624-628.
4. Sehgal A, Pulido JS, Mashayekhi A, Milman T, Deák GG. Diagnosing vitreoretinal lymphomas: an analysis of the sensitivity of existing tools. *Cancers (Basel)*. 2022;14(3):598.
5. Carbonell D, Mahajan S, Chee SP, et al. Consensus recommendations for the diagnosis of vitreoretinal lymphoma. *Ocul Immunol Inflamm*. 2021;29(3):507-520.
6. Albadri ST, Pulido JS, Macon WR, Garcia JJ, Salomao DR. Histologic findings in vitreoretinal lymphoma: learning from enucleation specimens. *Retina*. 2020;40(2):391-398.
7. Stacey AW, Pulido JS. The concept of minimal residual disease in the treatment and staging of vitreoretinal lymphoma. *Retina*. 2020;40(7):1213-1214.
8. Castellino A, Pulido JS, Johnston PB, et al. Role of systemic high-dose methotrexate and combined approaches in the management of vitreoretinal lymphoma: a single center experience 1990–2018. *Am J Hematol*. 2019;94(3):291-298.

CHAPTER 65

Familial Dense Vitreous Floaters in a Man

George Skopis ■ Jennifer I. Lim

History of Present Illness

We present a 36-year-old man with an unremarkable medical history referred for floaters of the left eye. He endorsed mild blurry vision of the left eye and denied any vision loss, flashes, or floaters of the right eye. He has no history of ocular conditions or ocular surgery.

OCULAR EXAMINATION FINDINGS

Visual acuity with correction was 20/20 in the right eye and 20/25 in the left eye. The anterior segment examination was normal in each eye, and intraocular pressures were 15 mmHg. Dilated fundus examination of the right eye was unremarkable. In contrast, dilated fundus examination of the left eye revealed dense vitreous opacities overlying the optic nerve and posterior pole and multiple, circumscribed, glass wool–like vitreous opacities in the periphery (Fig. 65.1). No retinal hemorrhages or scars were seen.

Questions to Ask

- Does the patient have a history of known autoimmune/inflammatory conditions? Various inflammatory/autoimmune conditions can manifest in the eye as vitreous inflammatory cells, vitreous haze, and vitreous opacities. It is also important to obtain a thorough review of systems to evaluate for systemic manifestations of autoimmune disease.
  - No
- Does the patient have a history of travel outside of the country, or has the patient been treated for any prior infections? Infectious sources of inflammation (e.g., syphilis, tuberculosis, toxoplasmosis) can present as vitreous opacities.
  - No
- Does the patient have a history of prior or current malignancy? Lymphoma or leukemia may present with vitreous opacities.
  - No
- Does the patient have a history of diabetes mellitus or hypertension? Inquiring about diseases associated with common causes of vitreous hemorrhage, such as diabetic neovascularization, retinal vein occlusions, and macroaneurysms, is indicated because vitreous opacities may result from dehemoglobinized vitreous hemorrhage.
  - No
- Does the patient have a history of ocular trauma, which can be associated with old vitreous hemorrhage?
  - No

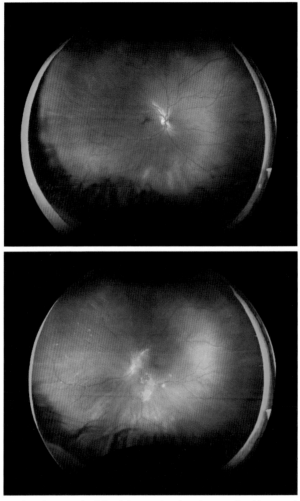

Fig. 65.1   (A) Color fundus photograph of the right eye showing clear media with normal optic nerve, retinal vessels, and retinal periphery. (B) Color fundus photograph of the left eye shows glass wool–like vitreous opacity over the optic nerve and parts of the posterior pole with more circumscribed vitreous opacities peripherally. Optic nerve, retinal vessels, and retinal periphery are normal.

- Is there a family history of eye disease? Amyloidosis can result in dense vitreous opacities that may require pars plana vitrectomy.
  - Yes. The patient's mother had vitreous floaters that required surgical removal.

Assessment

- This is a case of a 36-year-old man with no medical, ocular, or ocular surgical history who presented with floaters of the left eye and was found to have significant vitreous opacities in the left eye.

Differential Diagnosis

- Neoplastic: lymphoma, leukemia, melanoma, metastasis
- Infectious: syphilis, tuberculosis, toxoplasmosis
- Inflammatory: sarcoidosis or other uveitis
- Vitreous hemorrhage: diabetic retinopathy, sickle cell retinopathy, old central or branch retinal vein occlusion
- Asteroid hyalosis: usually asymptomatic in patients, and the opacities are round to oval, white to yellow-white, mobile particles that tend to return to their original positions, suspended in the vitreous
- Cholesterolosis bulbi or synchysis scintillans: usually asymptomatic in patients, small, flat crystalline (cholesterol crystals), yellow to gold, shiny, highly refractile particles that are not attached to the vitreous and thus sink to the inferior vitreous cavity in a "snow globe"–like manner; typically associated with chronic eye disease (chronic retinal detachment, chronic uveitis, trauma, hypermature cataract) or chronic vitreous hemorrhage
- Amyloidosis: visually significant, glass wool appearing, whitish, wispy vitreous opacities (Fig. 65.2).[1] If the retinal vessels are visible, the glass wool–like opacities may be seen emanating from the retinal vessels[2] (Fig. 65.3). Retinal neovascularization and vitreous hemorrhage may occur in this condition because of increased vascular endothelial growth factor production (Figs. 65.2, 65.3).[2,3]

Workup/Diagnosis

- Further history revealed the patient's mother had been diagnosed with amyloidosis and had undergone pars plana vitrectomy for dense, symptomatic floaters.
- A diagnostic/therapeutic pars plana vitrectomy was performed on this patient. The vitreous sample sent to pathology showed positive staining with Congo red and apple-green birefringence in polarized light. (An example of this is shown in Fig. 65.4.)
- A diagnosis of amyloidosis was made.

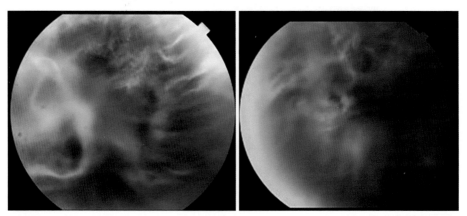

Fig. 65.2 *(Left)* Fundus photograph of patient's right eye before vitrectomy, showing severe vitreous amyloid deposition. *(Right)* Preoperative fundus photograph of patient's left eye with evidence of vitreous hemorrhage.(Reproduced with permission from *British Journal of Ophthalmology*. Originally Fig. 1 from O'Hearn TM, Fawzi A, He S, Rao NA, Lim JI. Early onset vitreous amyloidosis in familial amyloidotic polyneuropathy with a transthyretin Glu54Gly mutation is associated with elevated vitreous VEGF. *Br J Ophthalmol.* 2007;91(12):1607-1609.)

Multimodal Testing and Imaging

- Fundus photographs
  - On fundus examination dense and sheet like or wispy vitreous opacities may be seen, as well as retrolental white, well-circumscribed opacities with attached strands that can be traced posteriorly[1] (Figs. 65.1, 65.2). When the retinal vessels are visible, the glass wool–like opacities may be seen emanating from the retinal vessels (Fig. 65.3). Retinal neovascularization and vitreous hemorrhage have been described in this condition.
- Optical coherence tomography (OCT)
  - Findings on OCT include retinal surface deposits with a needle-shaped pattern extending from the internal limiting membrane into the vitreous[4] (Fig. 65.5).

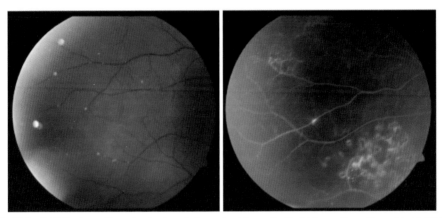

Fig. 65.3 *(Left)* Postoperative color fundus photograph of the patient's right eye, illustrating areas of retinal vascular abnormality and fine deposits of amyloid associated with retinal vessels. *(Right)* Fluorescein angiogram of the same eye showing areas of endolaser and a small tuft of neovascularization. (Reproduced with permission from *British Journal of Ophthalmology*. Originally Fig. 2 from O'Hearn TM, Fawzi A, He S, Rao NA, Lim JI. Early onset vitreous amyloidosis in familial amyloidotic polyneuropathy with a transthyretin Glu54Gly mutation is associated with elevated vitreous VEGF. *Br J Ophthalmol*. 2007;91(12):1607-1609.)

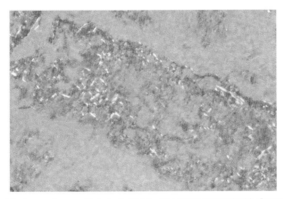

Fig. 65.4 Histological features of an undiluted vitrectomy specimen stained with Congo red and illuminated with polarized light, showing yellow-green birefringence characteristic of amyloid deposits. (Reproduced with permission from *British Journal of Ophthalmology*. Originally Fig. 3 from O'Hearn TM, Fawzi A, He S, Rao NA, Lim JI. Early onset vitreous amyloidosis in familial amyloidotic polyneuropathy with a transthyretin Glu54Gly mutation is associated with elevated vitreous VEGF. *Br J Ophthalmol*. 2007;91(12):1607-1609.)

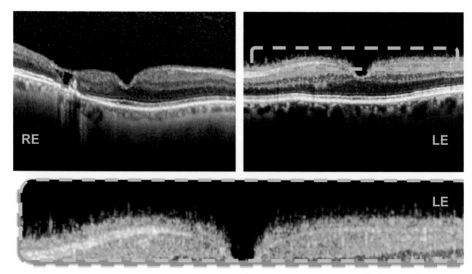

Fig. 65.5 Optical coherence tomography scans of the right eye (RE) showing mild thickening of the internal limiting membrane and of the left eye (LE) showing needle-shaped deposits on the retinal surface. (From Tasiopoulou A, Ong D, Lightman S. Characteristic needle-shaped pattern seen on OCT in a patient with ocular amyloidosis. *Ophthalmol Retina.* 2021;5(1)99-101.)

- Optical coherence tomography angiography (OCTA)
  - OCTA has shown reduced or absent density in the superficial and deep retinal capillaries and the choroidal capillaries, showing that the accumulation of amyloid can cause reduction in both the retinal and choroidal capillary circulations.[5]
- Fluorescein angiography (FA)
  - In some cases, areas of peripheral retinal neovascularization can develop. FA may be helpful in identifying this cause hemorrhage associated with the amyloid vitreous opacities.[3]

Management

- A diagnostic and therapeutic vitrectomy was performed on our patient. Vitreous samples were sent for histopathologic examination and were found to have positive staining with Congo red dye and apple-green birefringence in polarized light.
- Pars plana vitrectomy is a safe method of treatment,[6] but patients are at higher risk for iatrogenic retinal breaks because of tight vitreoretinal adhesions.[7] In addition, postoperatively recurrence of amyloid can occur, and patients may also develop glaucoma. Patients require regular and long-term follow-up for these recurrences and potential complications related to amyloidosis.[8]
- There have been reports in the literature of panretinal photocoagulation preventing progression of amyloid deposition.[9]
- Genetic testing is useful for diagnostic confirmation and for testing of asymptomatic at-risk family members. Our patient was heterozygous for a pathological gene variant of the *TTR* gene, confirming hereditary amyloidosis.
- Ocular amyloid may be a manifestation of systemic amyloidosis, and patients should be referred to their primary care physician for appropriate evaluation and referral.

Follow-up Care

- There are no previously established guidelines for follow-up.
- After standard postsurgical follow-up, patients need to be intermittently evaluated to monitor for recurrence.
- Most patients have bilateral but asymmetrical involvement. If the patient initially has unilateral involvement, frequent follow-up to monitor the other eye is needed, as it is likely to develop in the fellow eye over time.
- Our patient was seen 5 years later with new symptomatic floaters in the right eye due to amyloid deposits. He subsequently underwent pars plana vitrectomy in that eye.

Algorithm 65.1: Vitreous Opacity Flowchart

Key Points

- Consider amyloidosis in the differential diagnosis of vitreous opacities, especially when retrolenticular plaques and glass-wool opacities are present.
- Pars plana vitrectomy is both diagnostic and therapeutic. However, long-term follow-up is needed as opacities can recur.
- Amyloid deposition in the eye may be a part of a systemic syndrome. Genetic testing and appropriate referral are indicated for further evaluation.

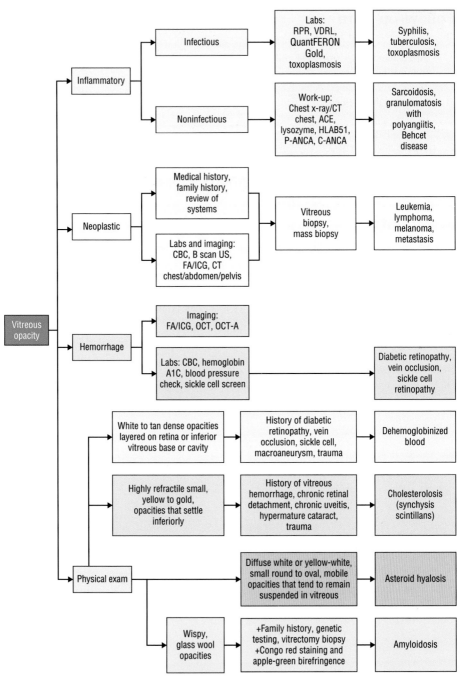

Algorithm 65.1   Vitreous opacity flowchart. *ACE,* angiotensin-converting enzyme; *CBC,* complete blood cell count; *CT,* computed tomography; *FA/ICG,* fluorescein angiography/indocyanine green angiography; *HLA-B51,* human leukocyte antigen-B51; *OCT,* optical coherence tomography; *OCTA,* optical coherence tomography angiography; *P-ANCA,* perinuclear anti-neutrophil cytoplasmic antibody; *RPR,* rapid plasma reagin; *US,* ultrasound; *VDRL,* Venereal Disease Research Laboratory.

References

1. Hitchings RA, Tripathi RC. Vitreous opacities in primary amyloid disease: a clinical, histochemical, and ultrastructural report. *Br J Ophthalmol.* 1976;60(1):41-54.
2. O'Hearn TM, Fawzi A, He S, Rao NA, Lim JI. Early onset vitreous amyloidosis in familial amyloidotic polyneuropathy with a transthyretin Glu54Gly mutation is associated with elevated vitreous VEGF. *Br J Ophthalmol.* 2007;91(12):1607-1609.
3. Savage DJ, Mango CA, Streeten BW. Amyloidosis of the vitreous: fluorescein angiographic findings and association with neovascularization. *Arch Ophthalmol.* 1982;100(11):1776-1779.
4. Tasiopoulou A, Ong D, Lightman S. Characteristic needle-shaped pattern seen on OCT in a patient with ocular amyloidosis. *Ophthalmol Retina.* 2021;5(1):99-101.
5. Tei M, Maruko I, Uchimura E, Tomohiro I. Retinal and choroidal circulation determined by optical coherence tomography angiography in patient with amyloidosis. *BMJ Case Rep.* 2019;12(2):e228479.
6. Koga T, Ando E, Hirata A, et al. Vitreous opacities and outcome of vitreous surgery in patients with familial amyloidotic polyneuropathy. *Am J Ophthalmol.* 2003;135(2):188-193.
7. You J. Vitrectomy for vitreous amyloidosis. *Int J Ophthalmol.* 2011;4(3):307-310.
8. Thiagasorupan P, Barreau E, Gendron G, et al. Specific postoperative complications of vitrectomy in hereditary transthyretin amyloidosis. *Eur J Ophthalmol.* 2022;32(2):1149-1156.
9. Kawaji T, Ando Y, Hara R, Tanihara H. Novel therapy for transthyretin-related ocular amyloidosis: a pilot study of retinal laser photocoagulation. *Ophthalmology.* 2010;117(3):552-555.

CHAPTER 66

Asymptomatic Bilateral Retinal White Spots

Kelly Bui ■ William F. Mieler

History of Present Illness

A 17-year-old female patient presents for a retinal examination given skin findings, referred by dermatology. She has no ocular history. There are skin lesions on her face, neck, trunk, and lower extremities.

Questions

- What is her medical history?
- Are there any known hereditary ocular conditions?
- Is there a family history of genetic or inflammatory conditions?
- Are the retinal spots single or multifocal?
- Are the retinal spots unilateral or bilateral?
- In which layer(s) of the retina are the lesions located?
- Is there associated ocular inflammation?

Medical History

- Multiple skin lesions: ash leaf spots on trunk and lower extremities, angiofibromas on face
- Asthma
- No history of seizures
- Normal intelligence
- Medications: none
- Family history: unremarkable
- Examination:
  - Visual acuity: right eye (OD), 20/20-; left eye (OS), 20/25 +3
  - Pupils: no relative afferent pupillary defect
  - Intraocular pressure: OD, 19 mm Hg; OS, 19 mm Hg
  - Anterior segment exam (ASE): within normal limits (WNL)
  - Posterior segment exam (PSE): (see Figs. 66.1–66.3)

Assessment

- Young female patient with an undiagnosed genetic condition who presents with skin and retinal lesions. The retinal lesions are multifocal, bilateral, and superficial, without calcifications. There is no associated ocular inflammation or retinal vascular abnormalities.[1-5]

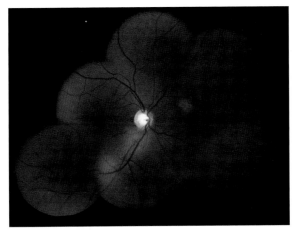

Fig. 66.1 Multiple retinal astrocytic hamartomas in the right eye, along the inferotemporal arcade and the nasal retina.

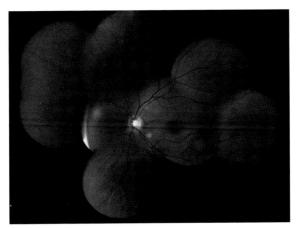

Fig. 66.2 Multiple retinal astrocytic hamartomas in the left eye, along the inferotemporal arcade, nasal retina, and midperiphery.

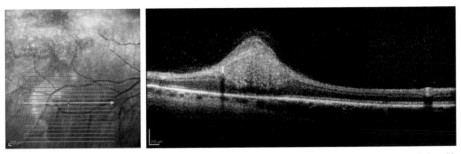

Fig. 66.3 Optical coherence tomography through a retinal astrocytic hamartoma demonstrates glial proliferation in the nerve fiber layer.

Differential Diagnosis

- Myelinated nerve fiber layer
- Cotton wool spot
- Pseudoneoplastic gliosis of the retina
- Presumed solitary circumscribed retinal astrocytic proliferation
- Retinoblastoma
- Astrocytoma
- Astrocytic hamartoma
  - Related to tuberous sclerosis complex (TSC) 1–3
  - Related to neurofibromatosis (NF)
  - Sporadic occurrence

Workup

- Brain magnetic resonance imaging (MRI): multiple cortical hamartomas with one calcified subependymal nodule
- Retroperitoneal ultrasound: bilateral angiomyolipomas
- Cardiac workup and genetics evaluation were pending

Diagnosis

Astrocytic hamartomas in a patient with TSC
- Glial proliferative in the retinal nerve fiber layer (RNFL)
- Three variants based on fundus appearance:
  - Type 1: flat, white and translucent, found above the retinal vessels
  - Type 2: raised, yellow, calcified "mulberry" lesions
  - Type 3 (mixed lesion): flat, translucent base with elevated, calcified center
- Typically has no associated vascular abnormalities
- Four variants based on optical coherence tomography (OCT) findings:
  - Type 1: Flat and confined within the RNFL
  - Type 2: Elevated with associated retinal traction
  - Type 3: "Moth-eaten" appearance related to calcification
  - Type 4: Optically empty cavities within lesions

Atypical Lesions

- They may grow in size.
- They can transform from type 1 to type 2 variant.
- Rarely have been associated with retinal exudation, serous retinal detachment, choroidal neovascularization, vitreous hemorrhage, and even neovascular glaucoma. These lesions may be more properly classified as giant cell astrocytoma, rather than astrocytic hamartoma.

Multimodal Imaging

- Fundus autofluorescence: lesions may either exhibit hyper- or hypo-autofluorescence (hyper-AF if calcifications are present).
- Fluorescein angiography: early, hypofluorescence with late mild leakage

- OCT angiography: plexus of capillary vessels within lesions, rarely associated with a feeder vessel
- B scan: medium internal reflectivity tumors, with high internal reflectivity if calcification is present

Management

- Workup and referrals to other medical subspecialties for associated genetic disorder (dermatology, neurology, nephrology, pulmonary, cardiology, and genetic counseling). Obtain appropriate imaging (such as brain MRI, abdominal MRI, electroencephalogram, pulmonary function test, echocardiogram).[4]
- Serial monitoring for retinal lesion growth and transformation.
- Treatment with laser photocoagulation or photodynamic therapy may be necessary for associated retinal exudation and/or cystoid macular edema.[6-9]

Algorithm 66.1: Algorithm for Retinal White Spot

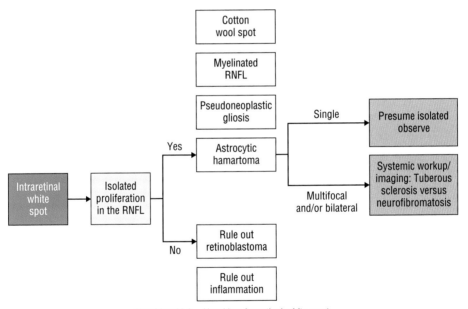

Algorithm 66.1 Algorithm for retinal white spot.

Key Points

- Retinal lesion(s) correspond to glial proliferation of the nerve fiber layer on OCT
- Bilateral and multifocal lesions are often associated with TSC or NF[10]
- *Differentiate from retinoblastoma,* particularly in younger patients with type 2 lesions
- Workup for TSC or NF
- Serial retinal examinations are recommended to monitor for lesion growth and transformation

References

1. Hodgson N, Kinori M, Goldbaum MH, Robbins SL. Ophthalmic manifestations of tuberous sclerosis: a review. *Clin Exp Ophthalmol.* 2016;45:81-86.
2. Rowsley SA, O'Callaghan FJ, Osborne JP. Ophthalmic manifestations of tuberous sclerosis: a population based study. *Br J Ophthalmol.* 2001;85:420-423.
3. Abdolrahimzadeh S, Plateroti AM, Recupero SM, Lambiase A. An update on the ophthalmologic features in the phakomatoses. *J Ophthalmol.* 2016;2016:3043026.
4. Northrup H, Krueger DA. Tuberous sclerosis complex diagnostic criteria update: recommendations of the 2012 International Tuberous Sclerosis Complex Consensus Conference. *Pediatr Neurol.* 2013;49:243-254.
5. Shields CL. Retinal pigment epithelial depigmented lesions associated with tuberous sclerosis complex. *Arch Ophthalmol.* 2012;130:387-390.
6. Zipori AB, Tehrani NN, Ali A. Retinal astrocytoma regression in tuberous sclerosis patients treated with everolimus. *J AAPOS.* 2018;22:76-79.
7. Saito W, Kase S, Ohgami K, Mori S, Ohno S. Intravitreal anti-vascular endothelial growth factor therapy with bevacizumab for tuberous sclerosis with macular oedema. *Acta Ophthalmol.* 2010;88:377-380.
8. Bloom SM, Mahl CF. Photocoagulation for serous detachment of the macula secondary to retinal astrocytoma. *Retina.* 1991;11:416-422.
9. Eskelin S, Tommila P, Palosaari T, Kivelä T. Photodynamic therapy with verteporfin to induce regression of aggressive retinal astrocytomas. *Acta Ophthalmol.* 2008;86:794-799.
10. Bui KM, Leiderman YI, Lim JI, Mieler WF. Multifocal retinal astrocytic hamartomas: a case series and review of the literature. *Retin Cases Brief Rep.* 2013;7:9-13.

CHAPTER 67

Unilateral Decreased Vision Associated With a Peripheral Mass in a Young Male Patient

Ivy Zhu ▓ William F. Mieler

History of Present Illness

A 28-year-old male patient was referred by an outside ophthalmologist for subacute vision loss in the right eye associated with a peripheral mass. The vision loss was reported to be painless and constant.

OCULAR EXAM FINDINGS

Initial evaluation revealed best-corrected visual acuity of 20/40 in the right eye and 20/20 in the left eye. Intraocular pressures, pupils, confrontational visual fields, and extraocular motility were within normal limits. The anterior segment of both eyes was unremarkable. Dilated fundus examination of the right eye revealed vitreous debris and a yellowish-pink mass with overlying retinal vessels, exudate, and associated subretinal fluid located in the inferotemporal periphery (Fig. 67.1). The fundus of the left eye was unremarkable.

IMAGING

Optical coherence tomography (OCT), fluorescein angiogram (FA), and B-scan ultrasonography were then obtained. OCT was normal and showed an intact foveal contour without evidence of macular edema or epiretinal membrane in either eye. FA revealed early filling and leakage of the retinal vessels overlying the elevated mass lesion (Figs. 67.2 and 67.3). The vessels were mildly dilated, nontortuous, and slightly increased in number compared with normal. In the late frames, there was extensive leakage from the inferotemporal lesion. There was also peripheral leakage with early termination of retinal vessels noted in both eyes. B-scan ultrasonography revealed an elevated lesion with maximal height of 4.02 mm of homogenous composition and medium to high internal reflectivity without shadowing (Fig. 67.4).

Questions to Ask

- Are there any current or previous kidney or neurological problems?
  - The review of systems for the patient was normal, and he denied any medical problems.
- Does the patient have any family members with inherited medical conditions or kidney or neurological problems?
  - The patient denied any inherited familial conditions, ocular or otherwise.

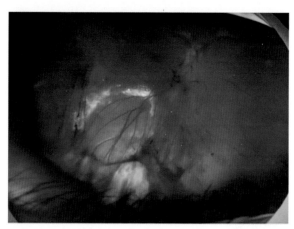

Fig. 67.1 Wide-field color fundus photograph of the right eye showing a large inferotemporal peripheral elevated mass with overlying retinal vessels and exudates at its posterior border. There was significant sub-retinal fluid leading to a localized exudative retinal detachment.

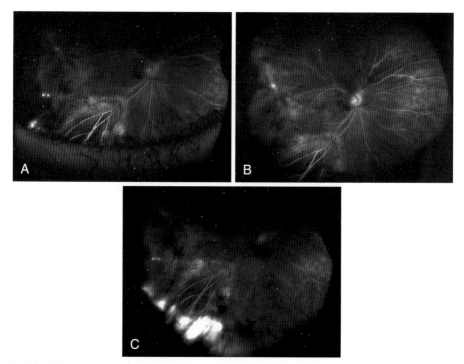

Fig. 67.2 Wide-field fluorescein angiogram of the right eye showing an inferotemporal mass. (A) An early frame demonstrating early filling of slightly dilated peripheral retinal vessels of increased number overlying an elevated lesion with leakage. There is some blockage that is seen throughout the study representing vitreous debris (likely hemorrhage). (B) A middle frame showing early termination of the peripheral temporal retinal vessels with abnormal branching and leakage. There is also some mild nasal peripheral vessel leakage. (C) A late frame showing extensive vessel leakage and hyperfluorescence at the anterior margin of the lesion.

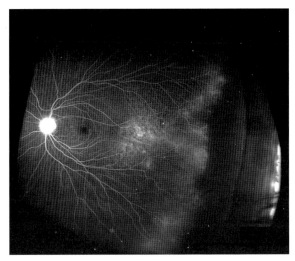

Fig. 67.3 Widefield fluorescein angiogram of the left eye showing early termination of the temporal peripheral retinal vessels with abnormal end branching and leakage. There is prominent nonperfusion anterior to the leaking vessels.

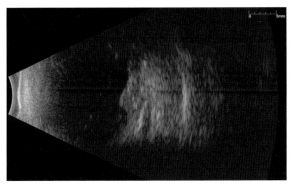

Fig. 67.4 A B-scan ultrasound of the right eye showing an elevated lesion 4.02 mm in height with homogenous composition and medium to high internal reflectivity.

- Are there any other ocular conditions or episodes of eye pain or inflammation?
  - The patient denied any ocular history, including episodes of eye pain or inflammation.
- Was the patient born prematurely?
  - The patient had a normal birth and delivery.

Assessment

- A 28-year-old male patient without known medical, ocular, or familial history presents with subacute decreased vision of the right eye and is found to have an inferotemporal mass lesion with mildly dilated overlying retinal vessels, exudates, and associated retinal detachment. FA demonstrated extensive leakage of these retinal vessels in the right eye and early termination of the temporal retinal vessels in both eyes. B-scan demonstrated a raised lesion of medium to high internal reflectivity.

Differential Diagnosis

- Vasoproliferative retinal tumor, primary or secondary
- Retinal capillary hemangioblastoma, sporadic or familial (von Hippel–Lindau disease)
- Amelanotic melanoma
- Coats disease (retinal telangiectasis)
- Retinal or choroidal granuloma
- Choroidal metastasis
- Retinoschisis

Working Diagnosis

- The inferotemporal pink-yellow lesion with overlying retinal vessels and surrounding exudates is consistent with a vasoproliferative tumor (VPT), likely secondary to undiagnosed familial exudative vitreoretinopathy (FEVR), which was seen in both eyes as early termination of temporal retinal vessels with vascular dragging and peripheral ischemia. The vessels are not extensively dilated or tortuous as would be seen in a retinal hemangioblastoma. The ultrasound is less likely amelanotic choroidal melanoma given its medium to high internal reflectivity.

Multimodal Testing and Results

- Color fundus photograph: Fundus photography often reveals a pink-red elevated lesion with overlying retinal vessels in the preequatorial retina, commonly in the inferotemporal quadrant. Frequently, there are surrounding exudates. Visualization of the lesion can be obscured by hemorrhage covering the tumor surface or within the vitreous.[4]
- OCT: OCT of the macula can reveal secondary epiretinal membrane or cystoid macular edema, which can lead to vision loss.
- FA: FA shows minimally dilated feeding vessels with extensive leakage of the lesion. FA can be helpful in defining the lesion and highlighting any other retinal vascular abnormalities.
- B-scan ultrasound: B-scan shows an elevated lesion, usually ranging from 1.0 to 5.0 mm in height. The average height is 3.0 mm. The internal reflectivity is typically medium to high, though this can vary.

Management

- The leading differential diagnosis for VPT is retinal hemangioblastoma, with prominent dilated and tortuous associated retinal vessels distinguishing VPT from retinal hemangioblastoma. In cases of diagnostic uncertainty, tumor biopsy may be indicated.
- VPT can be primary (idiopathic) or secondary to another ocular condition. Reported associated conditions include intermediate uveitis, retinitis pigmentosa, Coats disease, ocular toxocariasis, FEVR, and retinopathy of prematurity. Additional testing should be taken as indicated to evaluate for any associated conditions.[1]
- There currently exists no standard of care for treating VPTs. Management can include observation, cryotherapy, laser photocoagulation, photodynamic therapy, brachytherapy, intravitreal bevacizumab injection, intravitreal or periocular steroid injection, local resection, or any combination thereof. Management typically varies based on the size and features of the tumor.[2-5]
- In general, patients with small, asymptomatic tumors can be closely observed until symptoms develop or the tumor shows growth. Patients with vision-threatening complications require prompt treatment.

Follow-up Care

- Patients should be followed closely to monitor for tumor progression and the development of sequelae that can lead to vision loss. This patient did receive several anti-VEGF injections OD and peripheral scatter photocoagulation OU. The vasoproliferataive tumur has remianed stable for 5 years, with VA of 20.30 OD. Genetic testing was offered, though the patient has refused thus far.

Algorithm 67.1: Differential Diagnosis

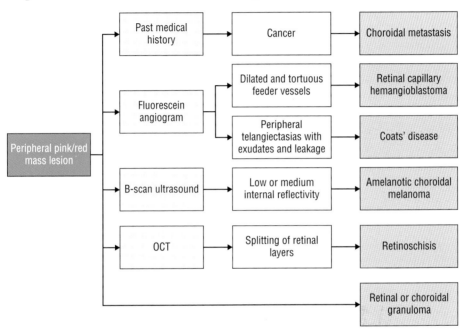

Algorithm 67.1   Differential diagnosis.

Key Points

- VPT is a rare, benign retinal lesion that has a pinkish-yellow appearance and is typically found anterior to the equator with surrounding exudates and minimally dilated feeding vessels, most commonly in the inferotemproal periphery.
- It can occur as a primary or idiopathic lesion, or it can be associated with other ocular conditions such as intermediate uveitis, retinitis pigmentosa, Coats disease, ocular toxocariasis, familial exudative vitreoretinopathy, and retinopathy of prematurity.
- FA demonstrates early and profound vessel leakage associated with the tumor. B-scan typically shows medium to high internal reflectivity. In cases of diagnostic uncertainty, tumor biopsy may be necessary. OCT may be used to detect and monitor for secondary complications such as cystoid macular edema or epiretinal membrane.
- Small asymptomatic lesions are frequently observed until patients develop symptoms or the lesion demonstrates growth.
- Reported treatment methods include cryotherapy, brachytherapy, laser photocoagulation, photodynamic therapy, intravitreal bevacizumab, intravitreal or periocular corticosteroid injection, local resection, or any combination thereof.

References

1. Jakobiec FA, Thanos A, Stagner AM, Grossniklaus HE, Proia AD. So-called massive retinal gliosis: a critical review and reappraisal. *Surv Ophthalmol.* 2016;61:339-356.
2. Shields JA, Decker WL, Sanborn GE, Augsburger JJ, Goldberg RE. Presumed acquired retinal hemangiomas. *Ophthalmology.* 1983;90:1292-1300.
3. Shields CL, Shields JA, Barrett J, De Potter P. Vasoproliferative tumors of the ocular fundus. Classification and clinical manifestations in 103 patients. *Arch Ophthalmol.* 1995;113:615-623.
4. Shields CL, Kaliki S, Al-Dahmash S, et al. Retinal vasoproliferative tumors: comparative clinical features of primary vs secondary tumors in 334 cases. *JAMA Ophthalmol.* 2013;131:328-334.
5. Cohen VM, Shields CL, Demirci H, Shields JA. Iodine I 125 plaque radiotherapy for vasoproliferative tumors of the retina in 30 eyes. *Arch Ophthalmol.* 2008;126:1245-1251.

CHAPTER 68

Peripheral Proliferative Retinal Lesion

Paul R. Parker ▪ Michael J. Heiferman ▪ William F. Mieler

Introduction

Presumed solitary circumscribed astrocytic retinal proliferation (PSCRAP) is a rare, benign retinal tumor that is typically discovered incidentally on examination. Usually, it is seen in White middle-aged male patients as an isolated lesion in the posterior pole. Although its location was originally thought to be the inner neurosensory retina, recent imaging studies with optical coherence tomography (OCT) angiography suggests it arises from the deep retina or retinal pigment epithelium (RPE).[1,2] Vision is usually preserved, and patients are asymptomatic. PSCRAP shows stability in size, but sometimes it can regress spontaneously.[3,4] Here we present a case of isolated PSCRAP in a patient referred for an incidental asymptomatic retinal finding.

History of Present Illness and Examination

A 74-year-old White male patient with mild chronic obstructive pulmonary disease and hyperopia was referred for retina evaluation. The patient denied any visual symptoms including photopsias, floaters, nyctalopia, or metamorphopsia.

OCULAR EXAM FINDINGS

On examination the visual acuity was 20/20 in the right eye and 20/25 in the left eye, intraocular pressure was 15 mm Hg in both eyes, and there was mild nuclear sclerosis in both eyes. Dilated fundus examination of the right eye revealed a well-circumscribed, elevated solid white lesion that was 3 mm temporal to the macula and appeared to be emanating from the retina (Fig. 68.1). The lesion was surrounded by a rim of pigment mottling that measured 1.0 mm circumferentially. Additionally, there was a choroidal nevus with overlying drusen in the inferonasal midperiphery measuring 5 mm × 6 mm. The left fundus was normal without retinal lesions, drusen, or pigmentary changes.

Differential Diagnosis

- Astrocytic hamartoma
- Retinoblastoma
- Retinocytoma
- Simple congenital RPE hamartoma
- Myelinated retinal nerve fibers
- Granuloma
- Reactive gliosis

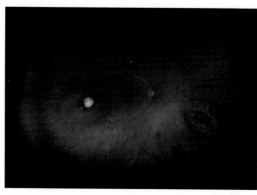

Fig. 68.1 Fundus photograph of the right eye, demonstrating the lesion temporal to the macula.

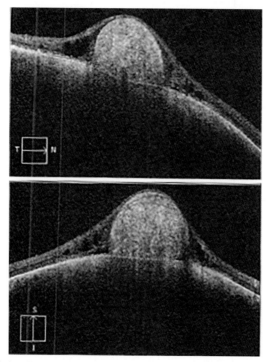

Fig. 68.2 Spectral domain optical coherence tomography demonstrating photographs showing the lesion temporal to the macula in the transverse nasotemporal (top) and superoinferior (bottom) planes.

Work up and Imaging

OCT revealed an elevated lesion arising from the junction of the inner neurosensory retina and RPE (Fig. 68.2). The fluorescein angiogram showed early blockage with a rim of mottled staining surrounding the lesion (Fig. 68.3). Ultrasonography showed a 1.75-mm thick homogenous lesion (Fig. 68.4) with medium internal reflectivity and no detectable spontaneous vascular activity or shadowing. Humphrey 24-2 visual field testing revealed a small nasal defect corresponding to the lesion temporal to the macula (Fig. 68.5).

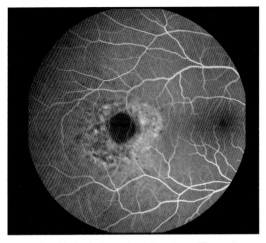

Fig. 68.3 Fluorescein angiography of lesion in the recirculation phase. The angiogram showed early blockage with a rim of mottled late staining surrounding the lesion.

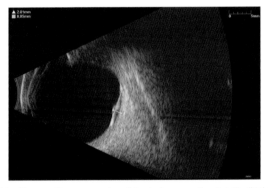

Fig. 68.4 B-scan ultrasonography of the lesion seen in a longitudinal plane.

Follow-up

The lesion was deemed to have no concerning features, and the patient was scheduled for follow-up every 6 months. The lesion has been followed for 4 years and has shown no change in size, color, or characteristics. Systemic health remains unchanged and stable.

Discussion

This case report highlights the clinical and diagnostic imaging features of PSCRAP, a rare, often incidentally discovered lesion in the posterior pole. First described in 2011,[3] the lesion has important distinguishing characteristics, such as opaque coloration that prevents visualization of the underlying retina, distinct borders, absence of calcification, and nondilated, nontortuous vessels that pass through or around the lesion.[3] It typically remains stable in size with no growth, though regression is possible; one case series showed regression in one out of seven cases,[3] and another case report described regression to a normal appearing retina within 8 months.[5] Most recently, multifocal lesions have been reported in the same eye.[6] All cases reported previously, as well as the present case, were solitary in presentation, as the name of the entity implies.

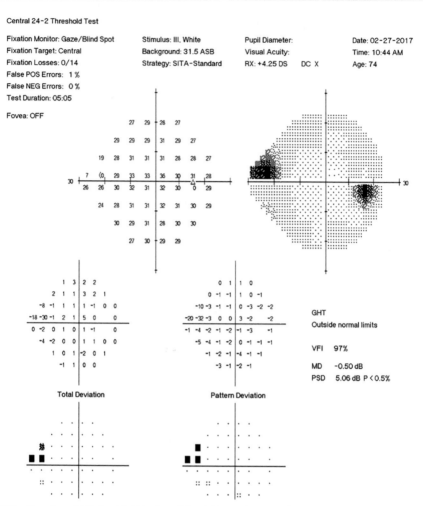

Fig. 68.5 Humphrey 24-2 visual field testing of the right eye demonstrating a nasal scotoma slightly above midline. The testing fixation losses and error rates show the test is reliable.

The pathogenesis is poorly understood, though some believe it to arise from astrocytes, as its name implies. Oligodendrocytes are also postulated to be a potential source, though neoplasia of these cells is more common in primary central nervous system pathology.[3] Many diagnostic imaging modalities have been used to characterize PSCRAP. Fluorescein angiography typically shows mild early hyperfluorescence in the venous phase and late fluorescence in the recirculation phase.[7] However, our patient's angiogram revealed early and late blockage with mottled staining. In fundus autofluorescence, both hyper- and hypoautofluorescence have been described, although hypoautofluorescence tends to be more common.[7]

The differential diagnosis is limited to both benign and malignant retinal proliferative tumors, such as astrocytic hamartoma, retinoblastoma, retinocytoma, simple congenital RPE hamartoma, myelinated retinal nerve fibers, granuloma, and reactive gliosis.[3] Also, it is important to consider a turbid pigment epithelial detachment, which can have a yellowish, raised appearance, caused by a subtle, underlying choroidal nevus.[5] The most clinically similar tumor is an astrocytic hamartoma (AH), seen in the inherited condition tuberous sclerosis. Both lesions can have hyper- and hypoautofluorescence;

however, PSCRAP is typically solitary and seen in middle-aged White men, whereas the multiple AH of tuberous sclerosis are seen more often in children. The important distinction clinically between PSCRAP and AH is that PSCRAP tends to be solitary and opaque, thus preventing a view of the posterior retina, and has no calcifications.[3] In terms of retinoblastoma, these present much earlier in life, contain calcifications, and are much more malignant in size and appearance.

As the lesion is very rare and benign by nature, there are no established guidelines on the management of PSCRAP. However, proper diagnosis is essential to confirm the benign nature of this rare lesion. It is important to rule out other more serious diagnoses, based on clinical findings and multimodal imaging characteristics of the lesion. Observation and close follow-up are recommended so as to avoid an incorrect diagnosis.

Algorithm 68.1: Algorithm of Steps Involved in Diagnosing and Managing Asymptomatic Fundus Lesions

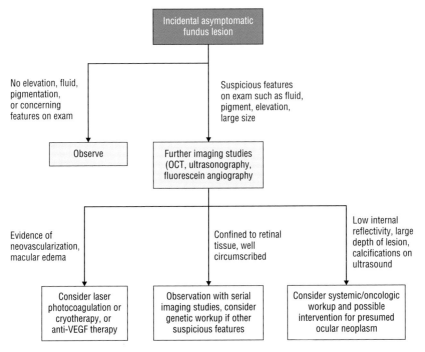

Algorithm 68.1   Algorithm of steps involved in diagnosing and managing asymptomatic fundus lesions. Primary decision-making in further diagnostic studies and intervention should be based on features seen on examination and imaging findings. *OCT,* Optical coherence tomography; *VEGF,* vascular endothelial growth factor.

Conclusion and Key Points

- We present a case a 74-year-old White male patient with an incidentally found solitary, white lesion in the retina. Our patient is found to have diagnostic features of PSCRAP: a rare, benign retinal tumor.
- Our patient has been monitored every 6 months for 3 years, and all aspects of the lesion and clinical examination have remained stable and unchanged.
- Further case series would be useful to better characterize the pathogenesis and features of this lesion, while also providing more established guidelines on clinical management.

References

1. Goldberg RA, Raja KM. Presumed solitary circumscribed retinal astrocytic proliferation in the fovea with OCT angiography: a misnomer. *Ophthalmic Surg Lasers Imaging Retina.* 2018;49(3):212-214.
2. Schwartz SG, Harbour JW. Spectral-domain optical coherence tomography of presumed solitary circumscribed retinal astrocytic proliferation versus astrocytic hamartoma. *Ophthalmic Surg Lasers Imaging Retina.* 2015;46(5):586-588.
3. Shields JA, Bianciotto CG, Kivela T, Shields CL. Presumed solitary circumscribed retinal astrocytic proliferation: the 2010 Jonathan W. Wirtschafter lecture. *Arch Ophthalmol.* 2011;129(9):1189-1194.
4. Asensio-Sánchez VM. Presumed solitary circumscribed retinal astrocytic proliferation: a lesion that can regress. *Int Med Case Rep J.* 2019;12:85-88.
5. Perez B, Shields CL, Shields JA. Large turbid retinal pigment epithelial detachment camouflaging an underlying choroidal nevus. *Retin Cases Brief Rep.* 2009;3(2):147-149.
6. McKay BR, Krema H, Yan P, Weisbrod D. A case of multifocal presumed solitary circumscribed retinal astrocytic proliferation lesions in the same eye. *Can J Ophthalmol.* 2021;56(2):e62-e64.
7. Dubey D, Shanmugam M, Ramanjulu R. Presumed solitary circumscribed retinal astrocytic proliferation. *Indian J Ophthalmol.* 2019;67(12):2052-2053.

CHAPTER 69

Bilateral Severe Vision Loss in a Middle-Aged Woman With Constitutional Symptoms

Maura Di Nicola ▧ Basil K. Williams Jr.

History of Present Illness

We present a case of a 64-year-old female patient who presented to the emergency department (ED) with progressive weakness, weight loss, dizziness, and dyspnea. The ophthalmology team was consulted because of severe visual decline that had started about 6 months prior. The patient had been previously evaluated elsewhere and had undergone cataract surgery in the left eye (OS) but continued to experience visual decline in both eyes (OU). Her past ocular history was otherwise insignificant. Her past medical history included type 2 diabetes mellitus, hypertension, and coronary artery disease.

OCULAR EXAMINATION FINDINGS

Best-corrected visual acuity (BCVA) was 20/400 OU. Intraocular pressure was within normal limits. External and slit lamp examination showed multiple iris nevi OU, moderate cataract in the right eye (OD), and posterior chamber intraocular lens OS. Dilated fundus examination showed a large area of choroidal hyperpigmentation at the posterior pole OU with multiple overlying orange deposits. There was a discrete pigmented choroidal lesion in the inferonasal midperiphery OD and in the superior periphery OS. Shallow exudative retinal detachments were also present OU.

IMAGING

Fundus photos captured ophthalmoscopic findings of diffuse choroidal hyperpigmentation with multiple overlying patches of orange subretinal deposits, most prominent at the posterior pole in both eyes, as well as pigmented choroidal lesions in the inferonasal midperiphery OD and in the superior periphery OS (Fig. 69.1A, B). Fundus autofluorescence (FAF) demonstrated alternating zones of hypo- and hyperautofluorescence, corresponding to areas of retinal pigment epithelium (RPE) loss and RPE thickening secondary to lipofuscin deposition, respectively (Fig. 69.1C, D). On fluorescein angiography (FA), these areas appeared hyperfluorescent due to window defects and hypofluorescent due to blockage (Fig. 69.1E). Indocyanine green angiography (ICGA) similarly revealed alternating zones of hypo- and hyperfluorescence and demonstrated hypofluorescence of the superior choroidal lesion OS (Fig. 69.1F). Optical coherence tomography (OCT) of the macula revealed alternating areas of RPE atrophy with increased signal transmission and irregular RPE thickening. Shallow subretinal fluid was noted OU (Fig. 69.1G, H).

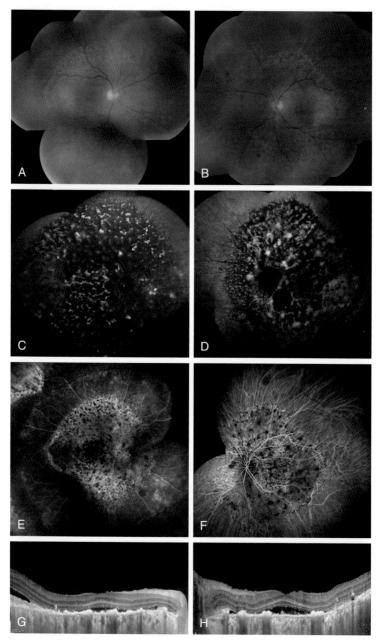

Fig. 69.1 (A, B) Fundus photographs demonstrating diffuse choroidal hyperpigmentation with overlying patches of lipofuscin, as well as pigmented choroidal lesions in the inferonasal midperiphery in the right eye (OD) and in the superior periphery in the left eye (OS). (C, D) Fundus autofluorescence shows the typical giraffe pattern with alternating zones of hypo- and hyperautofluorescence. (E) Fluorescein angiography shows a similar but reversed pattern OD. (F) Indocyanine green angiography demonstrating hypofluorescence of the superior choroidal lesion OS. (G, H) Optical coherence tomography of the macula shows alternating areas of retinal pigment epithelium (RPE) atrophy with increased signal transmission and irregular RPE thickening, with shallow subretinal fluid in both eyes.

Labs obtained in the ED revealed anemia, likely explaining the referred weakness, dizziness, and dyspnea. Computed tomography (CT) of the abdomen and pelvis revealed a pelvic mass, for which the patient was admitted and underwent endometrial biopsy revealing high-grade endometrial carcinoma.

Questions to Ask

- How quickly did the patient notice visual decline? Bilateral diffuse uveal melanocytic proliferation (BDUMP) usually presents with bilateral, rapid-onset, progressive, painless vision loss.[1,2]
  - Patient noticed significant visual decline about 6 months before presenting to the ED. She was evaluated elsewhere and underwent cataract surgery OS but continued to experience visual decline OU after surgery.
- How severe is vision loss? BDUMP often causes progressive, profound vision loss.
  - BCVA was 20/400 OU, despite previous cataract surgery OS.
- What is the age of the patient? BDUMP typically occurs in patients in their 50s through 80s and affects both sexes equally.[1]
  - Patient is a 64-year-old woman.
- Does the patient have a history of rapidly evolving cataracts? Patients with BDUMP experience rapid development of cataracts, reported in up to 73% of cases. Many patients undergo cataract surgery, but the expected visual improvement is not typically obtained after surgery.[1]
  - Patient developed visually significant cataracts within 2 to 3 months, but there was very limited visual improvement after surgery OS.
- Are there any other identifiable causes of vision loss? The clinical scenario most frequently encountered with BDUMP is that of sudden, bilateral vision loss in a middle-aged person with no clear underlying etiology. Visual function is usually disproportionate to fundus findings.[1]
  - Patient developed rapid, bilateral vision loss and fundus was remarkable for subtle background hyperpigmentation with overlying orange, subretinal patches. No other causes of vision loss could be identified.
- Does the patient report any systemic symptoms of an underlying malignancy (e.g., weakness, fatigue, weight loss, respiratory/gastrointestinal/neurological symptoms)? BDUMP often precedes the diagnosis of cancer by months to years, so the ophthalmologist might be the first person to assess the patient and should investigate associated symptoms suggestive of malignancy.[2]
  - Patient reported weakness, dizziness, and dyspnea and was found to have severe anemia upon workup in the ED.

Assessment

- This is a case of a 64-year-old female patient with bilateral severe vision loss, areas of choroidal thickening and hyperpigmentation, overlying orange subretinal lesions, and bilateral shallow exudative retinal detachment on OCT in the context of constitutional symptoms and presence of an abdominal mass.

Differential Diagnosis

- Multifocal choroidal nevi
- Multifocal choroidal melanoma
- Metastatic cutaneous melanoma

- BDUMP
- Uveal melanocytosis
- Uveal effusion syndrome
- Multifocal congenital hypertrophy of the RPE

Working Diagnosis

- BDUMP
  - Alternative name: bilateral diffuse melanocytic uveal hyperplasia

Multimodal Testing and Results

- Fundus photography
  - Fundus photography in patients with BDUMP shows diffuse hyperpigmentation with multiple orange patches of subretinal lipofuscin.
  - Multiple focally elevated pigmented and nonpigmented tumors can also be seen and documented on fundus photography.
- FAF
  - FAF often demonstrates nummular patches of alternating hypo- and hyperautofluorescence, most prominent at the posterior pole.[8]
  - Hyperautofluorescence corresponds to areas of lipofuscin pigment deposition, whereas hypoautofluorescence corresponds to areas of RPE loss.[8]
  - This pattern has been described as a "giraffe pattern," and it is considered typical for BDUMP.[2]
- OCT
  - OCT is helpful in demonstrating the alternating areas of RPE atrophy with increased signal transmission and RPE hypertrophy, corresponding to the alternating pigmented and orange subretinal patches seen ophthalmoscopically.[2]
  - Subretinal fluid is frequently found in BDUMP and can be easily detected on OCT.
  - Enhanced-depth imaging OCT and swept source OCT allow for better visualization of diffuse choroidal thickening and discrete elevated choroidal tumors, when present.[3]
- FA
  - Multifocal areas of early hyperautofluorescence corresponding to the nummular patches seen on fundus examination are considered typical of BDUMP.[4]
  - FA demonstrates a reversed pattern compared with autofluorescence, with hyperfluorescent areas corresponding to regions of RPE loss and hypofluorescent areas corresponding to lipofuscin accumulation.[2]
- ICGA
  - ICGA can be helpful in delineating the uveal melanocytic tumors, which appear hypofluorescent when present.[3]
- Ultrasonography (B-scan)
  - B-scan ultrasonography is helpful in demonstrating choroidal thickening, as well as uveal melanocytic tumors, when present.
- Ultrasound biomicroscopy (UBM)
  - UBM is helpful in documenting the presence of iris pigment epithelium cysts and angle closure, two rare findings described in some cases of BDUMP.[1]

- Systemic imaging
  - CT scan of the chest, abdomen, and pelvis, magnetic resonance imaging of the brain, and positron emission tomography (PET) should be considered to identify an underlying malignancy.

Management

- No standard of care exists for BDUMP. Several management strategies have been attempted, with variable results.
- Ocular radiation, intraocular surgery with drainage of the subretinal fluid, and intravitreal anti–vascular endothelial growth factor injections seem to be ineffective.[5]
- Local and systemic corticosteroids have been used in several reported cases but showed limited improvement in a small number of cases.[5,6]
- To date, the most effective treatments have been plasmapheresis and plasma exchange, along with treatment of the underlying malignancy. It is believed that plasmapheresis effectively removes cultured melanocyte elongation and proliferation factor, which is ectopically produced by the underlying malignancy and is responsible for melanocyte proliferation.[6,7]
- It is important to remember that BDUMP might be the first manifestation of an underlying malignancy in almost half the cases.[6] The most commonly associated malignancies are urogenital cancer in women and lung cancer in men.[6] Therefore it is important to order systemic testing and appropriately refer the patient to hematology/oncology for further care.
  - Our patient underwent PET and CT, which revealed the presence of an abdominal mass, with possible involvement of the retroperitoneal and pelvic lymph nodes. She subsequently had an endometrial biopsy, which demonstrated high-grade endometrial carcinoma, and she underwent a hysterectomy and received oncologic follow-up elsewhere.

Follow-up Care

- There is no standardized follow-up protocol for BDUMP.
- Follow-up care varies based on the patient's symptoms and treatment course, as well as the systemic status of the patient.
- Although there is wide variability in the course of the disease, patients should be monitored regularly by the ophthalmologist, if their systemic status allows.
- Prognosis is poor, with a median survival of 12 to 18 months after diagnosis of BDUMP.[6]

Algorithm 69.1: Algorithm for Differential Diagnosis for Bilateral Diffuse Uveal Melanocytic Proliferation (*BDUMP*)

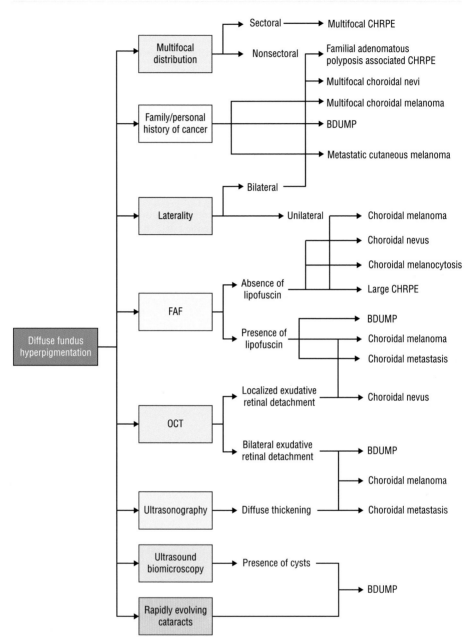

Algorithm 69.1 Algorithm for differential diagnosis for bilateral diffuse uveal melanocytic proliferation *(BDUMP)*. *CHRPE,* congenital hypertrophy of retinal pigment epithelium; *FAF,* fundus autofluorescence; *OCT,* optical coherence tomography.

Key Points

- BDUMP is a rare paraneoplastic syndrome that can cause sudden, profound, and otherwise unexplained visual loss in middle-aged individuals.
- It is characterized by the presence of diffuse choroidal thickening and hyperpigmentation with overlying orange lipofuscin deposition; development of multiple, slightly elevated melanocytic tumors with diffuse thickening of the uveal tract; exudative retinal detachment; and rapidly progressive cataracts.[4]
- FAF can demonstrate a typical giraffe pattern, with alternating hypo- and hyperautofluorescent areas, corresponding to regions of RPE loss and lipofuscin accumulation, respectively. This pattern is reversed on FA.[2]
- BDUMP can be the first manifestation of an underlying systemic malignancy in almost half of the cases; therefore it is important to order appropriate systemic imaging.[6]
- There is no standardized treatment and follow-up protocol for BDUMP, but the combination of plasmapheresis and treatment of the underlying cancer seems to be the most effective approach.[5,6]

References

1. O'Neal KD, Butnor KJ, Perkinson KR, et al. Bilateral diffuse melanocytic proliferation associated with pancreatic carcinoma: a case report and literature review of this paraneoplastic syndrome. *Surv Ophthalmol.* 2003;48(6):613-625.
2. Rahimy E, Sarraf D. Paraneoplastic and non-paraneoplastic retinopathy and optic neuropathy: evaluation and management. *Surv Ophthalmol.* 2013;58(5):430-458.
2. Rahimy E, Soheilian M. Giraffe pattern of bilateral diffuse uveal melanocytic proliferation. *Ophthalmology.* 2016;123(3):483.
3. Naysan J, Pang CE, Klein RW, Freund KB. Multimodal imaging of bilateral diffuse uveal melanocytic proliferation associated with an iris mass lesion. *Int J Retina Vitreous.* 2016;2:13.
4. Gass JD, Gieser RG, Wilkinson CP, et al. Bilateral diffuse uveal melanocytic proliferation in patients with occult carcinoma. *Arch Ophthalmol.* 1990;108(4):527-533.
5. Moreno TA, Patel SN. Comprehensive review of treatments for bilateral diffuse uveal melanocytic proliferation: a focus on plasmapheresis. *Int Ophthalmol Clin.* 2017;57(1):177-194.
6. Klemp K, Kiilgaard JF, Heegaard S, et al. Bilateral diffuse uveal melanocytic proliferation: case report and literature review. *Acta Ophthalmol.* 2017;95(5):439-445.
7. Miles SL, Niles RM, Pittock S, et al. A factor found in the IgG fraction of serum of patients with paraneoplastic bilateral diffuse uveal melanocytic proliferation causes proliferation of cultured human melanocytes. *Retina.* 2012;32(9):1959-1966.

CHAPTER 70

Diffuse Choroidal Thickness in a Patient With Migraine Headaches

Sayena Jabbehdari ▦ William F. Mieler

History of Present Illness

A 28-year-old female patient was referred by the outside retina practice for evaluation of a possible mass lesion in the left eye. The patient reported occasional headaches and pressure sensation without any systemic manifestation. The ocular mass lesion was initially detected on a computed tomography (CT) scan for the assessment of migraine headaches. Although the CT scan was negative for brain masses or lesions, it showed a 1.3 cm × 0.7 cm × 0.5 cm ovoid, well-circumscribed homogeneous mass in the left posterior upper aspect of the globe (Fig. 70.1). In addition, ocular melanoma and ocular metastasis were ruled out by a radiologist. Ocular history included mildly decreased vision in the left eye since childhood, without any recent acute vision changes. The patient had a medical history of migraine headaches, medically controlled hypertension, and glaucoma. There was no medical history of trauma, cancer, or infectious, inflammatory, or autoimmune conditions. She had no known drug allergies and was not taking any medications except a brimonidine eye drop in her left eye and medication for controlling hypertension. Reviews of systems and family and social history were unremarkable.

Questions to Ask

- What is the result of the ocular examination?
- What is the result of spectral domain optical coherence tomography (SD-OCT) and B-scan?
- Does the patient have any history of facial hemangioma?

Assessment

On ocular examination, the best-corrected visual acuity was 20/20 in the right eye and 20/60 in the left eye, with an element of amblyopia, but without any improvement with refraction. Extraocular movements were intact, the pupils were round and reactive, and there was a relative afferent pupillary defect only in the left eye. The refraction in the right eye was −4.00, whereas in the left eye it was +1.50, +2.00 × 90. Intraocular pressure by applanation was 14 mm Hg in the right eye and 24 mm Hg in the left eye while the patient was on brimonidine eye drop for her left eye. Visual field was full. Anterior and posterior segment examinations were unremarkable except for dilated episcleral vessels (Fig. 70.2A), glaucomatous optic nerve (Fig. 70.2B), and alteration of choroidal color in the left eye.

Differential Diagnosis

The differential diagnosis for ill-defined diffuse choroidal thickening includes choroidal melanoma, choroidal metastasis, choroidal osteoma, choroidal hemangioma, posterior uveitis, central

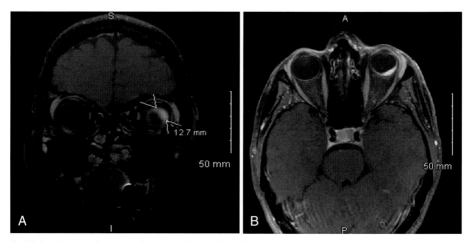

Fig. 70.1 Computed tomography scan of the brain without contrast demonstrating a 1.3 cm × 0.7 cm × 0.5 cm ovoid, well-circumscribed homogeneous mass in the left posterior upper aspect of the globe.

serous chorioretinopathy, Vogt-Koyanagi-Harada syndrome, and hypotony maculopathy/retinopathy (Fig. 70.3).

Multimodal Testing and Results

SD-OCT revealed normal retinal architecture without retinal pigment epithelium atrophy, retinal exudation, or subretinal fluid (Fig. 70.2D). B-scan echography of the left eye was subsequently performed revealing diffuse choroidal thickening with moderate homogeneity (Fig. 70.2C).

Working Diagnosis

Reviewing the patient's childhood photographs demonstrated the presence of left facial hemangioma with left upper eyelid involvement. In accordance with this history (Fig. 70.4) and the characteristic "tomato ketchup" appearance, the diagnosis of unilateral diffuse choroidal hemangioma in the setting of Sturge-Weber syndrome (SWS) was made. Choroidal hemangiomas are benign and rare vascular hamartomas that are associated with uveal tract abnormality in patients with SWS.[1,2] They are classified as either circumscribed choroidal hemangiomas (CCHs), which are more common in nonsyndromic cases, or diffuse choroidal hemangiomas (DCHs),[3-5] which sometimes manifest as asymptomatic, ill-defined choroidal masses with unclear borders.[3] In addition, exudative retinal detachment with subretinal fluid is seen in 50% of patients with DCH and SWS.[6,7]

Management

Treatment options for diffuse choroidal hemangioma in the setting of SWS include observation, photodynamic therapy (PDT),[7,8] anti–vascular endothelial growth factor (VEGF) (reported for CCH),[9] radioactive plaque therapy,[5,10] low-dose external beam radiation therapy (EBRT),[3] oral propranolol, thermal laser photocoagulation,[7] and transpupillary thermotherapy. Classically EBRT is used in the treatment of DCH with exudative retinal detachment, which often requires 3 to 4 weeks of treatment.[3] In general, EBRT, radioactive plaque therapy, PDT with verteporfin,

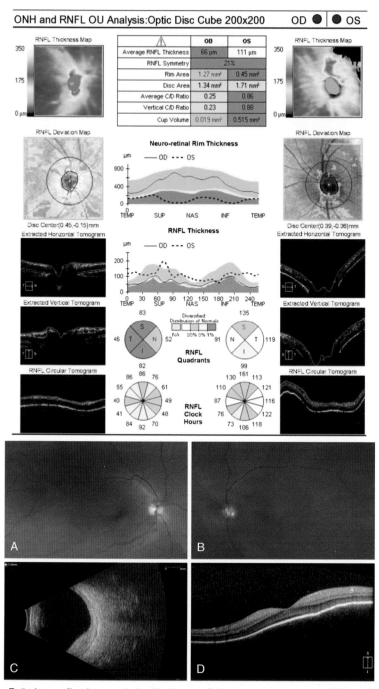

Fig. 70.2 Retinal nerve fiber layer analysis of both eyes. Color fundus photographs of (A) the right eye and (B) the left eye. (C) B-scan photograph of the left eye demonstrating diffuse choroidal thickening with moderate homogeneity. (D) Spectral-domain optical coherence tomography image of the macula in the left eye.

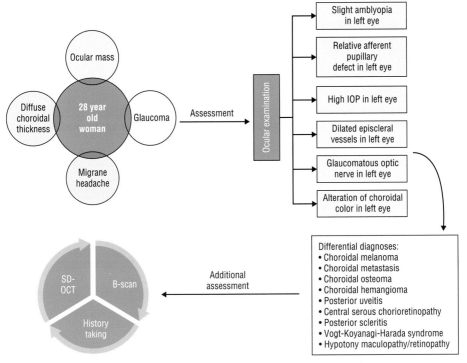

Fig. 70.3   Flow chart representation of differential diagnosis. *IOP,* Intraocular pressure.

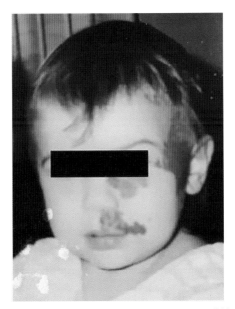

Fig. 70.4   Presence of facial hemangioma with left upper eyelid involvement.

PDT, or thermal laser photocoagulation is in combination with a VEGF inhibitor should be considered in cases with exudative retinal detachment or cystoid macular edema (CME).[7-10]

Although our patient did not have any CME, intra- or subretinal fluid, and/or retinal detachment, our management consisted of close observation with serial dilated fundus examinations.

Follow-up

Our management consisted of close observation with serial dilated fundus examinations. Our patient was extensively informed about her condition and prognosis. At her most recent follow-up appointment at 3 year postpresentation, the patient's visual acuity and examination were stable.

Algorithm 70.1: Algorithm for Management of Diffuse Choroidal Hemangiomas

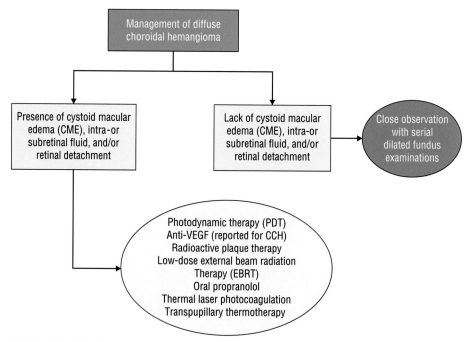

Algorithm 70.1   Algorithm for management of diffuse choroidal hemangiomas. *CCH,* Circumscribed choroidal hemangioma; *VEGF,* vascular endothelial growth factor.

Key Points

- Although the main concern of DCH is vision loss that is often secondary to nonrhegmatogenous retinal detachments, amblyopia, cystoid degeneration, and/or CME, cases with no evidence of retinal detachment or macular involvement should be monitored closely with periodic observation.
- Given that the lesion was not proximal to the fovea and had no CME or subretinal fluid, there was no indication for PDT, anti-VEGF antibodies, or EBRT.

References

1. Gottlieb JL, Murray TG, Gass JD. Low-dose external beam irradiation for bilateral diffuse choroidal hemangioma. *Arch Ophthalmol*. 1998;116(6):815-817.
2. Arevalo JF, Arias JD, Serrano MA. Oral propranolol for exudative retinal detachment in diffuse choroidal hemangioma. *Arch Ophthalmol*. 2011;129(10):1373-1375.
3. Scott IU, Alexandrakis G, Cordahi GJ, Murray TG. Diffuse and circumscribed choroidal hemangiomas in a patient with Sturge-Weber syndrome. *Arch Ophthalmol*. 1999;117(3):406-407.
4. Higueros E, Roe E, Granell E, Baselga E. Sturge-Weber syndrome: a review. *Actas Dermosifiliogr*. 2017;108(5):407-417.
5. Arepalli S, Shields CL, Kaliki S, Emrich J, Komarnicky L, Shields JA. Diffuse choroidal hemangioma management with plaque radiotherapy in 5 cases. *Ophthalmology*. 2013;120(11):2358-2359.e1-2.
6. Madreperla SA, Hungerford JL, Plowman PN, Laganowski HC, Gregory PT. Choroidal hemangiomas: visual and anatomic results of treatment by photocoagulation or radiation therapy. *Ophthalmology*. 1997;104(11):1773-1778.
7. Bains HS, Cirino AC, Ticho BH, Jampol LM. Photodynamic therapy using verteporfin for a diffuse choroidal hemangioma in Sturge-Weber syndrome. *Retina*. 2004;24(1):152-155.
8. Schmidt-Erfurth UM, Michels S, Kusserow C, Jurklies B, Augustin AJ. Photodynamic therapy for symptomatic choroidal hemangioma: visual and anatomic results. *Ophthalmology*. 2002;109(12):2284-2294.
9. Mandal S, Naithani P, Venkatesh P, Garg S. Intravitreal bevacizumab (avastin) for circumscribed choroidal hemangioma. *Indian J Ophthalmol*. 2011;59(3):248-251.
10. Chao AN, Shields CL, Shields JA, Krema H. Plaque radiotherapy for choroidal hemangioma with total retinal detachment and iris neovascularization. *Retina*. 2001;21(6):682-684.

CHAPTER 71

Vascularized, Pigmented Macular Lesion

Alexis Warren ▪ William F. Mieler

History of Present Illness

We present a case of a 6-year-old male patient with decreased vision and strabismus. Parents reported a normal birth history. Medical history is otherwise unremarkable.

OCULAR EXAMINATION FINDINGS

Visual acuity was 20/200 in the right eye and 20/30 in the left eye. Intraocular pressure was normal. The patient did exhibit a right exotropia. Dilated fundus examination exhibited a solitary and elevated gray tumor in the inferior macula with tortuous intrinsic vessels in the right eye. The periphery of the right eye was normal. The fundus of the left eye was normal throughout.

IMAGING

Fluorescein angiography (FA) highlighted the vascular tortuosity and prominence within the lesion, and late-phase photographs exhibited significant vascular leakage throughout the macula.

Questions to Ask

- Does the patient have any systemic symptoms or health conditions? Combined hamartomas can be associated with systemic syndromes, most commonly neurofibromatosis type 2, but also neurofibromatosis type 1, Gorlin syndrome, and even branchio-oculo-facial syndrome.
  - No
- What is the internal reflectivity of the macular lesion? Combined hamartomas are often misdiagnosed as choroidal melanomas. However, these hamartomas tend to have high-medium reflectivity, whereas choroidal melanomas have low-medium internal reflectivity.
  - High-medium internal reflectivity

Assessment

- This is a case of a young, otherwise healthy male patient with decreased vision, strabismus, and a unilateral gray elevated macular lesion involving all retinal layers with associated epiretinal membrane (ERM). The patient was assessed for possible neurofibromatosis, though the assessment was negative

Differential Diagnosis

- Choroidal melanoma
- Choroidal nevus
- Morning glory syndrome
- Retinoblastoma
- Retinal pigment epithelium adenoma or adenocarcinoma
- Melanocytoma
- Toxocara or toxoplasmosis infection
- Combined hamartoma of the retina and retinal pigment epithelium (CHRRPE)

Working Diagnosis

- Combined hamartoma of the retina and retinal pigment epithelium (CHRRPE)

Multimodal Testing and Results

- Fundus photographs
  - On fundus examination, these lesions can involve the macula or optic disc (Fig. 71.1). These lesions are often elevated and somewhat pigmented with prominent vessels within the tumor (Fig. 71.2). They are also often associated with an overlying ERM.[1]

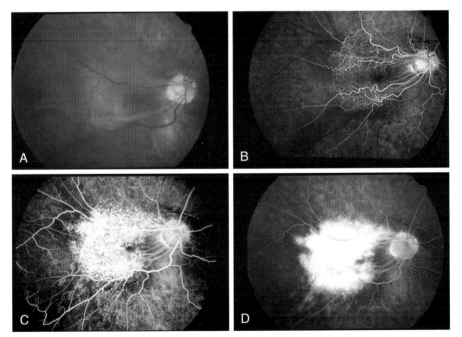

Fig. 71.1 (A) Fundus photography of the right eye with a pale gray macular lesion extending from the optic nerve. (B–D) Fluorescein angiography of the right eye showing early vascular prominence within the lesion and late leakage.

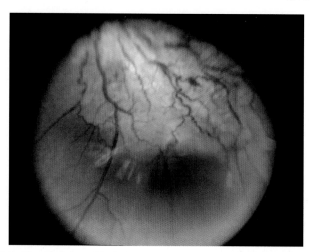

Fig. 71.2   Magnified view of the intrinsic vascularity and tortuosity of a similar lesion.

- Optical coherence tomography (OCT)
  - OCT findings of these alterations include preretinal membranes with associated retinal striae, disorganization of all retinal layers, and photoreceptor attenuation.[2]
  - More specifically, these tumors have been further described by the following terms:[3]
    - Minipeak: vertical vitreoretinal traction
    - Maxi-peak: folding of the inner retinal layers
    - Sawtooth or omega sign: distortion of the outer plexiform layer
- FA
  - These tests can be somewhat diagnostic for these lesions. Early phases exhibit prominence of the fine capillaries and vessels within the tumor with subsequent late phases showing leakage of these vessels (Fig. 71.1B-D).[1]
- OCT angiography (OCTA)
  - OCTA confirms the vascularity abnormalities in these lesions. Vascular tortuosity and traction have been documented in the superficial and deep layers within the retinal tumor.[4]

Management

- Although these lesions can present somewhat variably, vision loss in these patients is most often linked with a macular location of the lesion. However, even peripheral lesions can present with other vision-threatening consequences such as vitreous hemorrhage, choroidal neovascularization, ERMs, macular edema, and even retinal detachment.[5]
- Given these patients often present as children, amblyopia therapy should be considered, where appropriate, to improve visual acuity.
- Successful photodynamic therapy has been documented; however, most recently intravitreal anti–vascular endothelial growth factor (anti-VEGF) has become the mainstay for treatment of CHRRPE-related choroidal neovascularization.[5]
- Surgery for these lesions is somewhat controversial; however, there has been noted success and vision improvement for those lesions with significant ERMs and vitreoretinal traction after pars plana vitrectomy.[6]

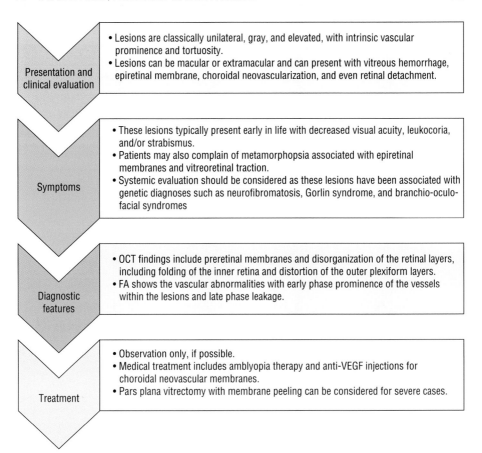

Presentation and clinical evaluation
- Lesions are classically unilateral, gray, and elevated, with intrinsic vascular prominence and tortuosity.
- Lesions can be macular or extramacular and can present with vitreous hemorrhage, epiretinal membrane, choroidal neovascularization, and even retinal detachment.

Symptoms
- These lesions typically present early in life with decreased visual acuity, leukocoria, and/or strabismus.
- Patients may also complain of metamorphopsia associated with epiretinal membranes and vitreoretinal traction.
- Systemic evaluation should be considered as these lesions have been associated with genetic diagnoses such as neurofibromatosis, Gorlin syndrome, and branchio-oculo-facial syndromes

Diagnostic features
- OCT findings include preretinal membranes and disorganization of the retinal layers, including folding of the inner retina and distortion of the outer plexiform layers.
- FA shows the vascular abnormalities with early phase prominence of the vessels within the lesions and late phase leakage.

Treatment
- Observation only, if possible.
- Medical treatment includes amblyopia therapy and anti-VEGF injections for choroidal neovascular membranes.
- Pars plana vitrectomy with membrane peeling can be considered for severe cases.

Fig. 71.3 Flow chart showing combined hamartoma of the retina and retinal pigment epithelium. *FA,* Fluorescein angiography; *OCT,* optical coherence tomography; *VEGF,* vascular endothelial growth factor.

Follow-up Care

- As this diagnosis is relatively rare, there are not established guidelines for follow-up care.
- Our patient is followed on a biannual basis by the pediatric and retina services.
- Specific follow-up care and scheduling should be based upon specific patient factors including presence of amblyopia, progression of vision loss, vitreoretinal traction/preretinal membranes, and presence of choroidal neovascularization.

Flow Chart

For a flow chart on CHRRPE, please see Fig. 71.3.

Algorithm 71.1: Algorithm for Pigmented Lesions in the Posterior Pole

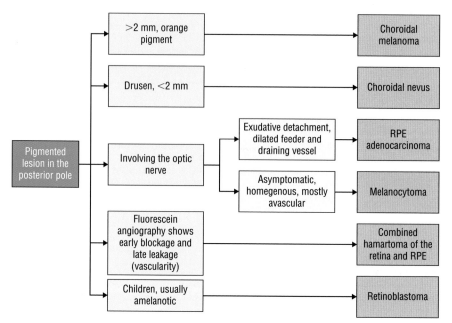

Algorithm 71.1 Algorithm for pigmented lesions in the posterior pole. *RPE,* Retinal pigment epithelium.

Key Points

- CHRRPEs are benign lesions that can present as extramacular or macular lesions, typically in younger patients.
- These lesions can be unilateral or bilateral and have been associated with some systemic genetic syndromes, most classically neurofibromatosis type 2.
- These lesions can be associated with choroidal neovascularization and may be treated with anti-VEGF therapy.
- Surgery may be warranted in these patients to alleviate vitreoretinal traction.

CHRRPEs are benign unilateral or bilateral lesions most often presenting in childhood as gray vascularized lesions in the macula.[1] These patients can may present with symptomatic decreased vision, metamorphopsia, or amblyopic strabismus.[1] These lesions can rarely develop choroidal neo-vascularization requiring anti-VEGF injections, and therefore are often only observed.[5] In rare cases surgery may be considered to improve ERMs and traction; however, this remains a debated topic.[6]

References

1. Agarwal A, ed. *Gass' Atlas of Macular Diseases.* 5th ed. Elsevier Saunders; 2012.
2. Shields CL, Mashayekhi A, Dai VV, Materin MA, Shields JA. Optical coherence tomographic findings of combined hamartoma of the retina and retinal pigment epithelium in 11 patients. *Arch Ophthalmol.* 2005;123(12):1746-1750.
3. Gupta R, Fung AT, Lupidi M, et al. Peripapillary versus macular combined hamartoma of the retina and retinal pigment epithelium: imaging characteristics. *Am J Ophthalmol.* 2019;200:263-269.
4. Scupola A, Grimaldi G, Sammarco MG, Sasso P, Marullo M, Blasi MA. Multimodal imaging evaluation of combined hamartoma of the retina and retinal pigment epithelium. *Eur J Ophthalmol.* 2020;30(3):595-599.
5. Schachat AP, Wilkinson CP, Hinton DR, Sadda SR, Wiedemann P. Combined hamartoma of the retina and retinal pigment epithelium. In: Schachat AP, Wilkinson CP, Hinton DR, Sadda SR, Wiedemann P, eds. *Ryan's Retina.* 6th ed. Elsevier; 2018.
6. Sun LS, Raouf S, Rhee D, Ferrone PJ. Surgical outcomes of epiretinal membrane removal due to combined hamartoma of the retina and RPE. *Ophthalmic Surg Lasers Imaging Retina.* 2020;51(10):546-554.

CHAPTER 72

Unilateral Macular Lesion in a Young Man

Michael T. Andreoli ■ William F. Mieler

History of Present Illness

A 21-year-old male patient with an unremarkable medical history was referred for a macular finding on routine examination.

OCULAR EXAMINATION FINDINGS

Visual acuity was 20/20 in each eye. Intraocular pressures were normal. Dilated fundus examination showed a small pigmented parafoveal lesion in the left eye.

IMAGING

Optical coherence tomography (OCT) showed a hyperreflective protuberance from the inner retina with dense posterior shadowing.

Questions to Ask

- Does the patient have a history of malignancy?
  - No
- Has this finding been noted previously?
  - No

Assessment

- This is a case of a 21-year-old male patient with no pertinent medical history with a very well-delineated, pigmented parafoveal macular lesion.

Differential Diagnosis

- Choroidal nevus
- Choroidal melanoma
- Combined hamartoma of the retina and retinal pigment epithelium (RPE)
- Congenital hypertrophy of the RPE
- Congenital simple hamartoma of the RPE

Working Diagnosis

- Congenital simple hamartoma of the RPE

Multimodal Testing and Results

- Fundus photographs
  - On fundus examination, a heavily pigmented, well-circumscribed parafoveal mass is typically seen (Fig. 72.1).[1,2]
- OCT
  - OCT of the mass shows hyperreflectivity of a nodule extending from the inner retina, with dense shadowing through the full thickness of the retina. An adjacent epiretinal membrane is common (Fig. 72.2).[3]
- Fluorescein angiography (FA)
  - FA typically shows focal blockage without leakage.[4]

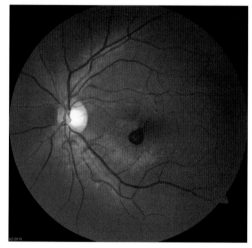

Fig. 72.1 Fundus photograph: posterior pole photograph demonstrates a small, well-circumscribed hyperpigmented parafoveal lesion.

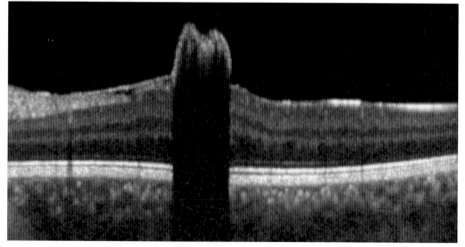

Fig. 72.2 Optical coherence tomography shows a nodular hyperreflective protuberance from the inner retina with dense posterior shadowing obscuring the full thickness of the retina.

Management

■ No treatment is indicated. An occasional case may require vitrectomy with membrane peel for associated epiretinal membrane.

Follow-up Care

■ Periodic surveillance is recommended.

Algorithm 72.1: An Algorithm for the Differential Diagnosis of Congenital Simple Hamartoma of the Retinal Pigment Epithelium

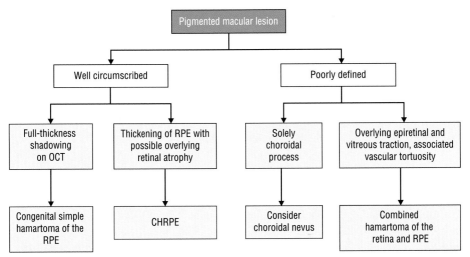

Algorithm 72.1 An algorithm for the differential diagnosis of congenital simple hamartoma of the retinal pigment epithelium. *CHRPE*, Congenital hypertrophy of the retinal pigment epithelium; *OCT*, optical coherence tomography; *RPE*, retinal pigment epithelium.

Key Points

■ Congenital simple hamartoma of the RPE is a rare diagnosis, but it is important to recognize to avoid unnecessary diagnoses of malignancy.
■ Congenital simple hamartoma of the RPE may be safely observed.
■ There may be an associated epiretinal membrane that seldom may require surgical intervention.

References

1. Shields CL, Shields JA, Marr BP, Sperber DE, Gass JD. Congenital simple hamartoma of the retinal pigment epithelium: a study of five cases. *Ophthalmology.* 2003;110(5):1005-1011.
2. Grant LW, Seth RK. Congenital simple hamartoma of the retinal pigment epithelium. *Semin Ophthalmol.* 2014;29(4):183-185.
3. Barnes AC, Goldman DR, Laver NV, Duker JS. Congenital simple hamartoma of the retinal pigment epithelium: clinical, optical coherence tomography, and histopathological correlation. *Eye (Lond).* 2014;28(6):765-766.
4. López JM, Guerrero P. Congenital simple hamartoma of the retinal pigment epithelium: optical coherence tomography and angiography features. *Retina.* 2006;26(6):704-706.

CHAPTER 73

A Young Boy Who Failed Routine School Screening With Unilateral Decreased Vision and an Irregular Reddish Macular Lesion

Katherine G. Chen ■ William F. Mieler

History of Present Illness

A 6-year-old male patient presented for ocular evaluation after failing his school visual screening examination. Visual acuity was 20/200 in the right eye (OD) and 20/20 in the left eye (OS). The left eye was entirely normal. Intraocular pressure was within normal limits in both eyes (OU), and anterior segment examination OU was unremarkable. Dilated fundus examination OD revealed a clear vitreous cavity but was notable for a retinal lesion (Fig. 73.1). As noted, the fundus examination OS was normal.

Questions to Ask

- Are there any additional ocular symptoms (e.g., diplopia, any noted ocular misalignment by parents)?
- What is the patient's ocular history (e.g., strabismus, amblyopia, ocular trauma)?
- Does the patient have a family history (e.g., of other ocular diseases, but specifically of similar retinal lesions)?
- Are there any neurological symptoms (e.g., seizures, headaches, visual disturbances)?
- Are there any skin findings?
- What is the patient's complete medical history?
  - Medical history and birth history
  - Surgical history
  - Allergies
  - Social history
  - Review of systems

Assessment

- Our patient had no additional ocular symptoms, neurological or skin findings, and no family history of retinal lesions. Additional imaging with fluorescein angiography (FA) was obtained and demonstrated early hypofluorescence of the lesion with delayed and incomplete filling of aneurysms in the mid-late phases (Fig. 73.2).

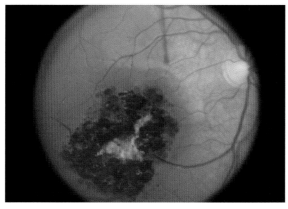

Fig. 73.1 Fundus photograph of the right eye. Retinal lesion characterized by a large cluster of aneurysms filled with dark red blood in the inferotemporal macula. White/gray fibroglial membranes can be seen centrally overlying a small portion of the lesion.

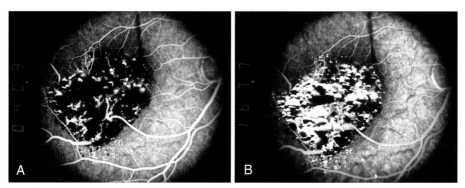

Fig. 73.2 Fluorescein angiography of the right eye. (A) Early phase showing generalized hypofluorescence of the tumor mass with early focal filling within the saccular aneurysms (B) Midphase of the angiogram, showing progressive slow and incomplete filling of the aneurysms with plasma-erythrocytic filling of the saccular aneurysms.

Differential Diagnosis

- Retinal cavernous hemangioma (RCH)
- Retinal capillary hemangioma (von Hippel–Lindau disease)
- Retinal telangiectasias (Coats disease, Leber miliary aneurysm)

Additional characteristics of these diagnoses are described and summarized below.

Working Diagnosis

- Given this patient's incidental finding with no symptoms, clinical presentation on dilated fundus examination, and findings on FA, this patient was diagnosed with an RCH.

Discussion

Retinal cavernous hemangioma (RCH) is a rare benign congenital retinal vascular harmartoma.[1-3] The etiology is unknown, and most cases are sporadic; however, few cases of familial autosomal dominant inheritance have been reported.[1,4,5] A review by Wang et al.[2] reported 96 cases published in the literature and found no gender or racial predilection. Although RCH is a congenital lesion, patients are mostly asymptomatic, and therefore the lesion is usually found incidentally on routine examination. The median age of presentation is 21 years of age, with 70% presenting between the ages of 7 and 40 years.[2]

RCHs are unilateral in 90% of cases. The location of the tumor is most commonly in the retinal periphery; however, macular (10–13% of cases)[2,3] and optic nerve head lesions may also occur. Patients with macular lesions can experience mild vision disturbances, and those with lesions over the optic nerve head generally have good vision but can have an enlarged blind spot or scotomas. Other clinical symptoms include occasional vitreous hemorrhage (VH), subretinal hemorrhage, retinal detachment, strabismus, and diplopia. Although RCHs are typically isolated findings, they may rarely represent a phakomatosis with associated central nervous system (CNS) and/or skin hemangiomas. Those with CNS involvement can also have neurological symptoms including seizures, headaches, and transient visual disturbances.

On ophthalmological examination, RCHs appear as clusters of saccular aneurysms filled with dark blood, described as a "cluster of grapes". They fill very slowly on angiography, and there may be layering of the plasma and red blood cells within the aneurysms, which is a consequence of the slow blood flow through the tumor. White or gray fibroglial membranes may eventually develop overlying the tumor. Occasionally, VH may occur, though it is thought that this is due to contracture of the fibroglial membranes and not from increased or enhanced blood flow. VH due to an RCH is often minimal and spontaneously resolves. The surrounding retinal vasculature is usually not affected, there are no feeder vessels, and exudation is extremely rare.

Although our patient has characteristic findings of RCH on the clinical examination and imaging, his presentation is unusual given his young age.

Other differential diagnoses, summarized below, are unlikely:

- Retinal capillary hemangioma (von Hippel–Lindau disease)
    - Retinal capillary hemangiomas are benign vascular tumors that arise from the retina or optic disc. They can be isolated lesions or associated with von Hippel–Lindau disease. Patients generally present with blurred vision or visual field (VF) loss. Clinical examination shows a small, round, orange-red tumor with a prominent dilated feeding artery and draining vein (Fig. 73.3A). These characteristic feeder vessels and leakage can be seen on FA (Fig. 73.3B). RCHs, in contrast, do not have feeder vessels, do not affect normal retinal vasculature, and rarely have exudation or leakage.

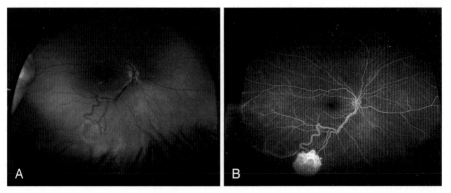

Fig. 73.3 *(Left)* (A) Color fundus photograph and *(right)* (B) fluorescein angiography from a different patient, showing a red-orange capillary hemangioma with dilated feeding artery and draining vein.

- Retinal telangiectasias (Coats disease, Leber miliary aneurysms)
  - Coats disease and Leber miliary aneurysms both exhibit idiopathic retinal telangiectasias. Retinal telangiectasias are also generally unilateral and are characterized by progressive vascular dilation with intraretinal and subretinal exudation. Individual aneurysms are often found along retinal vessels in contrast to the cluster of saccular aneurysms seen in RCHs.

Multimodal Imaging and Testing

- FA
  - RCHs demonstrate early hypofluorescence of the main tumor with delayed, slow, incomplete filling in later phases on FA. The plasma-erythrocytic separation can also be visualized in the late phases, with fluorescein collecting in the superior portion of the aneurysms as blood cells that layer inferiorly block accumulation of the dye. Retinal circulation demonstrates normal perfusion, and leakage is rarely seen.
- B-scan ultrasonography
  - B-scan ultrasonography is used in patients who present with VH obscuring the view of the fundus. This is rarely necessary but would show pedunculated, irregular surface lesions without acoustic solidity and an absence of choroidal excavation.
- Optical coherence tomography (OCT)
  - OCT would show the aneurysms of the RCH arising from the inner retinal layers and can also demonstrate fibrous membranes overlying the tumor.[2,6] OCT is rarely necessary in helping to establish the diagnosis.
- VF testing
  - VF testing is performed in patients with optic nerve head lesions to evaluate for enlarged blind spots or scotomas.

Management

RCHs are nonprogressive in nature and rarely increase in size. Therefore the standard of care is periodic observation with routine follow-up.

The most common cause of acute vision loss in RCH is secondary to VH or, as in this case, when the RCH is macular in location. However, VH related to RCH is often minimal and usually spontaneously resolves. Pars plana vitrectomy can be considered in cases with significant VH. Cryotherapy and laser photocoagulation have also been used in early cases to treat vitreous and/or subretinal hemorrhages; however, they are rarely used today. Reported adverse effects from these treatments include secondary VH and tumor enlargement.[1,7]

Patients with neurological symptoms should undergo neuroimaging to evaluate for CNS hemangiomas and cerebral involvement.

Follow-up Care

- Patients should have periodic and routine follow-up with return precautions if they develop acute vision loss or other vision changes. The vascular lesion in this patient did not show any appreciable change over time.

Algorithm 73.1: The Diagnosis of a Retinal Cavernous Hemangioma is Generally Straightforward

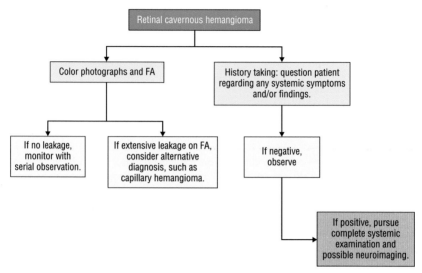

Algorithm 73.1 The diagnosis of a retinal cavernous hemangioma is generally straightforward. Complete history taking, color photographs, and a fluorescein angiogram *(FA)* suffice to establish the diagnosis and provide documentation of the features.

Key Points

- RCH is a rare benign vascular hamartoma that is usually unilateral and nonprogressive in nature.
- Most cases are sporadic; few reported familial autosomal dominant inheritance.
- RCH is characterized by clusters of thin-walled saccular aneurysms filled with dark venous blood (often described as a cluster of grapes).
- It is usually asymptomatic unless located in or adjacent to the macula.
- Systemic associations may occasionally include CNS and cutaneous hemangiomas. CNS hemangiomas can present with neurological symptoms (seizures, headaches, and transient visual disturbances).
- Patients should undergo routine periodic examination to monitor the lesion.
- Vitrectomy can be considered in cases of significant VH.

References

1. Gass JD. Cavernous hemangioma of the retina: a neuro-oculo-cutaneous syndrome. *Am J Ophthalmol.* 1971;71(4):799-814.
2. Wang W, Chen L. Cavernous hemangioma of the retina: a comprehensive review of the literature (1934–2015). *Retina.* 2017;37(4):611-621.
3. Agarwal A, Sternberg P. Cavernous hemangioma. In: Schachat AP, Sadda SR, Widemann P, Hinton DR, Wilkinson CP, eds. *Ryan's Retina.* 6th ed. Elsevier; 2017:2421-2426.
4. Goldberg RE, Pheasant TR, Shields JA. Cavernous hemangioma of the retina. A four-generation pedigree with neurocutaneous manifestations and an example of bilateral retinal involvement. *Arch Ophthalmol.* 1979;97(12):2321-2324.
5. Dobyns WB, Michels VV, Groover RV, et al. Familial cavernous malformations of the central nervous system and retina. *Ann Neurol.* 1987;21(6):578-583.
6. Li J, Li Y, Li H. New interpretation of multimodality fundus imaging for retinal cavernous hemangioma. *Curr Eye Res.* 2019;44(4):423-427.
7. Klein M, Goldberg MF, Cotlier E. Cavernous hemangioma of the retina: report of four cases. *Ann Ophthalmol.* 1975;7(9):1213-1221.

CHAPTER 74

Unilateral Loss of Vision With a Vascular Retinal Lesion

Michael J. Heiferman ▪ William F. Mieler

History of Present Illness

A 37-year-old female patient presented with no significant medical history. The patient was referred by an outside ophthalmologist for a red retinal lesion in her right eye. One month before presentation, she noted decreased vision in her right eye described as a white/gray shadow in her vision. This vision change has remained stable since onset, and she has no other associated symptoms including flashes, new floaters, pain, redness, or photophobia. She has no ocular, medical, or surgical history. She takes no medications, including eye drops, and she has no known drug allergies. The patient smokes a pack of cigarettes per day, and she does not drink alcohol or use illicit drugs. She has no family history of medical problems, including ocular disease, and a review of systems is only positive for anxiety.

OCULAR EXAM FINDINGS

On examination, the patient's uncorrected vision was 20/20 in both eyes. Intraocular pressure was 17 in both eyes. Confrontational visual fields and extraocular movements were full. The anterior slit lamp examination was unremarkable in both eyes. Posterior examination of the right eye revealed clear media, a sharp disc with 0.2 cup-to-disc ratio, and retinal thickening with hard exudates in the inferior macula. In the inferior midperiphery, there was an elevated red lesion 3 mm in diameter with large, dilated feeder vessels coursing off the inferior arcade (Fig. 74.1). Posterior examination of the left eye was unremarkable without vascular abnormalities or retinal lesions.

IMAGING

- The right eye showed exudates in the inferior macula and an elevated red lesion (about 3 mm in diameter) in the inferior midperiphery. There were large, dilated feeder vessels coursing off the inferior arcade (Fig. 74.1A).
- Fluorescein angiography of the right eye showed a hyperfluorescent lesion with minimal leakage and large feeder vessels (Fig. 74.1B).

Questions to Ask

- Does the patient have any skin cavernous hemangiomas currently? Did she have any as a child?
- Is there any family history of renal cell carcinoma, cerebellar hemangioblastoma, or pheochromocytoma?

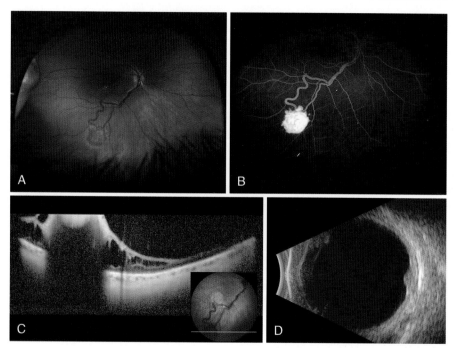

Fig. 74.1 (A) Ultrawide-field pseudocolor photograph of the right eye with exudates in the inferior macula and an elevated red lesion 3 mm in diameter in the inferior midperiphery with large, dilated feeder vessels coursing off the inferior arcade. (B) Fluorescein angiography of the right eye with a hyperfluorescent lesion with minimal leakage and large feeder vessels. (C) Optical coherence tomography demonstrating cystoid macular edema in the inferior macula with associated hard exudates. The lesion is hyperreflective emanating from the inner retina. Inlay infrared reflectance map. (D)B scan ultrasonography measuring the thickness of the lesion as 2.52 mm, with medium echogenicity.

Assessment

■ This is a 37-year-old female patient with 1 month of decreased vision in the right eye found to have inferior macular edema and an elevated red retinal lesion in her inferior midperiphery with dilated feeder vessels (Algorithm 74.1).

Differential Diagnosis

■ Retinal capillary hemangioma
■ Dilated feeder vessels and associated exudation can be related to von Hippel–Lindau syndrome
■ Retinal vasoproliferative tumor
■ Inferotemporal peripheral location, feeder vessels slightly dilated/tortuous (but less so than capillary hemangioma)
■ Retinal cavernous hemangioma
■ "Cluster of grapes" appearance, usually asymptomatic
■ Retinal arteriovenous malformation
■ Large, dilated tortuous vessels from arteriovenous communications with no intervening capillaries, usually no exudation, subretinal fluid, or masses
■ Coats disease (retinal telangiectasis)
■ Aneurysmal dilation of blood vessels with prominent subretinal exudate, no masses

Working Diagnosis

A working diagnosis of retinal capillary hemangioma was made based on history and examination. Further retinal imaging, magnetic resonance imaging (MRI) of the brain, computed tomography (CT) of the abdomen/pelvis, and genetic testing for von Hippel–Lindau syndrome were obtained.

Retinal capillary hemangiomas are benign vascular tumors that arise from the retina or optic disc. The average age of detection is 15 to 35 years old, and they can be isolated or associated with von Hippel–Lindau syndrome.[1,2] Patients with multiple lesions or bilateral involvement are more likely to have von Hippel–Lindau syndrome, although all patients should undergo systemic evaluation.

Von Hippel–Lindau syndrome is an autosomal dominant disorder caused by a mutation in a tumor suppressor gene on chromosome.[3] Other associated systemic manifestations include cavernous hemangiomas of the skin; renal cell carcinoma; pheochromocytoma; cysts of the kidney, pancreas, and liver; and hemangioblastomas in the cerebellum, medulla, pons, and spinal cord.

Multimodal Testing and Results

- Optical coherence tomography demonstrated cystoid macular edema in the inferior macula with associated hard exudates. The lesion was hyperreflective emanating from the inner retina.
- Fluorescein angiography showed a hyperfluorescent lesion with minimal leakage and large feeder vessels.
- Ultrasonography measured the thickness of the lesion as 2.52 mm with medium echogenicity.
- MRI brain and CT abdomen/pelvis were unremarkable.
- Genetic testing was negative for genes associated with von Hippel–Lindau syndrome.

Management

- Three months after the patient's initial presentation, she returned with a decrease in her right eye vision to 20/40. The decision was made to proceed with planned focal laser directly to the lesion with the following parameters: power 650 mW, duration 0.6 seconds, size 400 μm, and 154 applications to an end point of whitening the entire surface of the lesion while avoiding the feeder vessels.[4]
- Four months after the initial presentation, the patient's vision remained 20/40 with scant vitreous hemorrhage overlying the lesion. The decision was made to repeat the focal laser with similar parameters as above.
- The patient underwent a total of five focal laser therapy sessions over 5 months.
- Other treatment options for retina capillary hemangiomas include cryotherapy, plaque radiotherapy, photodynamic therapy, and, rarely, pars plana vitrectomy with surgical excision.[1–3]

Follow-up Care

Nine months after the initial presentation, the patient's visual acuity was 20/25 +1 in the right eye. On examination, the macular edema had resolved, the lesion had regressed in size, and there was minimal overlying vitreous hemorrhage. Ultrasonography measured the thickness of the lesion to be 1.36 mm compared with 2.52 mm on initial presentation. The decision was made to observe with the plan to follow up in 2 months.

Algorithm 74.1: Algorithm for Vascular Lesion Diagnosis

Hemangioma has a vascular tumor while AVM does not (the absence of vascular tumor and no exudation is a double negative).

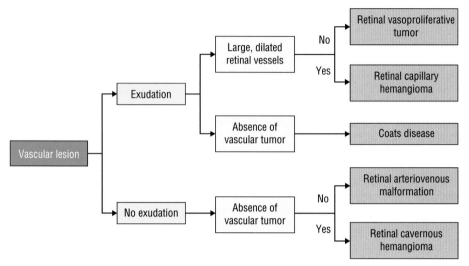

Algorithm. 74.1   Algorithm for vascular lesion diagnosis.

Key Points

- Retinal capillary hemangiomas are vascular lesions with dilated feeder vessels and associated exudation, and they can be associated with von Hippel–Lindau syndrome.
- A systemic workup should accompany the diagnosis of retinal capillary hemangiomas including MRI of the brain, CT of the abdomen/pelvis, and genetic testing for von Hippel–Lindau syndrome.
- Primary treatment of retinal capillary hemangiomas includes multiple sessions of focal laser or cryotherapy with the end points of lesion regression and resolution of exudation.

References

1. Shields JA, Decker WL, Sanborn GE, Augsburger JJ, Goldberg RE. Presumed acquired retinal hemangiomas. *Ophthalmology.* 1983;90:1292-1300.
2. Maher ER, Yates JR, Harries R, et al. Clinical features and natural history of von Hippel–Lindau disease. *Q J Med.* 1990;77:1151-1163.
3. Singh AD, Shields CL, Shields JA. von Hippel–Lindau disease. *Surv Ophthalmol.* 2001;46:117-142.
4. Blodi CF, Russell SR, Pulido JS, Folk JC. Direct and feeder vessel photocoagulation of retinal angiomas with dye yellow laser. *Ophthalmology.* 1990;97:791-797.
5. Welch RB. The recognition and treatment of early angiomatosis retinae and use of cryosurgery as an adjunct to therapy. *Trans Am Ophthalmol Soc.* 1970;68:367-424.
6. Atebara NH. Retinal capillary hemangioma treated with verteporfin photodynamic therapy. *Am J Ophthalmol.* 2002;134:788-790.
7. Gaudric A, Krivosic V, Duguid G, Massin P, Giraud S, Richard S. Vitreoretinal surgery for severe retinal capillary hemangiomas in von Hippel–Lindau disease. *Ophthalmology.* 2011 Jan 1;118(1):142-9.

Page numbers followed by *f* represent figures.

X

X-linked retinoschisis (XLR), 25
  algorithm for, 29, 29f
  assessment for, 24
  differential diagnosis of, 25
  follow-up care for, 28
  history of, 24
  management of, 28
  multimodal testing and results of, 25–28, 25f,
    26f, 27f
  ocular examination findings in, 24
  questions on, 24
  workup and diagnosis of, 25

Y

Yellow macular spots, 1–8
  algorithm for, 7, 7f
  assessment for, 4
  diagnosis of, 4
  differential diagnosis of, 4
  follow-up care for, 7
  history of, 2
  imaging for, 2, 3f, 4f
  management of, 6–7
  multimodal testing and results of, 5–6, 6f
  ocular examination findings in, 2, 3f
  questions on, 2–3